Case Studies in Ophthalmology

Case Studies in Ophthalmology

Editor: Clayton Mason

AMERICAN
MEDICAL PUBLISHERS
www.americanmedicalpublishers.com

AMERICAN
MEDICAL PUBLISHERS
www.americanmedicalpublishers.com

Cataloging-in-Publication Data

Case studies in ophthalmology / edited by Clayton Mason.
p. cm.
Includes bibliographical references and index.
ISBN 979-8-88740-621-3
1. Ophthalmology. 2. Eye--Diseases. 3. Eye--Diseases--Treatment. I. Mason, Clayton.
RE46 .C55 2023
617.7--dc23

American Medical Publishers,
41 Flatbush Avenue,
1st Floor, New York,
NY 11217, USA

ISBN 979-8-88740-621-3 (Hardback)

Contents

Preface

Ophthalmology is a specialized area within medicine which focuses on the diagnosis, treatment and prevention of disorders related to the eyes and visual system. The eyes are complex organs responsible for vision, and maintaining their health is crucial for optimal visual function. Some of the eye conditions which are dealt with under this field are refractive errors, cataracts, glaucoma, macular degeneration and diabetic retinopathy. It also addresses other eye conditions, such as dry eye syndrome, eye infections, corneal disorders, retinal detachments, and ocular tumors. It makes use of various diagnostic tools and techniques, including visual acuity tests, slit-lamp examinations, fundus photography, optical coherence tomography (OCT), and angiography, to assess and diagnose eye disorders accurately. This book includes some of the vital pieces of work being conducted across the world, on various topics related to opthalmology. It will serve as a valuable source of reference for graduate and postgraduate students.

The researches compiled throughout the book are authentic and of high quality, combining several disciplines and from very diverse regions from around the world. Drawing on the contributions of many researchers from diverse countries, the book's objective is to provide the readers with the latest achievements in the area of research. This book will surely be a source of knowledge to all interested and researching the field.

In the end, I would like to express my deep sense of gratitude to all the authors for meeting the set deadlines in completing and submitting their research chapters. I would also like to thank the publisher for the support offered to us throughout the course of the book. Finally, I extend my sincere thanks to my family for being a constant source of inspiration and encouragement.

Editor

1

Ocular Hypotonia and Transient Decrease of Vision as a Consequence of Exposure to a Common Toad Poison

Renato Pejic,[1] **Marija Simic Prskalo**,[1] **and Josip Simic**[2]

[1]*University Clinical Hospital Mostar, Department of Ophthalmology, Bosnia and Herzegovina*
[2]*Faculty of Health Studies, University in Mostar, Bosnia and Herzegovina*

Correspondence should be addressed to Renato Pejic; renato.pejic@gmail.com

Academic Editor: Stephen G. Schwartz

The common toad produces venom (bufotoxin) that is produced in the parotid gland of the toad as well as in the skin. This toxic compound is a potent inhibitor of Na^+/K^+-ATPase activity. Physiological effects of bufotoxin are similar to those of digitalis and cause increased heart rate and muscle contractions. Ocular toxicity was described. A 67-year-old female patient was admitted to the emergency service because of sudden vision loss and a burning sensation in both eyes after she had been exposed to the poison of a toad. Slit lamp examination showed conjunctival hyperaemia and signs of ocular hypotonia. Topical antibiotic treatment was administered, and after 24 hours, corneal oedema and ocular hypotonia were in remission. Inhibition of Na^+/K^+-ATPase is a well-known effect of the toad venom. Na^+/K^+-ATPase is a part of corneal endothelial cells, ciliary body, and iris, and its inhibition caused by exposure to bufadienolides induces corneal dysfunction, decreased vision, and ocular hypotonia. Effects of bufadienolides on the decrease of ocular pressure appear to be very strong, with quick action. This rarely described effect of the bufotoxin can be used as a basis for further research of toad venom and its pharmacological potential. *Purpose.* To present a case of a 67-year-old female patient who experienced a sudden decrease in vision after exposure to the poison from a common toad (*Bufo bufo*).

1. Introduction

The common toad, or European toad (*Bufo bufo*), is an amphibian found in almost all of Europe (with the exception of Iceland, Ireland, and some Mediterranean islands) and in parts of North Asia and North-west Africa. It can live up to 50 years in captivity, and its age is counted by growth rings on their phalanges [1]. It has green-gray-brown skin covered with lumps that produce bufadienolides. Bufadienolides are produced in parotid glands and the skin of a toad [2]. These toxic compounds are potent inhibitors of Na^+/K^+-ATPase activity, and toads use these as a natural repellent against predators and also as an immune defence against pathogens [3, 4]. Bufadienolides are divided into bufagenins, the smaller, hydrolysed molecules which have stronger cardiotoxic effects, and bufotoxins, the larger bufadienolide molecules with an amino-acid side chain [5]. Some research suggests that the ratio of bufadienolides depends of environmental factors [6]. Bufotoxin was first isolated by Hienrich Wieland in 1922, and its structure was described by the same team 20 years later ($C_{40}H_{60}N_4O_{10}$) [7]. The physiological effects of bufotoxin are similar to those of digitalis and causes increased heart rate and muscle contractions. Therefore, it is used worldwide in traditional medicine as an aphrodisiac [8] or as an anti-inflammatory agent [9]. Exposure to large amounts of toxin may cause cardiovascular and respiratory symptoms, such as paralysis and seizures, increased salivation, vomiting, hyperkalemia, cyanosis, and hallucinations [10]. Cases of poisoning of children were described after kissing a frog [11]. Ocular toxicity was also described [12, 13].

2. Case Report

A 67-year-old female patient was admitted to the emergency service because of sudden vision loss and a burning sensation in both eyes after she had been exposed to the poison of a common toad. The patient stated that she had been working in a garden when she noticed something moving under a cabbage leaf. She found a frog under the leaf, got scared, and instinctively stabbed the frog with a knife that she had in her hand. Right after she stabbed the frog, she got a spray of aerosol from the frog's skin on her face. She immediately felt a burning sensation in her eyes and eyelids, ran away to a washroom, and washed her face with a tap water. She noticed that her eyes were red and that her vision was very blurry.

One hour after, she had been examined by an ophthalmologist in a medical center. BCVA (*Best Corrected Visual Acuity*) was 0.3 in her right eye (RE) and 0.2 in the left eye (LE). Slit lamp examination showed conjunctival hyperaemia, slight oedema, and folds of the Descemet membrane of the cornea indicating ocular hypotonia. The anterior eye chamber was clear, and pupillary reactions were normal. Cataract was found on both eyes (grade CO2N1P0 in a LOCS III (*Lens Opacities Classification System*)). Hypotonia was confirmed by Goldmann aplanation tonometry with IOP (*intraocular pressure*) 9 mmHg in the right eye and 10 mmHg in the left eye. The fundus of both eyes was normal. After examination, eyes were washed with 0.9% saline solution and topical antibiotic ointment was administered (tobramicin 5 mg/4 times a day). After one hour, IOP increased to 10 mmHg in the right eye and 12 mmHg in the left eye. The patient was examined again after 6 hours, and regression of corneal oedema was found, as well as the improvement of vision; BCVA RE was 0.7 and BCVA LE was 0.5. IOP pressure also increased to 13 mmHg in both eyes. After 12 hours, BCVA improved to 0.8 in the right eye and 0.6 in the left eye. IOP pressure was 14 mmHg in the right eye and 15 mmHg in the left eye and Descemet membrane folds, as well as corneal oedema, were in remission.

3. Discussion

The toxic effect of bufadienolides on the cornea with consequential corneal oedema and ocular hypotension was probably caused by the inhibition of Na^+/K^+-ATPase, which is a well-known effect of the toad's venom [14]. Na^+/K^+-ATPase is a part of corneal endothelial cells and has an important role in maintaining corneal clarity through active pumping [15, 16]. It is also a part of the ciliary body epithelium and iris where it controls the rate of aqueous humor formation. It consists of $\alpha 1$ and $\alpha 2$ subunits which are present in the ciliary body epithelium. The $\alpha 1$ subunit is present on the basolateral surface of the pigmented epithelium, while the $\alpha 2$ subunit is located in the nonpigmented epithelium on the side facing the aqueous humor [17]. Some studies have suggested that the Na^+/K^+ ATPase $\alpha 1$ subunit might control overall sodium secretion to the aqueous humor, while the $\alpha 2$ may be responsible for the entry of sodium to the ciliary epithelium bilayer across the basolateral surface of the pigmented epithelium [18–20]. Inhibition of Na^+/K^+-ATPase in these tissues caused by exposure to bufadienolides was the most obvious reason for corneal dysfunction that caused a transient decrease of vision, and also for a hypotonia as a result of ciliary body dysfunction and disturbed control of aqueous humor production. The improvement in IOP after a few hours was probably not caused by the administered topical antibiotic treatment but rather by time passed from the exposure, where the irrigation of the ocular surface helped to remove the remaining toxin and inhibited continuous exposure, which resulted in ciliary function recovery and IOP improvement.

In conclusion, the poison of a common toad can cause ocular hypotonia and corneal oedema. Effects of bufadienolides on a decrease of ocular pressure appear to be very strong, with quick action and caused by Na^+/K^+ ATPase inhibition in corneal endothelium cells, ciliary body, and iris. This rarely described effect of bufadienolides could be used as a basis for further research of a toad's venom and its effects on ocular surface and pharmacological potential.

References

[1] A. S. M. Hemelaar and J. J. Van Gelder, "Annual growth rings in phalanges of *Bufo bufo* (Anura, Amphibia) from the Netherlands and their use for age determination," *Netherlands Journal of Zoology*, vol. 30, no. 1, pp. 129–135, 1979.

[2] R. Shine, "The ecological impact of invasive cane toads (*Bufo marinus*) in Australia," *The Quarterly Review of Biology*, vol. 85, no. 3, pp. 253–291, 2010.

[3] B.-I. Henrikson, "Predation on amphibian eggs and tadpoles by common predators in acidified lakes," *Ecography*, vol. 13, no. 3, pp. 201–206, 1990.

[4] K. Barnhart, M. E. Forman, T. P. Umile et al., "Identification of bufadienolides from the boreal toad, *Anaxyrus boreas*, active against a fungal pathogen," *Microbial Ecology*, vol. 74, no. 4, pp. 990–1000, 2017.

[5] K. K. Chen and A. L. Chen, "Similarity and dis-similarity of bufagins, bufotoxins, and digitaloid glucosides," *Journal of Pharmacology and Experimental Therapeutics*, vol. 49, no. 4, pp. 561–579, 1933.

[6] V. Bókony, B. Üveges, V. Verebélyi, N. Ujhegyi, and Á. M. Móricz, "Toads phenotypically adjust their chemical defences to anthropogenic habitat change," *Scientific Reports*, vol. 9, no. 1, p. 3163, 2019.

[7] K. K. Chen, H. Jensen, and A. L. Chen, "Action of Bufotoxins," *Proceedings of the Society for Experimental Biology and Medicine*, vol. 29, no. 7, pp. 907–907, 1932.

[8] G. Ashok, Ramkumar, S. R. Sakunthala, and D. Rajasekaran, "An interesting case of cardiotoxicity due to bufotoxin (toad toxin)," *The Journal of the Association of Physicians of India*, vol. 59, pp. 737-738, 2011.

[9] J. Qi, C. K. Tan, S. M. Hashimi, A. H. M. Zulfiker, D. Good, and M. Q. Wei, "Toad glandular secretions and skin extractions as anti-inflammatory and anticancer agents," *Evidence-Based Complementary and Alternative Medicine*, vol. 2014, 9 pages, 2014.

[10] M. M. Sebastian, *Veterinary Toxicology*, Academic Press, 2007, MM S.

[11] K. Henricksen, "The danger of kissing toads: fire-bellied toad exposure and assessment parameters in children," *Journal of Emergency Nursing*, vol. 25, no. 3, pp. 235–237, 1999.

[12] J. M. Lopez-Lopez, M. R. Sanabria, and S. J. de Prada, "Ocular toxicity caused by toad venom," *Cornea*, vol. 27, no. 2, pp. 236-237, 2008.

[13] M. B. Forrester, "Pediatric exposures to *Bombina* toads reported to poison centers," *Pediatric Emergency Care*, vol. 34, no. 1, pp. 25-26, 2018.

[14] K. Shimada, K. Ohishi, H. Fukunaga, J. S. Ro, and T. Nambara, "Structure-activity relationship of bufotoxins and related

compounds for the inhibition of Na^{+},K^{+}-adenosine triphosphatase," *Journal of Pharmacobio-Dynamics*, vol. 8, no. 12, pp. 1054–1059, 1985.

[15] Z. Li, H. Duan, W. Li et al., "Nicotinamide inhibits corneal endothelial mesenchymal transition and accelerates wound healing," *Experimental Eye Research*, vol. 184, pp. 227–233, 2019.

[16] W. T. Ho, C. C. Su, J. S. Chang et al., "In vitro and in vivo models to study corneal endothelial-mesenchymal transition," *JoVE (Journal of Visualized Experiments)*, vol. 114, 2016.

[17] N. A. Delamere, "Ciliary body and ciliary epithelium," in *Advances in Organ Biology*, vol. 10, pp. 127–148, Elsevier, 2005.

[18] S. Ghosh, N. Hernando, J. M. Martín-Alonso, P. Martin-Vasallo, and M. Coca-Prados, "Expression of multiple Na^{+},K^{+}-ATPase genes reveals a gradient of isoforms along the nonpigmented ciliary epithelium: functional implications in aqueous humor secretion," *Journal of Cellular Physiology*, vol. 149, no. 2, pp. 184–194, 1991.

[19] X. Arakaki, P. McCleary, M. Techy et al., "Na,K-ATPase alpha isoforms at the blood-cerebrospinal fluid-trigeminal nerve and blood-retina interfaces in the rat," *Fluids and Barriers of the CNS*, vol. 10, no. 1, p. 14, 2013.

[20] I. González-Marrero, L. Hernández-Abad, E. Carmona-Calero, L. Castañeyra-Ruiz, J. Abreu-Reyes, and A. Castañeyra-Perdomo, "Systemic hypertension effects on the ciliary body and iris. An immunofluorescence study with aquaporin 1, aquaporin 4, and Na^{+},K^{+} ATPase in hypertensive rats," *Cells*, vol. 7, no. 11, p. 210, 2018.

2

Challenges in the Management of Upper Lid Keloid

Ruchi Goel,[1] **Samreen Khanam**,[1] **Shalin Shah**,[1] **and Ravindra Kumar Saran**[2]

[1]*Ophthalmology, Maulana Azad Medical College, New Delhi, India*
[2]*Pathology, Govind Ballabh Pant Hospital, New Delhi, India*

Correspondence should be addressed to Ruchi Goel; gruchi1970@gmail.com

Academic Editor: Stephen G. Schwartz

A middle-aged lady presented with a firm, nontender mass on the left upper lid and area behind the left ear following lid reconstruction with postauricular graft for cicatricial ectropion 11 months prior. She had a similar mass on the right shin. She was diagnosed as a case of multiple keloids. Intralesional injection of triamcinolone acetonide suspension and 5-Fluorouracil (5-FU) in the upper lid keloid resulted in ulceration of its surface. Surgical excision, injection of 5-FU in the keloid bed with temporal forehead flap reconstruction, was performed. Occurrence of inadvertent postoperative wound infection with *Acinetobacter baumannii* was treated with local dressing with colistimethate sodium. Adjuvant therapy with topical imiquimod cream 5% was given subsequently for 24 weeks with no recurrence of the lid keloid after 16 months. The patient was managed using a combination of conservative and surgical therapy and multidisciplinary team work and kept on a long term follow-up.

1. Introduction

Wound healing is a natural dynamic process involving a complex interplay between regulatory mediators and involves stages of inflammation, proliferation, and remodeling. The phase of remodeling, which usually begins 3 weeks after tissue injury and continues for months thereafter, is primarily responsible for variation in scar quality. Abnormal regulation of the healing process can result in pathological scarring in the form of keloids and hypertrophic scars [1]. Keloids as compared to hypertrophic scars, appear slowly over months, extend beyond the wound causing greater aesthetic disfiguration and discomfort [2].

The occurrence of keloids has strong racial and genetic influences, with higher incidence seen in individuals with African, Asian, and Native American ethnicity (ranging from 5% to 16%) [3]. Familial cases have also been observed, and a number of genes and genetic loci identified, although no one specific gene has been found to be associated. Melanocytes appear to play a contributory role in keloid development as its incidence is very low in Caucasians (approximately, 0.1%), and has rarely been reported in individuals with albinism [4].

Keloids are mostly seen in wounds experiencing high tensile forces. In the head and neck region, the common sites for keloid formation are ear lobe, postauricular area, occipital scalp, and upper neck [5].

Involvement of upper eyelids is rare, possibly due to its inherent characteristics of thinness and laxity of skin. Many of the conventional treatment protocols may not apply to this region. Herein, we describe the challenges faced during the management of the upper lid keloid.

2. Case Presentation

A middle-aged lady presented with the chief complaint of a progressively increasing mass on her left upper eyelid and behind the left ear for the past 7 months which caused discomfort in wearing spectacles. She had a history of road traffic accident 11 months back during which she sustained injury to both lids of the left eye and fracture of the right leg bones. Her records revealed left upper lid reconstruction with postauricular graft 10 months prior for upper lid cicatricial ectropion with lagophthalmos. Two months following

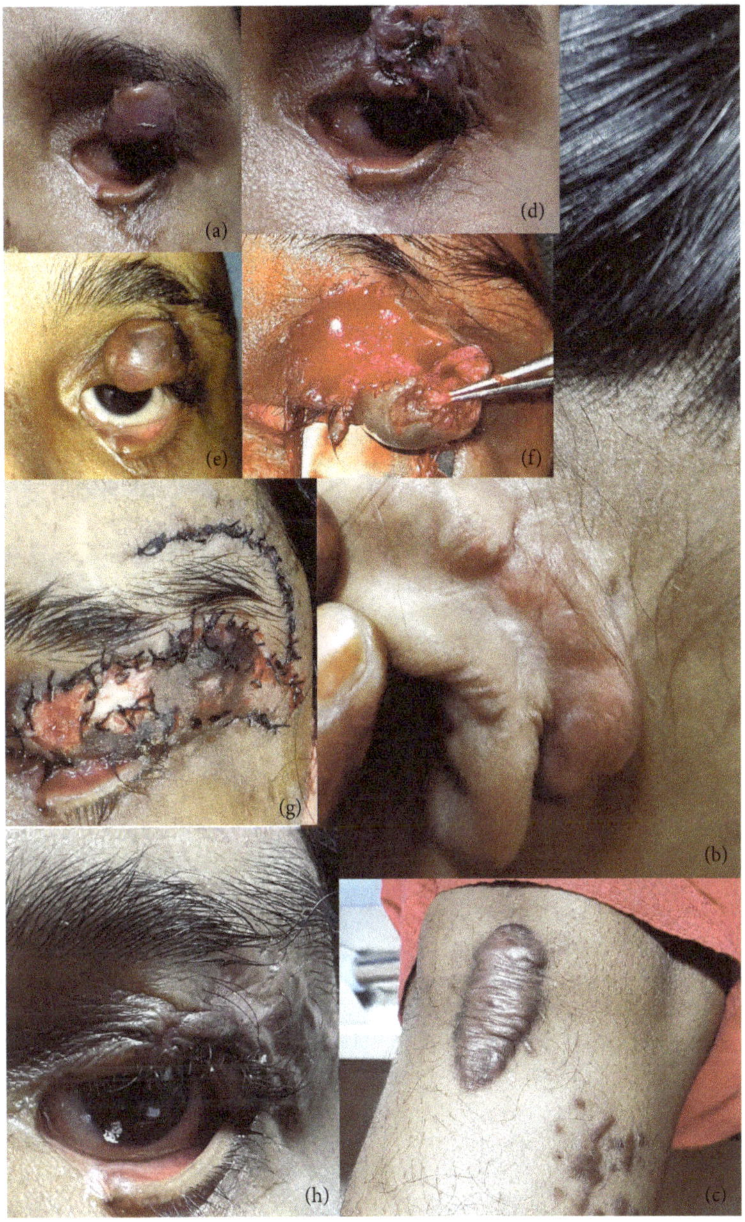

Figure 1: (a) A well-defined mass seen on the left upper lid (1.5 cm × 1.2 cm × 1 cm) involving the lid margin. (b) Thickened mass seen in the postauricular area. (c) Hyperpigmented lesions seen on the right leg. (d) Ulceration of keloid surface following intralesional 5-FU (50 mg/mL) and crystalline TAC (40 mg/mL) injection. (e) Regrowth of keloid after discontinuation of 5-FU (50 mg/mL) and crystalline TAC (40 mg/mL) injection. (f) Excision of keloid. (g) Development of postsurgical wound infection. (h) Clinical appearance after 16 months of upper lid keloid excision.

surgery, she started having itching, redness, and thickening of the left upper lid and postauricular region.

Upon presentation to our clinic, her best corrected visual acuity was 20/20 in both eyes. A thickened mass (1.5 cm × 1.2 cm × 1 cm) involving the lid margin was seen on the left upper lid (Figure 1(a)). It was nontender and firm in consistency with no overlying skin changes. There was limitation in the left eyelid excursion. The left lower eyelid had 1/3rd medial defect with canalicular injury and cicatricial ectropion. Syringing was patent through the upper punctum. Bell's phenomenon was good. The extraocular adenexa of the right eye as well as the anterior and posterior segments of both the eyes were unremarkable.

Firm lesions (4 cm × 5 cm × 5 cm) were seen in the left postauricular region and anterior aspect of the right leg (4 cm × 1.5 cm × 0.5 cm) and right medial leg (Figures 1(b) and 1(c)). There was no history of previous injury or ear piercing. Her father gave history of similar lesions on his chest wound 20 years back for which he had undergone excision with no further recurrence.

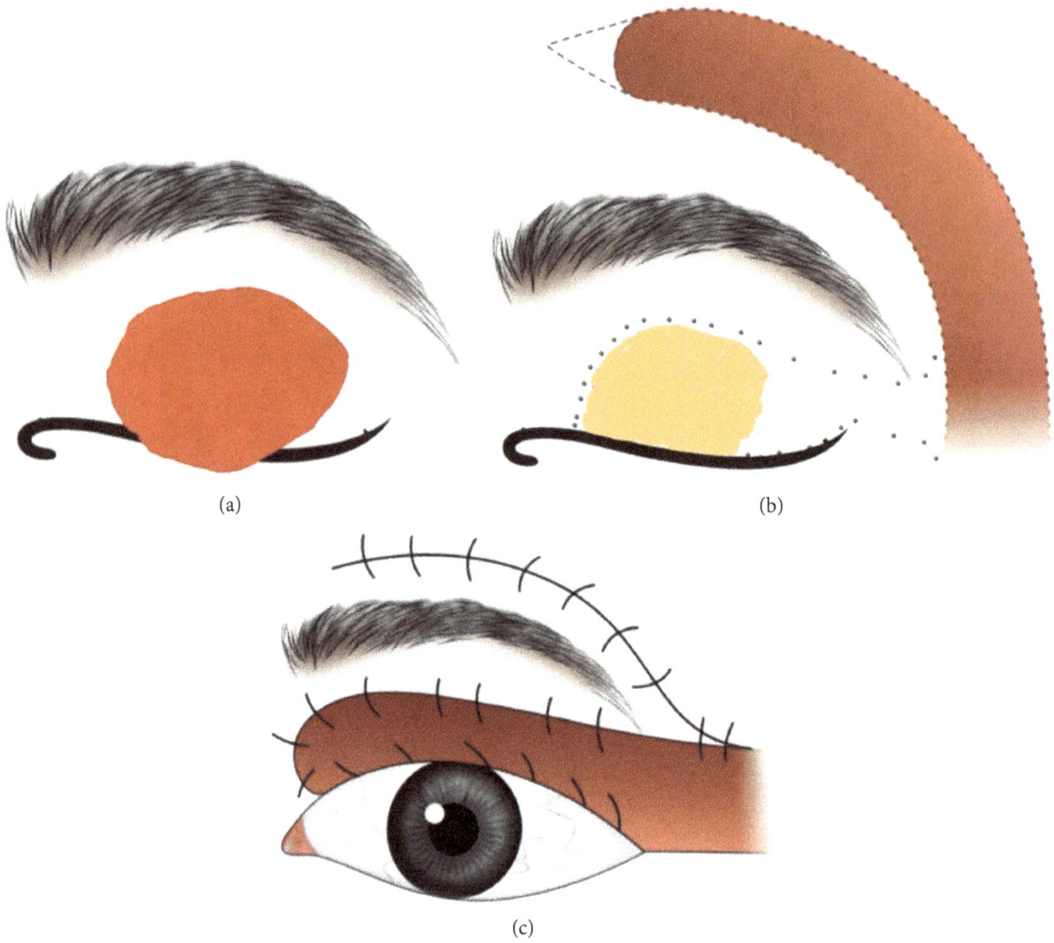

FIGURE 2: (a) A well-defined mass seen on the left upper lid involving the lid margin. (b) After excision of the mass, the skin was undermined to decrease the size of the anterior lamellar defect and a lateral forehead rotational flap was raised. (c) The lateral forehead flap was mobilized to cover the defect, and the wound was closed without tension on suture line.

Her blood group was A positive. Haemogram, blood sugar, and kidney function tests were within normal limit.

3. Treatment

A diagnosis of multiple keloids was made, and treatment was commenced for the upper lid lesion. She was advised to apply silicone gel (Scarend silicone gel, Mankind pharmaceuticals) twice a day for a month. Three doses of intralesional 5-Fluorouracil (5-FU) (50 mg/mL) and crystalline triamcinolone acetonide suspension (TAC) (40 mg/mL) in 3 : 1 ratio were then given at 3 weekly intervals. There was a shrinkage in the size of the lesion (1.3 cm × 1.2 cm × 0.5 cm), but further injections were stopped following development of ulceration on the keloid surface (Figure 1(d)). The ulcer healed in a month; however, the patient declined further injections. She returned 8 months later with increase in the size of the upper lid lesion (1.6 cm × 1.3 cm × 1.2 cm) (Figure 1(e)). Complete surgical excision of the eyelid keloid was performed, and the defect was closed with a lateral forehead rotational flap under asepsis (Figure 1(f), Figure 2). One millilitre of 5-FU (50 mg/mL) was injected at the wound site intraoperatively. She was discharged on tablet Augmentin 625 mg 8 hourly, tablet Ibuprofen 400 mg 8 hourly, and local application of tobramycin eye ointment twice daily.

Histopathological features of the excised lesion were suggestive of keloid. The interstitium showed focal positivity on transforming growth factor beta (TGF-β) marker. There were mature collagen fibres and absence of myofibroblasts in the marginal area (Figure 3).

In the follow-up visit on the 7th postoperative day, tissue discoloration and a pus point were noticed adjacent to the lid suture (Figure 1(g)). The discharge was sent for microbiological examination and *Acinetobacter baumanii,* sensitive to colistin, and tigecycline *was* isolated. Daily dressing with application of colistimethate sodium (CMS) (4.5 million IU) (Xylistin, Cipla) colistin powder was done for 14 days, which resulted in satisfactory wound healing. The patient was advised local application daily of imiquimod 5% cream for 24 weeks.

4. Outcome and Follow-Up

At 16 months of follow up, there was no evidence of recurrence of keloid on the left upper lid (Figure 1(h)). She was advised to keep a watch for symptoms suggestive of keloid

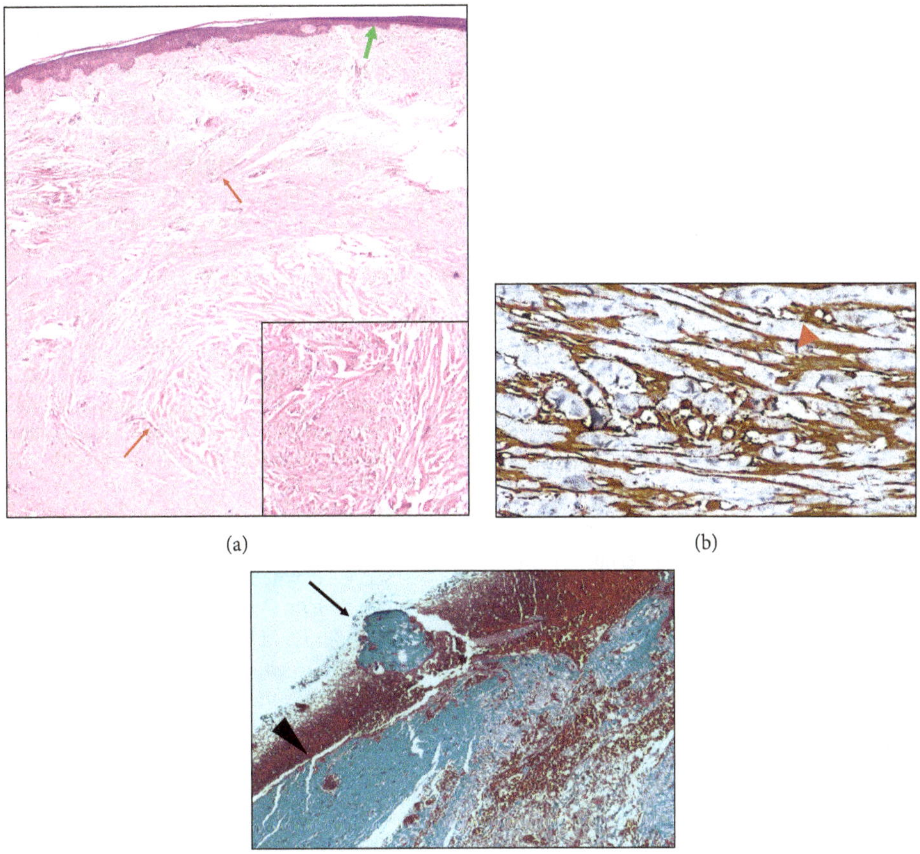

FIGURE 3: (a) Histopathology showing stretched out epithelium (green arrow), paucicellular thick collagen bundles, and few widely scattered blood vessels (red arrows) (hematoxylin-eosin stain-HE, 4x). Inset shows disorganised, large, hyalinised collagen fibres (HE, 20x). (b) TGF-β marker shows focal positivity (red arrowhead) in the interstitium suggesting active fibroblast activity (Immunohistochemistry, 40x). (c) Thick collagen bundles (black arrowhead) with a nodule of thick collagen fibres (black arrow) at the margin of the lesion (Masson-trichome stain, 10x).

recurrence such as firmness and redness of the scar or surrounding area and itching.

Her postauricular keloid was excised by the plastic surgery department. She was not inclined for treatment of her leg lesions or left lower lid ectropion.

5. Discussion

The development of keloid results in cosmetic disfigurement, pruritus, pain, and hyperesthesia resulting in impairment of health-related quality of life. It is usually seen in individuals between 10 and 30 years but can affect beyond sixth decade [6, 7]. Lesser frequency of scar formation in elderly is attributed to reduction in skin tension and sebaceous gland activity. Associated risk factors include dark skin pigmentation, positive family history, blood group A, and hormonal changes occurring during puberty or pregnancy [8].' Our patient was a quadragenarian, with brown skin colour, a positive family history, and blood group A.

Keloids most commonly affect upper arms, skin overlying joints, chest, shoulders, and ear lobes. High skin tension plays a critical role in scar formation. Tension across an incision tends to pull the skin edges apart and the wound, in response increases the collagen deposition. Areas with rich blood supply like face are known to heal with finer scars [1]. In our patient, possibly, in postinjury, there was a development of a large upper lid defect which led to extensive cicatrization. Closure of both donor and recipient site under tension during the reconstruction procedure, in a predisposed patient, could have led to keloid formation in both the donor and recipient area.

In the early stages of keloid maturation, corticosteroids, 5-Fluorouracil (5-FU), bleomycin, and verapamil have been used for treatment [9]. Application of silicone gel or hydrocolloid dressings prior to intralesional injection of 5FU or TAC results in scar softening [10]. Surgical excision is indicated in nonreactive refractory keloids and often combined with adjuvant therapy, such as corticosteroid, 5-FU, radiotherapy, 5% imiquimod application, or cryotherapy to lower the recurrence rates [11, 12].

TAC is the most widely used corticosteroid with reported recurrence rates varying from 33% to 50% when used alone [3]. 5-FU, a pyrimidine analog, inhibits the proliferation and differentiation of myofibroblasts. It is used as monotherapy or in combination with steroids. The reported side effects of intralesional steroid are pain, skin atrophy, alteration in skin pigmentation, and formation of telangiectasias. The 5-FU may cause local erythema, pain, hyperpigmentation, ulceration, a burning sensation, and sloughing [11, 13]. We used a combination therapy of 5-FU and TAC; however, following three doses of intralesional injection, though the volume decreased, an ulcer developed on the surface of keloid. Later, following discontinuation of injection, the keloid again increased in size.

Wide surgical excision of keloid is recommended to prevent regrowth [14]. Wide excision was not suitable for the upper lid keloid, as in our case. The clinically visible mass was thus excised, 5-FU was injected in the wound bed, and the wound meticulously closed after mobilization of temporal forehead flap to avoid skin tension. Intramarginal core excisions have low recurrence rates in mature keloids [15]. In general, recurrence rates of 0 to 44% have been reported with surgical excision without adjuvant therapy [2]. The plausible options after excision in our case included local injection of steroids, 5 FU, and interferon alpha-2b. Also, topical imiquimod cream 5% and application of an absorbent material soaked in 1 mg/mL of mitomycin C could have been used. Compressive therapy successfully used in ear keloids was not appropriate for upper lid. Radiation therapy, an effective adjunctive therapy after excision, is usually reserved for refractory keloids [5]. Since our patient was unwilling for injectables, topical imiquimod cream 5% (Imiquad, Mecoson labs private limited, India) was prescribed twice a day for 24 weeks after control of postoperative wound infection. The patient did not show recurrence of upper lid keloid till the last follow-up visit.

Despite detailed instructions to maintain wound hygiene, the patient developed postoperative infection with *Acinetobacter baumanii,* sensitive to colistin and tigecycline. Local application of colistin instead of systemic administration, in susceptible infections, prevents renal toxicity and reduces the treatment cost [16]. In our case also, the infection was successfully controlled with local application of colistimethate sodium; however, the wound healed with scarring of lid margin.

To conclude, keloid of the eyelid, a rarely reported clinical entity, can be managed by a combination of surgical and nonsurgical treatment modalities. Given the occurrence of keloid at multiple sites and unpredictable duration of recurrence, a multidisciplinary coordination and a long-term follow-up is required.

References

[1] D. Son and A. Harijan, "Overview of surgical scar prevention and management," *Journal of Korean Medical Science*, vol. 29, no. 6, pp. 751–757, 2014.

[2] U. Betarbet and T. W. Blalock, "Keloids: a review of etiology, prevention, and treatment," *The Journal of Clinical and Aesthetic Dermatology*, vol. 13, no. 2, pp. 33–43, 2020.

[3] M. Morelli Coppola, R. Salzillo, F. Segreto, and P. Persichetti, "Triamcinolone acetonide intralesional injection for the treatment of keloid scars: patient selection and perspectives," *Clinical, Cosmetic and Investigational Dermatology*, vol. - Volume 11, pp. 387–396, 2018.

[4] F. L. Gao, R. Jin, L. Zhang, and Y. G. Zhang, "The contribution of melanocytes to pathological scar formation during wound healing," *International Journal of Clinical and Experimental Medicine*, vol. 6, no. 7, pp. 609–613, 2013.

[5] K. Boahene, A. E. Brissett, and L. R. Jones, "Facial plastic surgery controversies: keloids," *Facial Plastic Surgery Clinics of North America*, vol. 26, no. 2, pp. 105–112, 2018.

[6] J. P. Andrews, J. Marttala, E. Macarak, J. Rosenbloom, and J. Uitto, "Keloids: The paradigm of skin fibrosis - pathomechanisms and treatment," *Matrix Biology*, vol. 51, pp. 37–46, 2016.

[7] K. Kassi, K. Kouame, A. Kouassi et al., "Quality of life in black African patients with keloid scars," *Dermatol Reports*, vol. 12, no. 2, p. 8312, 2020.

[8] N. Ojeh, A. Bharatha, U. Gaur, and A. L. Forde, "Keloids: current and emerging therapies," *Scars Burn Heal.*, vol. 6, p. 2059513120940499, 2020.

[9] J. A. Ledon, J. Savas, K. Franca, A. Chacon, and K. Nouri, "Intralesional treatment for keloids and hypertrophic scars: a review," *Dermatologic Surgery*, vol. 39, no. 12, pp. 1745–1757, 2013.

[10] G. V. de Oliveira and M. H. Gold, "Hydrocolloid dressings can be used to treat hypertrophic scars: an outpatient dermatology service devoted to treat keloids and challenging scars," *Journal of Cosmetic Dermatology*, vol. 19, no. 12, pp. 3344–3348, 2020.

[11] J. Y. Shin and J. S. Kim, "Could 5-Fluorouracil or triamcinolone be an effective treatment option for keloid after surgical excision? A meta-analysis," *Journal of Oral and Maxillofacial Surgery*, vol. 74, no. 5, pp. 1055–1060, 2016.

[12] M. H. Gold, M. McGuire, T. A. Mustoe et al., "International Advisory Panel on Scar Management. Updated international clinical recommendations on scar management: part 2–algorithms for scar prevention and treatment," *Dermatologic Surgery*, vol. 40, no. 8, pp. 825–831, 2014.

[13] S. F. Ekstein, S. P. Wyles, S. L. Moran, and A. Meves, "Keloids: a review of therapeutic management," *International Journal of Dermatology*, vol. 60, no. 6, pp. 661–671, 2021.

[14] K. T. Tan, N. Shah, S. A. Pritchard, D. A. McGrouther, and A. Bayat, "The influence of surgical excision margins on keloid prognosis," *Annals of Plastic Surgery*, vol. 64, no. 1, pp. 55–58, 2010.

[15] G. Lemperle, J. Schierle, K. E. Kitoga, K. Kassem-Trautmann, C. Sachs, and A. Dimmler, "Keloids: which types can be excised without risk of recurrence? A new clinical classification," *Plastic and Reconstructive Surgery. Global Open*, vol. 8, no. 3, p. e2582, 2020.

[16] S. Murali, A. V. Pillai, and R. Ramachandran, "Efficacy of colistimethate sodium as local application in necrotising fasciitis," *BML Case Reports*, vol. 12, no. 11, article e232354, 2019.

3

Intravitreal Brolucizumab for Choroidal Neovascularization Associated to Angioid Streaks

Somnath Chakraborty[1] and Jay Umed Sheth[2]

[1]*Retina Institute of Bengal, Siliguri, India*
[2]*Surya Eye Institute and Research Center, Mumbai, India*

Correspondence should be addressed to Somnath Chakraborty; somnathboom@gmail.com

Academic Editor: Stephen G. Schwartz

A 44-year-old-female with angioid streak- (AS-) associated choroidal-neovascularization (CNV) was treated with one dose of intravitreal brolucizumab (IB). At one-month, the patient's visual acuity (VA) improved from 20/120 to 20/40 with a dry macula on spectral-domain optical-coherence tomography (SD-OCT). After observation, the VA improved further to 20/32 with absence of any fluid on the SD-OCT at three months. No ocular or systemic adverse events were noted. In conclusion, intravitreal brolucizumab (IB) is an efficacious and safe therapeutic option for the management of CNV secondary to AS. Further prospective studies with a larger sample size, varied therapeutic regimens, and longer follow-up period are needed to corroborate our findings.

1. Introduction

Angioid streaks (AS) are linear cracks or dehiscence in an unusually weak or calcified Bruch's membrane [1]. They can be caused by systemic diseases such as pseudoxanthoma elasticum (PXE), Ehlers–Danlos syndrome, Paget's disease, or sickle cell disease, although up to 50% of patients may have no obvious systemic association [1]. One of the most significant complications of AS is choroidal neovascularization (CNV), which has been recorded in 70–86% of eyes [1, 2]. Over time, 71% of these patients also develop CNV in the contralateral eye [1, 2]. Subfoveal and juxtafoveal CNV in AS have been treated with photodynamic therapy (PDT) with suboptimal visual outcomes in the long term [3, 4]. Similarly, equivocal results with considerable recurrences have been observed in extrafoveal CNV treated with thermal laser (TL) photocoagulation [5, 6].

According to recent research, the use of antivascular endothelial growth factor (anti-VEGF) therapy is efficacious in the management of CNV secondary to AS [7–12]. The use of ranibizumab, bevacizumab, and aflibercept, among the existing anti-VEGF medications, has been documented for treating AS-related CNV [7–12]. The most recently FDA-approved treatment for neovascular age-related macular degeneration (nAMD) is the brolucizumab (Beovu ®; Novartis, Basel, Switzerland) molecule [13]. It has been successfully used in the management of recalcitrant diabetic macular edema (DME) as an off-label medication [13].

We herein report a novel case of AS-associated CNV which was successfully treated with intravitreal brolucizumab (IB).

2. Case Report

A 44-year-old female presented with a reduction in vision and metamorphopsia in the left eye (OS) for 3 months. Her best-corrected visual acuity (BCVA) was 20/20 in the right eye (OD) and 20/120 in OS. Both eyes (OU) anterior segments were unremarkable with normal intraocular pressure (IOP) of 18 mmHg. Fundus examination of OD was normal while OS showed the presence of AS with subretinal hemorrhage (SRH). On spectral-domain optical coherence tomography (SD-OCT), there was the presence of subretinal hyperreflectivity, subretinal fluid (SRF), and a thickened Bruch's membrane. A diagnosis of CNV secondary to AS was made and the patient underwent treatment with

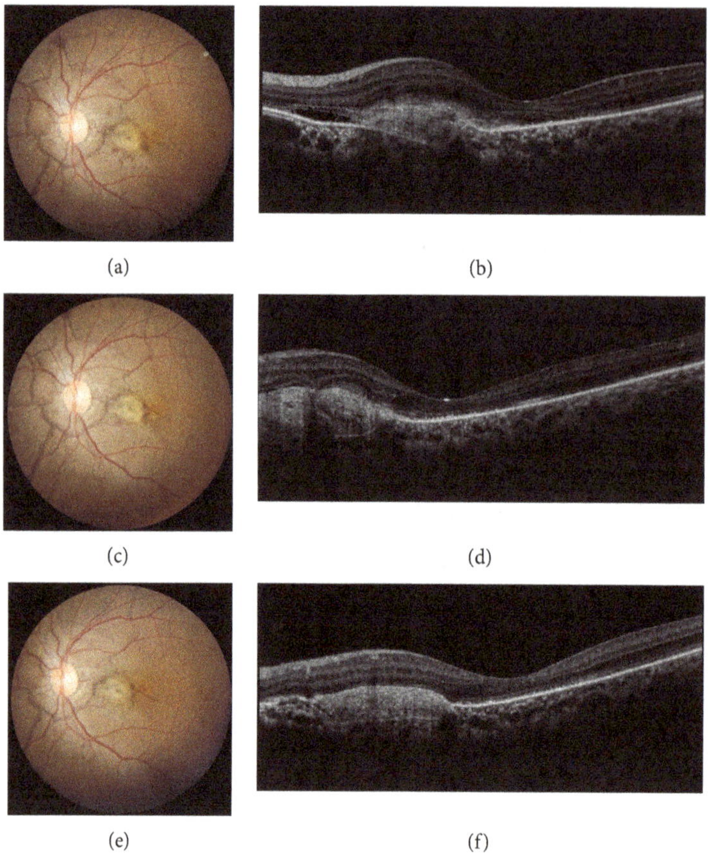

Figure 1: At baseline, the color fundus photograph (CFP) of the left eye (OS) showed the presence of angioid streaks (AS) with subretinal hemorrhage (SRH) suggestive of an underlying choroidal neovascularization (CNV) (a). Spectral-domain optical coherence tomography of the OS illustrated the presence of subretinal fluid (SRF) with subretinal hyperreflectivity and thickened Bruch's membrane (b). After undergoing intravitreal brolucizumab injection, the SRH reduced significantly at one month (c) and disappeared completely by three months (e) as noted on the CFP. The SD-OCT scans at months 1 (d) and 3 (f) demonstrated complete resolution of the fluid and a reduction in the subretinal hyperreflectivity.

intravitreal brolucizumab (IB) (6 mg/0.5 ml) following a discussion of all the therapeutic options. At one month, the patient's BCVA improved to 20/40 with a dry macula on SD-OCT. Trace SRH was present clinically, and the patient was observed. The trace SRH resolved completely by the end of three months with an improvement in BCVA to 20/32. The SD-OCT was dry at this stage too. There were no ocular or systemic adverse effects observed. Figure 1 depicts the changes in color fundus photograph (CFP) and SD-OCT in OU throughout the course of the treatment.

3. Discussion

In our case report, we describe a patient with AS who developed CNV which was successfully treated by brolucizumab injection. To date, although off-label, the use of brolucizumab for CNV management in AS has not been reported. In our case, we found no ocular or systemic adverse effects.

The AS is histologically characterized as cracks in the elastic lamina of the Bruch's membrane (BM) with accompanying calcification [1, 14]. The majority of AS are asymptomatic and need periodic fundus examination [1, 2]. AS can cause substantial vision impairment due to CNV development [2]. The risk factors for the development of CNV include advancing age and the length, width, and location of the AS [2, 14, 15]. Wider and longer AS have been linked to an increased likelihood of CNV in several studies [2, 15]. Moreover, if the AS is situated within one optic disc diameter of the foveola, the probability of CNV formation is significantly increased [15, 16]. Various therapeutic modalities, including PDT and TL, have been explored in the past but are no longer employed due to poor outcomes [3–6, 17]. After VEGF inhibitors were established in the treatment of CNV secondary to nAMD, they provided an effective therapeutic option for other chorioretinal disorders such as AS [1, 2].

Cases with AS and associated CNV are infrequent, and hence, there have been very few studies evaluating the efficacy of intravitreal anti-VEGF therapy in its management. Teixeira et al. initially reported the use of intravitreal bevacizumab injection in a patient with subfoveal CNV and AS [18]. Subsequently, the use of the other anti-VEGF molecules, including ranibizumab and aflibercept, has been reported in the literature [7, 8, 11, 12]. A retrospective series of 35 eyes with CNV secondary to AS treated with ranibizumab was evaluated by Mimoun et al. [19]. At a mean follow-up of 24.1 months, the authors noted an improvement or stabilization of BCVA in 30 eyes (85.7%), absence of leakage on fundus fluorescein angiography (FFA) in 23 eyes (65.7%), and reduction or stabilization of central macular thickness (CMT) in 18 eyes (51.5%) [19]. The Italian EYLEA-STRIE study was a multicentre, open-label, phase IIb study evaluating the safety and efficacy of intravitreal aflibercept therapy on a pro-re-nata basis in 23 eyes of 20 patients with CNV secondary to AS [11]. At 48 weeks, the authors observed an improvement in BCVA with visual stabilization within 15 letters in 81.8% of the eyes and a significant reduction in CMT [11]. According to Sekfali et al., switching to aflibercept injection was a good treatment choice for patients with CNV secondary to AS who had resistant or recurrent illness after at least 12 months of ranibizumab therapy [20]. The authors demonstrated an improvement in BCVA with a significant reduction in CMT, along with 71% of the eyes having no intraretinal (IRF)/SRF and 77% having no leakage on FFA among the 14 eyes [20]. However, the efficacy of brolucizumab injection in these cases, whether treatment-naïve or with recalcitrant/recurrent disease, has not been reported in the literature.

Brolucizumab is a single-chain humanized antibody fragment with a relatively small molecular size and a weight of only 26 kDa [13]. Brolucizumab's effective molar dose is 12-fold greater than aflibercept and 22-fold more than ranibizumab due to its low molecular weight, which is 1/1.8 of that of ranibizumab and 1/4 of that of aflibercept [13]. Smaller molecules, such as brolucizumab, have exhibited superior target-tissue penetration, resulting in longer durability, better efficacy, and reduced systemic exposure [21]. These molecular properties of brolucizumab can be advantageous in a condition such as AS which has thickened and calcified Bruch's membrane and an abnormal retinal pigment epithelium (RPE) [1, 14]. Theoretically, its smaller size and increased tissue penetration make it an ideal candidate to pass through this abnormal RPE-Bruch's membrane tissue complex and act on the CNV. With this backdrop, our patient received intravitreal brolucizumab (IB) and demonstrated promising visual and anatomical outcomes. Moreover, although intraocular inflammation (IOI) remains a concern with brolucizumab therapy, we did not note any ocular or systemic adverse event in our case up to three months [13].

In conclusion, this is the first reported case demonstrating the role of intravitreal brolucizumab injection in the management of CNV secondary to AS. Further prospective studies with a larger sample size and different therapeutic regimens are needed to validate our findings.

References

[1] I. Chatziralli, G. Saitakis, E. Dimitriou et al., "Angioid streaks," *Retina*, vol. 39, no. 1, pp. 1–11, 2019.

[2] I. Georgalas, D. Papaconstantinou, C. Koutsandrea et al., "Angioid streaks, clinical course, complications, and current therapeutic management," *Therapeutics and Clinical Risk Management*, vol. 5, no. 1, pp. 81–89, 2009.

[3] A. C. Browning, A. K. Chung, F. Ghanchi et al., "Verteporfin photodynamic therapy of choroidal neovascularization in angioid streaks: one-year results of a prospective case series," *Ophthalmology*, vol. 112, no. 7, pp. 1227–1231.e1, 2005.

[4] A. C. Browning, W. M. Amoaku, A. K. Chung et al., "Photodynamic therapy for angioid streaks," *Ophthalmology*, vol. 114, no. 8, pp. 1592–1592.e1, 2007.

[5] J. I. Lim, N. M. Bressler, M. J. Marsh, and S. B. Bressler, "Laser treatment of choroidal neovascularization in patients with angioid streaks," *American Journal of Ophthalmology*, vol. 116, no. 4, pp. 414–423, 1993.

[6] A. Pece, P. Avanza, L. Galli, and R. Brancato, "Laser photocoagulation of choroidal neovascularization in angioid streaks," *Retina*, vol. 17, no. 1, pp. 12–16, 1997.

[7] I. D. Ladas, A. I. Kotsolis, D. S. Ladas et al., "Intravitreal ranibizumab treatment of macular choroidal neovascularization secondary to angioid streaks: one-year results of a prospective study," *Retina*, vol. 30, no. 8, pp. 1185–1189, 2010.

[8] J. Tilleul, G. Mimoun, G. Querques et al., "Intravitreal ranibizumab for choroidal neovascularization in angioid streaks: four-year follow-up," *Retina*, vol. 36, no. 3, pp. 483–491, 2016.

[9] C. Alagöz, N. Alagöz, A. Özkaya et al., "Intravitreal bevacizumab in the treatment of choroidal neovascular membrane due to angioid streaks," *Retina*, vol. 35, no. 10, pp. 2001–2010, 2015.

[10] M. Sawa, F. Gomi, M. Tsujikawa, H. Sakaguchi, and Y. Tano, "Long-term results of intravitreal bevacizumab injection for choroidal neovascularization secondary to angioid streaks," *American Journal of Ophthalmology*, vol. 148, no. 4, pp. 584–590.e2, 2009.

[11] M. B. Parodi, M. V. Cicinelli, A. Marchese et al., "Intravitreal aflibercept for management of choroidal neovascularization secondary to angioid streaks: the Italian EYLEA-STRIE study," *European Journal of Ophthalmology*, vol. 31, no. 3, pp. 1146–1153, 2021.

[12] E. Esen, S. Sizmaz, and N. Demircan, "Intravitreal aflibercept for management of subfoveal choroidal neovascularization secondary to angioid streaks," *Indian Journal of Ophthalmology*, vol. 63, no. 7, pp. 616–618, 2015.

[13] D. Chakraborty, J. U. Sheth, S. Boral, and T. K. Sinha, "Off-label intravitreal brolucizumab for recalcitrant diabetic macular edema: a real-world case series," *American Journal of Ophthalmology Case Reports*, vol. 24, article 101197, 2021.

[14] J. S. Shilling and R. K. Blach, "Prognosis and therapy of angioid streaks," *Transactions of the Ophthalmological Societies of the United Kingdom*, vol. 95, no. 2, pp. 301–306, 1975.

[15] A. M. Mansour, N. H. Ansari, J. A. Shields, W. H. Annesley Jr., C. M. Cronin, and E. L. Stock, "Evolution of angioid streaks," *Ophthalmologica*, vol. 207, no. 2, pp. 57–61, 1993.

[16] A. M. Mansour, J. A. Shields, and W. H. Annesley Jr., "Macular degeneration in angioid streaks," *Ophthalmologica*, vol. 197, no. 1, pp. 36–41, 1988.

[17] V. Govindhari and J. Chhablani, "To laser or not?," *Indian Journal of Ophthalmology*, vol. 66, no. 3, pp. 463–466, 2018.

[18] A. Teixeira, N. Moraes, M. E. Farah, and P. P. Bonomo, "Choroidal neovascularization treated with intravitreal injection of bevacizumab (Avastin) in angioid streaks," *Acta Ophthalmologica Scandinavica*, vol. 84, no. 6, pp. 835-836, 2006.

[19] G. Mimoun, J. Tilleul, A. Leys, G. Coscas, G. Soubrane, and E. H. Souied, "Intravitreal ranibizumab for choroidal neovascularization in angioid streaks," *American Journal of Ophthalmology*, vol. 150, no. 5, pp. 692–700.e1, 2010.

[20] R. Sekfali, G. Mimoun, S. Y. Cohen et al., "Switching from ranibizumab to aflibercept in choroidal neovascularization secondary to angioid streaks," *European Journal of Ophthalmology*, vol. 30, no. 3, pp. 550–556, 2020.

[21] Q. D. Nguyen, A. Das, D. V. Do et al., "Brolucizumab: evolution through preclinical and clinical studies and the implications for the management of neovascular age-related macular degeneration," *Ophthalmology*, vol. 127, no. 7, pp. 963–976, 2020.

4

Paracentral Acute Middle Maculopathy and Central Retinal Venous Occlusion following Electrical Injury

Sahel Khazaei,[1] Mehrdad Motamed Shariati,[1] Naser Shoeibi,[1] Mohammad Arjmand,[2] and Seyedeh Maryam Hosseini[1]

[1]*Eye Research Center, Mashhad University of Medical Sciences, Mashhad, Iran*
[2]*Sabzevar University of Medical Sciences, Heshmatie Hospital, Sabzevar, Iran*

Correspondence should be addressed to Seyedeh Maryam Hosseini; smaryam_hosseini@yahoo.com

Academic Editor: Kevin J. Blinder

Purpose. To report a case of central retinal vein occlusion (CRVO) and paracentral acute middle maculopathy (PAMM) following electric shock injury. *Case Description.* A 45-year-old male presented with a significant painless decreased vision in the right eye following an electrical injury of the right hand in his workplace. The best-corrected visual acuity (BCVA) of the right eye was 20/40. Funduscopic examination of the right eye revealed diffuse superficial and deep intraretinal hemorrhages, mild venous tortuosity, and an area of the pale retina. Optical coherence tomography (OCT) demonstrated hyperreflective band-like lesions in the middle retinal layers. Patchy areas of vascular flow void in deep capillary plexus seen in OCT angiography of the right eye were compatible with PAMM. Fluorescein angiography of the right eye was indicative of delayed venous filling suggestive of CRVO. The left eye was completely normal on exam and imaging. *Conclusion.* This report illustrates the occurrence of CRVO associated with PAMM following electric shock injury. Electrical injury leads to a wide range of retinal manifestations. Clinicians need to pay attention to any hyperreflectivity and thinning of middle retinal layers in OCT in cases with the presentation of sudden visual loss following electrical injuries.

1. Introduction

Electrical injuries lead to a wide range of ocular manifestations, from the eyelid, conjunctival, corneal, and lens involvement to posterior segment manifestations. Complications such as vitreous hemorrhage, retinal detachment, retinal edema, chorioretinal rupture, macular hole, Purtscher-like retinopathy and retinal vascular occlusive diseases are examples of retinal pathologies reported following electrical injuries [1–3].

The severity of the electrical damage depends on the electric current intensity, the exposure time, and the tissue resistance to the electricity [4]. The optic nerve and retina are low resistance tissues and therefore easily damaged by electrical current [5].

Several mechanisms have been proposed to explain how tissue damage occurs following electrical injuries. These mechanisms include direct transmission of the current, heat effect, tissue ischemia, and mechanical injury from electrical shock waves [6]. The electric current passes through the retinal pigment epithelium (RPE) cells, then generates heat and causes tissue damage; the absorption of the energy by the RPE cells can cause damage to the overlying retina. Because of a higher concentration of melanin in the macula (RPE cells are thicker and more compact), it causes more heat production and thermal damage. In addition, although the macula is the most affected area, the entire retina may be affected [7]. Here, we describe a case of unilateral PAMM and non-ischemic CRVO following electrical injury.

2. Case Description

A 45-year-old male, an electrical technician by profession, presented to us with marked painless decreased vision in the right eye (RE) since the last day following an electrical injury in his workplace. A current of 400 V passed through his right hand before the presentation. There was no history

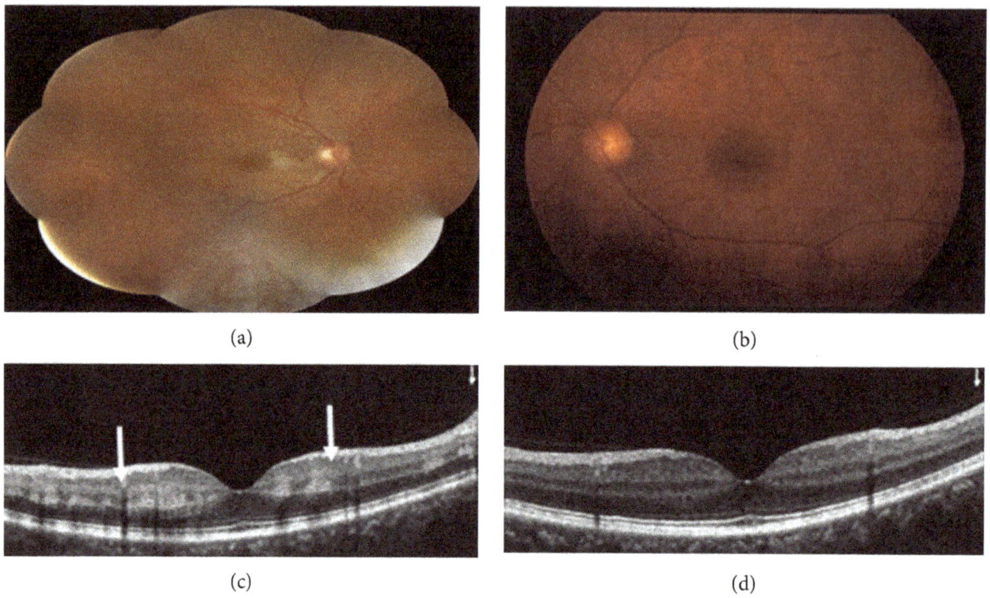

Figure 1: Color fundus photography (CFP) and spectral-domain optical coherence tomography (SD-OCT) of the right eye (a, c) and the left eye (b, d) at presentation. CFP of the RE (a) shows mild venous engorgement and widespread peripheral retinal hemorrhages located in all 4 quadrants and multiple small areas of pale retina in the macula. CFP of the left eye LE (b) does not show any retinal abnormalities. SD-OCT scan of the macula of the RE (c) shows hyperreflective band-like lesions in the middle retinal layers of the macula (arrows) of the RE and no abnormalities at the macula of the LE (d).

of unconsciousness or falling after injury. No significant family or past medical history was documented. His general physical examination was normal.

On ocular examination, his best-corrected visual acuity (BCVA) was 20/40 for the right eye (RE) and 20/20 for the left eye (LE). The pupil examination revealed round and reactive pupils and a negative relative afferent pupillary defect.

Extraocular movements were normal. Intraocular pressure measured 12 mmHg for the RE and 13 mmHg for the LE. Anterior segment examination was unremarkable. We found diffuse superficial and deep intraretinal hemorrhages and mild venous tortuosity compatible with CRVO and an area of the pale retina in the macula of the RE. The examination of the LE was entirely normal.

Multimodal imaging including spectral-domain optical coherence tomography (SD-OCT) (Heidelberg Eye Explorer version 1.9.13.0, Spectralis Viewing Module 6.5.2.0; Heidelberg Engineering), OCT angiography (Optovue, Inc., Fremont, CA, USA, software version: 2018,0,0,18), and fluorescein angiography (Heidelberg Eye Explorer version 1.9.13.0, Spectralis Viewing Module 6.5.2.0; Heidelberg Engineering) has been performed to make a more accurate diagnosis. SD-OCT of the RE showed no macular edema and hyperreflective band-like lesions in the middle retinal layers suggestive of paracentral acute middle maculopathy (PAMM). (Figure 1). OCT angiography (OCT-A) with a scanning area of 6∗6 mm of the RE was indicative of attenuation of vascular flow signal in the superficial capillary plexus and patchy areas of vascular flow void in the deep capillary plexus (Figure 2). In fluorescein angiography (FA) of the RE, delayed venous filling was observed (Figure 3). No abnormality was detected in the imaging of the LE.

Our patient's BCVA was 20/20 in both eyes after a month of follow-up, and no neovascularization of the retina or iris had developed.

3. Discussion

PAMM was first described in 2013 by Sarraf et al. as a hyperreflective band-shaped lesion in the inner nuclear layer (INL) and the outer plexiform layer (OPL), leading to thinning of the INL. PAMM first was considered as a variant of acute macular neuroretinopathy (AMN), but these are now known as two distinct entities. Unlike PAMM, AMN lesions are red wedge-shaped intraretinal lesions that point toward the fovea and are better seen with infrared reflectance images. On the other hand, AMN lesions in OCT are placed deeper than PAMM and involve the outer nuclear layers and the OPL and may lead to thinning and destruction of the outer retinal layers. Although the exact mechanism of PAMM is still under investigation, OCT-A findings have suggested vascular changes in the intermediate and deep capillary plexus due to hypoperfusion. The INL and OPL are located in the watershed area of the retinal blood supply. In a hypoperfusion state, the maximum blood flow is directed toward the superficial capillary plexus and choroid, so INL and OPL are more prone to ischemia [8]. Also, the high oxygen demand of the horizontal cells in the middle retina made this area more sensitive to ischemic damage [9].

Another mechanism that is responsible for INL damage in PAMM is reperfusion injury. Reperfusion occurred following a transient hypoperfusion results in increased production of reactive oxygen species, nitric oxide neurotoxicity, inflammation, and extravascular leakage. Reperfusion injury is associated with chronic changes of PAMM [10].

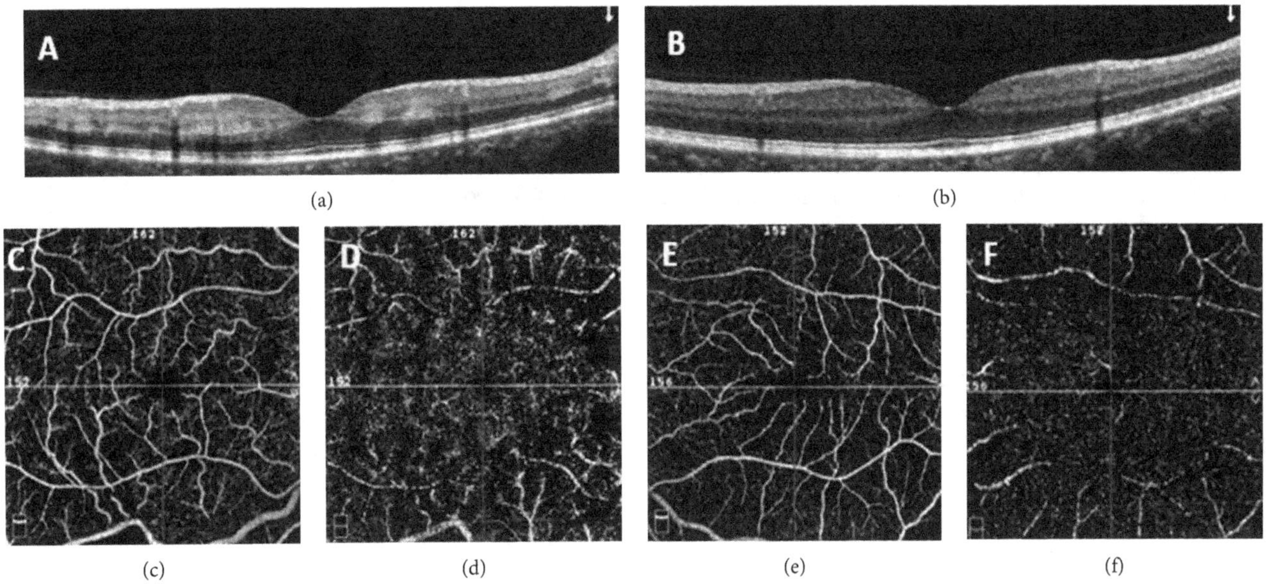

FIGURE 2: OCT angiography (OCT-A) with a scanning area of 6∗6 mm at presentation. OCT-A shows mild attenuation of the vascular flow signal in the superficial capillary plexus (SCP) (c) and patchy areas of vascular flow void in the deep capillary plexus (DCP) (d) of the RE and normal flow in the SCP (e) and DCP (f) of the LE.

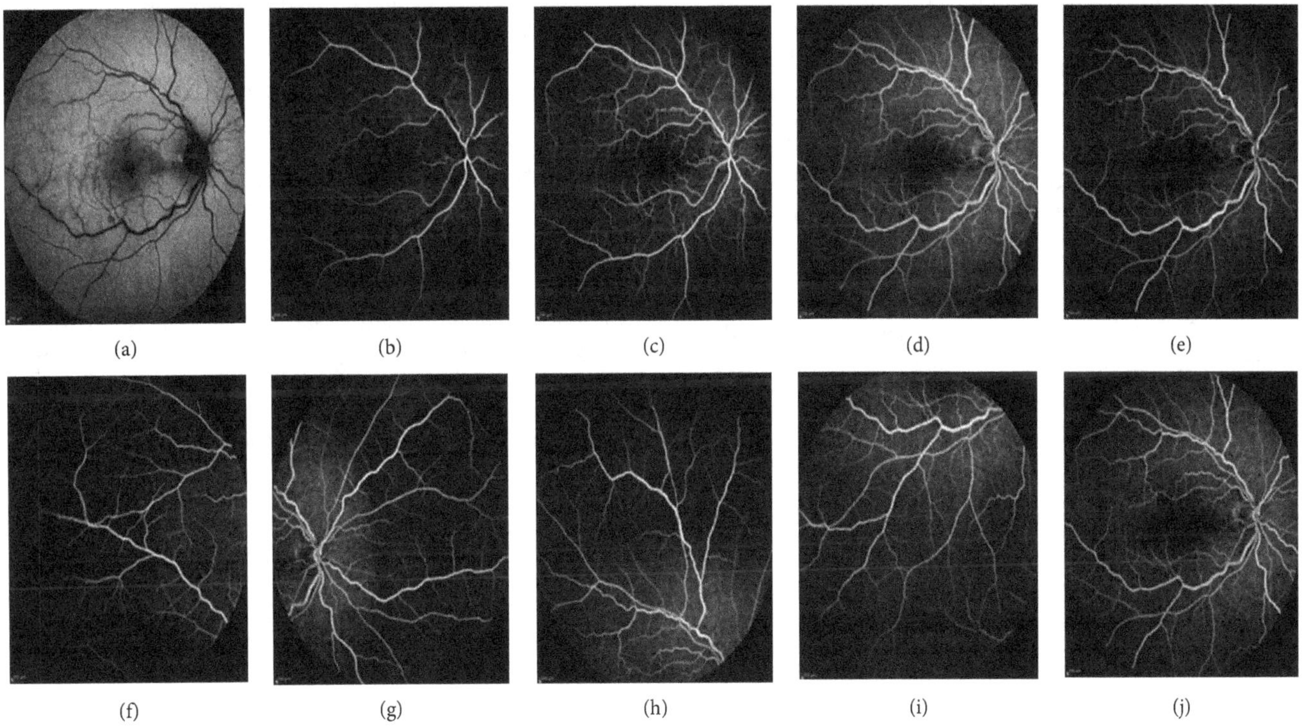

FIGURE 3: Fluorescein angiography frames of the right eye at presentation show delayed venous filling with the absence of macular edema or nonperfusion in the late phase of the angiogram.

Previous studies have shown the association between some retinal vascular diseases and PAMM including retinal artery and venous occlusion [11].

Electric current can damage tissue in several ways. The direct passage of electricity through the tissues leads to the destruction of the cell membrane and direct cell damage. Also, the heat produced by the conversion of electrical energy causes vascular contraction, resulting in tissue ischemia and eventually necrosis. Also, the direct mechanical injury caused by an electric shock wave is noted. The tissue conductivity of electrical current also affects the severity of the damage, so tissues such as the retina and optic nerve are more vulnerable to electrical injury. The macular region is more prone to electrical injury due to several reasons. The avascularity of the fovea makes it more sensitive to ischemic damage. Due to the greater accumulation of melanin in the macula, the heat produced in the macular region is higher, and the risk of tissue ischemia is more [4, 5].

It seems that in our patient, the transmission of electric current led to vascular constriction followed by tissue ischemia and presented with central retinal vein occlusion. Findings of the fundoscopic examination including diffuse superficial and deep intraretinal hemorrhages and mild venous engorgement and delayed venous filling in FA support the diagnosis. According to the abovementioned mechanisms, both hypoperfusion and reperfusion injury may disturb vascular flow toward the deep capillary plexus (DCP) and cause PAMM in this patient. Although FA has been the gold standard for the evaluation of retinal blood circulation, it is not able to show blood flow in the vascular layers of the retina separately. OCT-A is a noninvasive modality, which is helpful for this purpose. In our patient, hyperreflective, band-like lesions in the middle retinal layers of the macula in SD-OCT, and patchy areas of vascular flow void in the DCP in OCT-A are suggestive of PAMM.

There is yet to be a treatment that has been proved to reverse PAMM; thus, treatment should be focused on the underlying cause of PAMM when it is present [11]. In our case, CRVO was present as mentioned above. Intravitreal injections of antivascular endothelial growth factor (VEGF) and steroid implants are currently available treatments for macular edema secondary to CRVO. Patients with lower baseline VA (count finger or less) showed higher absolute improvement after treatment. Anti-VEGF injections, according to prior studies, are more preferable due to higher and more lasting visual outcome improvements as well as fewer side effects. Steroids would generally not be favored in individuals with an increased risk of glaucoma or younger phakic patients. On the other hand, more endophthalmitis rate is reported after intravitreal steroids compared to anti-VEGF injections [12]. Because there was no sign of macular edema in the physical examination or retinal imaging in the reported case and his baseline visual acuity was not particularly low, we decided on clinical follow-up without intervention.

As in our patient, the majority of PAMM cases have a good visual prognosis, with good final VA and no known neovascularization or rubeosis iridis in concomitant CRVO and CRAO cases [8].

4. Conclusion

The present case illustrates a patient with a sudden unilateral marked decrease in visual acuity following an electrical injury at the workplace. Findings of ocular examination and multimodal imaging support the diagnosis of PAMM and nonischemic CRVO. Electrical injuries lead to a wide range of retinal presentations that can be nonspecific. Ophthalmologists need to be familiar with the various ocular manifestations of electrical injuries. Paying attention to a history of electrical injury in an otherwise healthy person presented with PAMM may be helpful. This is the first report of PAMM following electric shock injury. Currently, this report does not prove any definite relationship between electrical injury and PAMM, and further studies are required for preparing a causal relationship.

Consent

Researchers ensure that they have obtained informed written consent from the patient for the publication of clinical examinations and retinal imaging.

References

[1] A. Sharma, Y. V. G. Reddy, A. P. Shetty, and S. M. A. Kader, "Electric shock induced Purtscher-like retinopathy," *Indian journal of ophthalmology.*, vol. 67, no. 9, pp. 1497–1500, 2019.

[2] H. R. Choe and U. C. Park, "Different types of maculopathy in eyes after a high-voltage electrical shock injury," *Case reports in ophthalmology.*, vol. 10, no. 1, pp. 19–23, 2019.

[3] E. Rishi, V. Indu, and U. Sharma, "Lightning Injuries of the Posterior Segment of the Eye," *Taiwan Journal of Ophthalmology*, 2021.

[4] A. Sanford and R. L. Gamelli, "Lightning and thermal injuries," *Handbook of clinical neurology.*, vol. 120, pp. 981–986, 2014.

[5] F. Ascaso, I. Bartolomé, J. Berniolles et al., "Electric shock-induced retinal vein occlusion: a propos of two cases," *Acta Ophthalmologica.*, vol. 94, 2016.

[6] J. Rajagopal, S. B. Shetty, A. G. Kamath, and G. G. Kamath, "Macular hole following electrical shock injury," *Canadian journal of ophthalmology Journal canadien d'ophtalmologie.*, vol. 45, no. 2, pp. 187-188, 2010.

[7] R. Ranjan, G. J. Manayath, P. Dsouza, and V. Narendran, "Spontaneous anatomical and functional recovery of bilateral electric shock maculopathy," *Indian journal of ophthalmology.*, vol. 65, no. 11, pp. 1256–1261, 2017.

[8] J. Scharf, K. B. Freund, S. Sadda, and D. Sarraf, "Paracentral acute middle maculopathy and the organization of the retinal capillary plexuses," *Progress in Retinal and Eye Research.*, vol. 81, article 100884, 2021.

[9] D. McLeod and S. Beatty, "Evidence for an enduring ischaemic penumbra following central retinal artery occlusion, with implications for fibrinolytic therapy," *Progress in retinal and eye research.*, vol. 49, pp. 82–119, 2015.

[10] X. Chen, S. J. Desai, and C. R. Baumal, "Paracentral acute middle maculopathy in pregnancy," *Retinal Cases and Brief Reports.*, vol. 14, no. 3, pp. 221–223, 2020.

[11] N. Moura-Coelho, T. Gaspar, J. T. Ferreira, M. Dutra-Medeiros, and J. P. Cunha, "Paracentral acute middle maculopathy—review of the literature," *Clinical and Experimental Ophthalmology.*, vol. 258, no. 12, pp. 2583–2596, 2020.

[12] R. Gale, C. Gill, M. Pikoula et al., "Multicentre study of 4626 patients assesses the effectiveness, safety and burden of two categories of treatments for central retinal vein occlusion: intravitreal anti-vascular endothelial growth factor injections and intravitreal Ozurdex injections," *British Journal of Ophthalmology.*, vol. 105, no. 11, pp. 1571–1576, 2021.

5

En Face Optical Coherence Tomography Imaging Ellipsoid Zone Regeneration in Laser-Induced and Solar Maculopathies

Jeanne M. Gunzinger,[1] Katrin Fasler,[1] Daniel Barthelmes,[1] Peter Maloca,[2,3,4,5] Pascal W. Hasler,[2,3,4] Christian Böni,[1] and Sandrine A. Zweifel[1]

[1]*Department of Ophthalmology, University Hospital Zurich, Zurich 8091, Switzerland*
[2]*Institute of Molecular and Clinical Ophthalmology Basel (IOB), Basel, Switzerland*
[3]*Department of Ophthalmology, University Hospital Basel, Basel 4056, Switzerland*
[4]*OCTlab, Department of Ophthalmology, University Hospital Basel, Basel, Switzerland*
[5]*Moorfields Eye Hospital, London, UK*

Correspondence should be addressed to Sandrine A. Zweifel; sandrine.zweifel@usz.ch

Academic Editor: Antonio Ferreras

The purpose of the study was to analyze imaging findings in spectral domain en face optical coherence tomography (SD OCT) in patients with laser-induced and solar maculopathies focusing on the possible regeneration of the ellipsoid zone. In a retrospective case series of 3 patients (4 eyes) with solar maculopathy and 2 patients (3 eyes) with laser-induced maculopathy who underwent a comprehensive ocular examination, ellipsoid zone (EZ) was segmented from SD OCT data. Evaluation of EZ in en face OCT revealed a hyporeflective lesion surrounded by a hyperreflective border. The area of EZ alteration was measured manually in en face OCT. All patients showed partial EZ regeneration. Mean EZ alteration decreased from 0.12 mm^2 (range: 0.05–0.32) at baseline to 0.07 mm^2 (range: 0.01–0.22) at last follow-up ($p = 0.018$, mean follow-up: 372 days; range: 115–592). Mean best visual acuity (BVA) improved from 20/36 at baseline to 20/30 ($p = 0.018$). In conclusion, en face OCT imaging clearly delineated the area of EZ alteration in patients with laser-induced and solar maculopathies. Follow-up showed significant reformation of the EZ as well as improvement of BVA.

1. Introduction

Laser- induced maculopathies as well as solar maculopathy are two rather rare photo-induced occurrences. Ex vivo histological examinations of solar retinopathy mainly show changes in the outer retina, more precisely in foveal and parafoveal photoreceptor cells (containing photo pigments) and retinal pigment epithelium (RPE, containing melanin, lipofuscin and retinoids) [1]. The parafoveal rod cells have pyknotic nuclei as a sign of inevitable death of these cells. Retinal pigment epithelium cells also show slight structural anomalies, suggesting possible cell death and detachment from Bruch's membrane. Furthermore, there are degenerative changes and loss of melanin granules of the RPE [2]. Minor damages to the RPE can be repaired by local division and/or cell sliding [1].The rather transparent cells of the inner retina are not directly involved in laser-induced or solar maculopathy [3].

The rapid development of optical coherence tomography (OCT) technology allows in vivo examinations of the different retinal and choroidal structures. Typical findings in patients with solar maculopathy include focal defects in the hyperreflective layers corresponding to the ellipsoid zone (EZ), the interdigitation zone, and the RPE [4, 5, 6]. These defects are mostly surrounded by a distinctive hyperreflective ring in en face OCT, presumably consisting of cellular debris [7]. The defect in the hyperreflective bands of the outer retina often disappears within weeks, which underlines the possibility of RPE recovery or regeneration mentioned above. Laser-induced maculopathies show similar patterns, but can present more extensive alterations including full thickness macular holes and/or retinal haemorrhage [8, 9]. Regeneration of the EZ after

Table 1: Patients characteristics, diagnosis, and visual acuity outcome.

Patient no.	Age (years)	Interval between exposure and presentation (days)	Eye involved	Diagnosis	Initial visual acuity (Snellen)	Last follow-up (days)	Last visual acuity (Snellen)
1	23	1	OD	Laser-induced maculopathy	20/33	249	20/20
			OS	Laser-induced maculopathy	20/33	24	20/20
2	19	7	OD	Laser-induced maculopathy	20/20	16	20/16
3	38	4	OD	Solar maculopathy	20/20	431	20/16
4	41	3	OD	Solar maculopathy	20/123	45	20/50
			OS	Solar maculopathy	20/123	45	20/60
5	72	1	OD	Solar maculopathy	20/20	592	20/20

laser-induced or solar maculopathy has also been documented, although several authors described persistent defects and concluded that this is due to an irreparable degeneration (as photoreceptors are post mitotic) [5, 6].

Laser-induced and solar maculopathies are both photic retinopathies which, although involving different pathogenetic types, often present similar clinical features and regeneration patterns. To further improve knowledge about the changes and regeneration of the EZ in both of these entities, we conducted a quantitative analysis using en face spectral domain (SD) OCT. We analysed short-term and long-term findings of two patients with laser-induced and three patients with solar maculopathy, who presented themselves within one week after the incident. Additionally, we looked for similarities and differences between laser-induced and solar maculopathies.

2. Materials and Methods

This retrospective chart review was approved by the local ethics committee. Five patients (seven involved eyes) who presented themselves at the emergency clinic of the Department of Ophthalmology of the University Hospital of Zurich with visual complaints due to sun or laser exposure within the prior week were identified. Each patient underwent history taking and extensive ocular examination including best visual acuity (BVA) using glasses and/or pinhole, anterior segment examination, dilated ophthalmoscopic examination of the macula and peripheral retina, OCT imaging, and fundus photography. The SD OCT images were obtained with the Heidelberg Spectralis (version 1.9.13.0) and analyzed with the Heidelberg software (Spectralis Viewing Module 6.5.2.0; Heidelberg Engineering, Heidelberg, Germany). In addition to the standard imaging protocol (Scan area was at least a $15 \times 25°$ rectangle centered on the macula covered by 49 B-scans) a dense raster scanning protocol (with a pattern size of at least 15×5 and a distance between B-Scans of $11\,\mu$m or $33\,\mu$m) or so-called transverse imaging was acquired in every patient. Automated OCT layer segmentation was checked and adjusted manually where necessary. Area, largest diameter, and diameter orthogonal to it of the alteration in the EZ – hypo- and/or hyperreflective areas—were measured by two independent readers using integrated measurement tool. In cases without distinctive loss of EZ, the hyperreflective area visible on OCT was considered as the presumed area of EZ alteration.

2.1. Statistical Methods. Data were codd in Excel and analyzed with SPSS version 23. Descriptive statistics such as mean and standard deviations were computed.

Differences of largest diameter, orthogonal, area and BVA logMAR between the last and the first visits were computed. Non-parametric paired Wilcoxon test was applied to investigate the decrease of measurements of EZ alteration and BVA with time. Two-way mixed intraclass correlation coefficient was used for evaluation of inter-reader reliability. The number of days between both measurements was computed. Non-parametric Spearman correlation investigated the association between the numbers of days and the decrease of EZ alteration and BVA parameters.

Results with p-value less than 5% were interpreted as statistically significant.

3. Results

An overview of patient's characteristics is given in Table 1. Patient's involved eyes showed a mean BVA of 20/36 (logMAR 0.25, SD $\pm$ 0.35) at first presentation and a mean BVA of 20/30 (logMAR 0.17 SD $\pm$ 0.37) at last follow-up.

Mean area of EZ alterations was $0.12\,mm^2$ (SD $\pm$ 0.10) at first presentation and $0.07\,mm^2$ (SD $\pm$ 0.08) at last follow-up for reader one (R1) and $0.21\,mm^2$ (SD $\pm$ 0.22) and $0.05\,mm^2$ (SD $\pm$ 0.04) for reader two (R2), inter-reader correlation (including all follow ups) was 0.914. Average

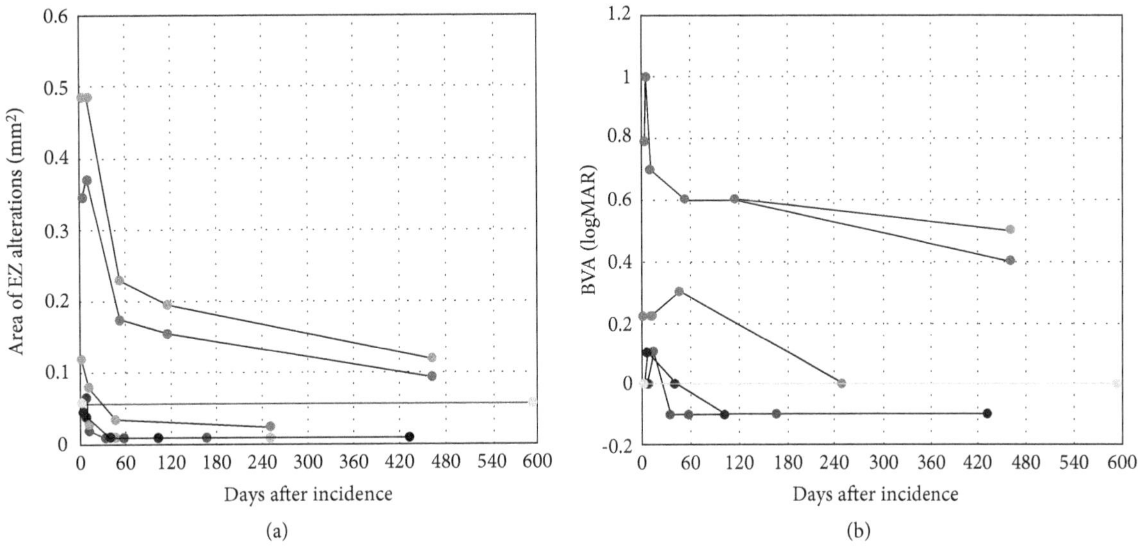

FIGURE 1: Plot of (a) area of ellipsoid zone (EZ) alterations (averages of both readers) and (b) best visual acuity (BVA) over time for all patients/eyes. Most of EZ alteration reduction and improvement of BVA occurred within first two month. Correlation between size of EZ alterations and BVA was significant (0.855, $p < 0.001$).

follow-up time was 372 (range 161–592) days. Statistical analysis showed a mean increase in BVA of approximately one line in Snellen (logMAR −0.17 SD ± 0.37, $p = 0.027$) and a mean decrease in the area of EZ alterations of $0.09\,mm^2$ (SD ± 0.06, $p = 0.018$) comparing baseline examination and last follow-up for R1 and $0.16\,mm^2$ (SD ± 0.19, $p = 0.027$) for R2. Further, the largest diameter of the EZ alterations as well as the diameter orthogonal to this showed significant reduction from first to last follow-up for both R1 and R2 (p -values 0.018–0.028, inter-reader correlations 0.966–0.968). All patients showed a decrease in the EZ alteration measurements and six out of seven eyes showed an increase in BVA, whereas the seventh eye showed a stable BVA of 20/20 (Figures 1 and 2).

Correlation of area of EZ alteration and BVA was significant (0.852, $p < 0.001$ for R1; 0.859, $p < 0.001$ for R2), using Spearman's rho. Most improvement in both EZ alterations and BVA occurred within first 2 months.

3.1. Report of Cases. Patient 1 (Figure 3) was a 23-year-old male who looked directly into a green laser pointer light with each eye individually, presumably out of curiosity. He presented himself one day after the incident with vision loss and central scotoma in both eyes. BVA at first consultation was 20/33 in both eyes. Anterior segment examination was normal. Dilated ophthalmoscopic examination showed a central yellow spot in both eyes (Figure 3(a)). A hyperreflective band reaching from the RPE to the outer plexiform layer as well as a hyporeflective zone expanding from the EZ to the ELM (Figure 3(b)) could be observed on OCT. On last follow-up a distinct hyporeflective zone in the outer retina, boarded by intact ELM and RPE was noted. Early en face OCT on the level of the EZ showed a hyporeflective oval zone surrounded by an inner distinct hyperreflective ring and an outer faint hyporeflective zone (Figure 3(c)). Follow-up of en face OCT showed a pronounced hyporeflective defect in the EZ, reducing in size over several months. BVA dropped to 20/40 in both eyes at week six and improved to 20/20 in both eyes at last consultation 8 months after the incident.

Patient 2 was a 19-year-old woman who had looked directly into a laser show light projector of unknown strength on holidays abroad and experienced a small central scotoma in her right eye (Figure 4(a)). OCT showed a lamellar macular hole which resolved completely within 2 months. There was a small area of hyperautofluorescence at first presentation in the impact region (Figure 4(c)). Fluorescein angiography 10 days after the incident did not show any leakage or staining (Figure 4(d)). Indocyanine-green (ICG) angiography at the same time point did show minimal irregular hyper- and hypocyanescence in the region of impact in the late frames (Figure 4(e)). BVA first dropped to 20/25 ten days after the incident (while EZ alteration was already decreasing in size) and then improved to 20/15 after one month.

Patient 3 (Figure 4(b)) was a 38-year-old male who watched a solar eclipse without any protection, but he closed the eyes alternatively. He presented himself 4 days after the incident due to ongoing decreased vision in the right eye and small central scotoma. BVA at first consultation was 20/20 in both eyes. Anterior segment examination was normal. Dilated ophthalmoscopic examination of the right eye showed central pigment alteration. A hyperreflective band in the central fovea reaching from the RPE to the outer plexiform layer was noted on B-scan OCT. A hyporeflective zone in the outer retinal layers was not present at baseline, but appeared later during follow-up. En face OCT at the level of the EZ showed a mild hyperreflective ring, presumed as area of EZ alteration. A distinct hyporeflective defect in the EZ layer was seen one month after the incident, which then reduced in size but persisted until last follow-up. BVA dropped by one line to 20/25 in the right eye one week after the incident, improved again to 20/20 at one month and to 20/15 at 14 weeks and thereafter.

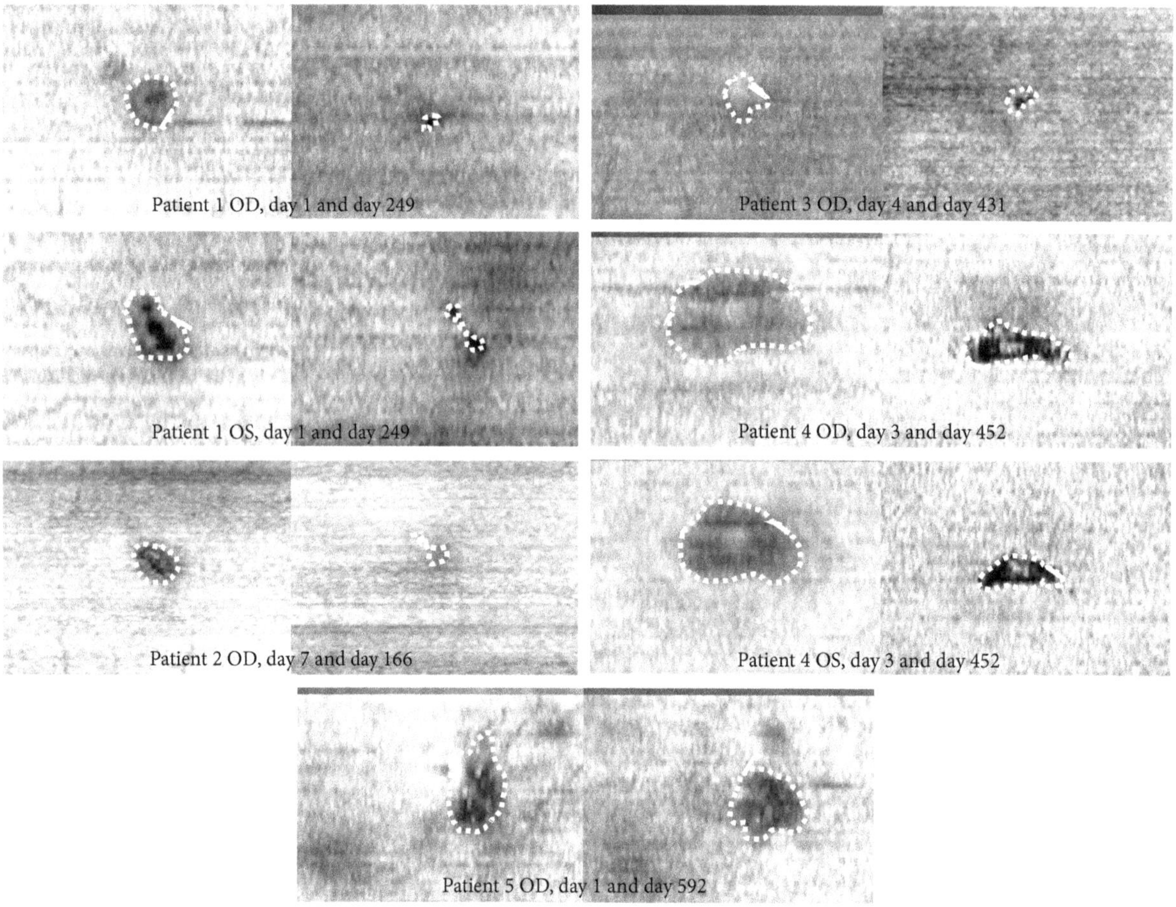

FIGURE 2: En face OCT of all patients at first and last visit. Patient 1 to 3 suffered laser injuries, patients 4 to 6 suffered solar maculopathy. Areas of EZ alterations are indicated by the dotted lines.

Patient 4 (Figure 5) was a 41-year-old male with a history of schizophrenia which was currently treated with escitalopram, a selective serotonin reuptake inhibitor, not known to have any effect on phototoxicity. He presented himself three days after sudden onset of vision loss and central scotoma in both eyes. On the day before onset of symptoms, he participated in a street parade. He denied sun gazing or drug abuse, but reconstruction of the events was difficult. At first consultation, BVA was 20/123 in both eyes. Anterior segment examination was normal. Dilated ophthalmoscopic examination showed a clearly yellow area at the fovea with a reddish centre in both eyes (Figure 5(a)). B-scan OCT demonstrated disruption of the RPE and the EZ and a wide hyperreflective band reaching from the outer nuclear layer to the outer plexiform layer (Figure 5(b)), similar to patient 1. En face OCT at the level of the EZ showed a hyporeflective defect surrounded by a hyperreflective ring (Figure 5(c)), which evolved into a central alteration with granular appearances and expanding in size before regressing to a clearly delineated EZ loss. BVA first dropped to 20/200 in both eyes 4 days after the incident, improved again to 20/100 in both eyes at 10 days, to 20/80 in both eyes at 2 months and was 20/50 in right and 20/60 in left eye at last follow-up. Initial presentation and evolution let presume a solar maculopathy.

Patient 5 was a 72-year-old woman experiencing a paracentral scotoma in the right eye, after observing a solar eclipse. OCT en face imaging showed only slight EZ regeneration (although followed for 592 days). BVA was always 20/20.

4. Discussion

Laser-induced and solar maculopathies are relatively rare events. These injuries often result in EZ alterations and decreased BVA. This case series demonstrates a significant reduction of EZ alterations over time after such an injury and that BVA is strongly correlated with the size of EZ loss.

In most patients, hyporeflective cavities on the level of the RPE and/or the EZ with an overlying hyperreflective band reaching up to the outer plexiform layer, appearing to follow the Henle fibers, could be detected. This is consistent with other reports [5, 6, 11] which described the primary defect site to be the RPE with involvement of the outer photoreceptor segments by photochemical and/or photothermal reactions in extended injuries [1, 12]. In laser-induced retinal injuries in zebra fish the early hyperreflectivity seen in OCT histologically correlates to an early edema, which is followed by disorganization of photoreceptors and loss of nuclei in the outer nuclear layer after one day [13], keeping in mind that OCT images are based on tissue reflectivity and not on tissue or cell types (while reflectivity is amongst other things depending on the complex refractive index of the cellular and extracellular components

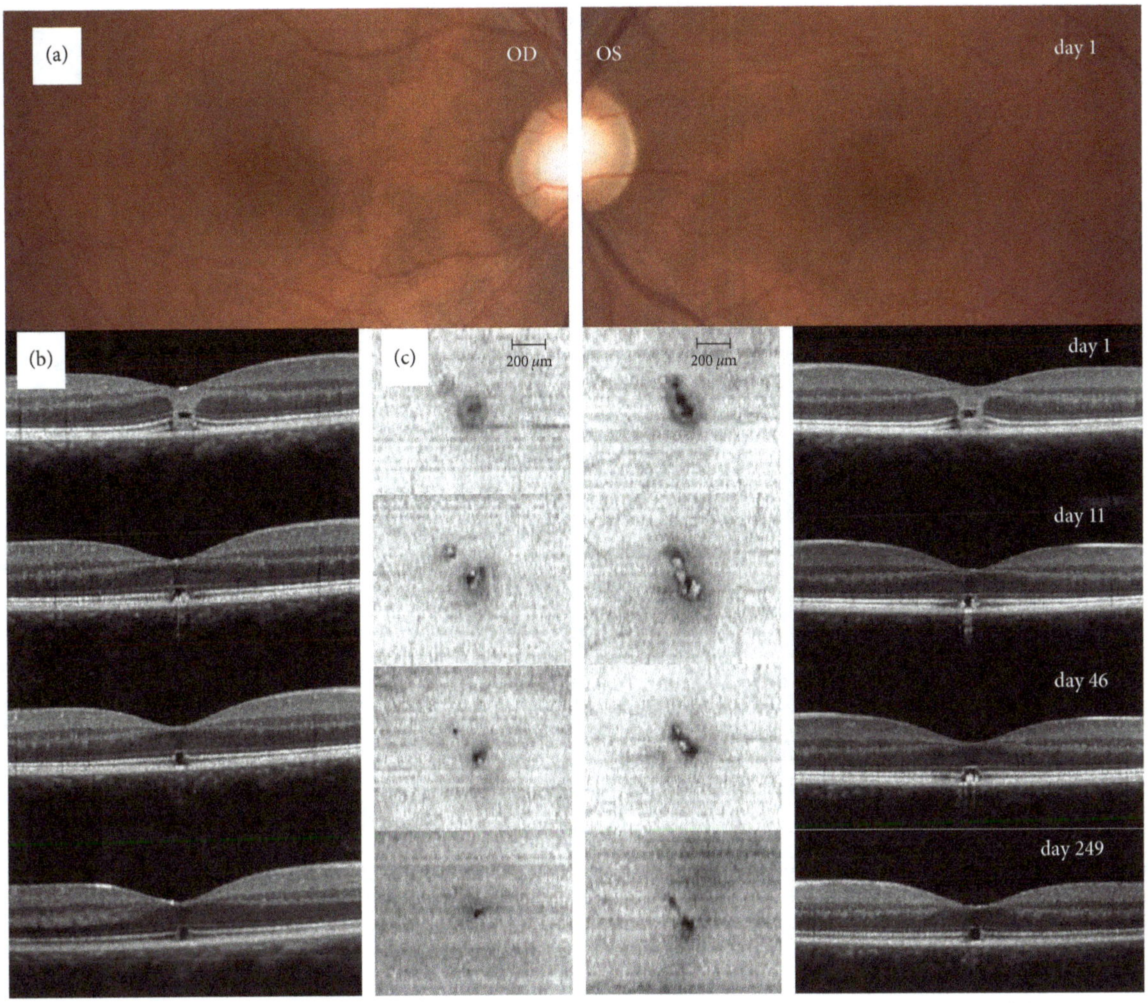

FIGURE 3: Regeneration of the ellipsoid zone in a patient with laser-induced maculopathy. (a) Fundus photography on day 1 after the accident showing small central lesion in both eyes of patient 1. (b) B-scan OCT images through the fovea of the right and left eye depicts a hyperreflective band reaching from the retinal pigment epithelium (RPE) to the outer plexiform layer extending slightly to the perifoveal region (assumingly following the Henle fibers) and a hyporeflective zone expanding from the ellipsoid zone (EZ) to the external limiting membrane (ELM) in both eyes on day 1. It also showed thickened subfoveal outer retinal layers and a hyporeflective zone expanding from the EZ to the ELM. These findings diminish over follow-up (day 11, 46, and 249). Last follow-up on day 249 showed only a distinct hyporeflective zone in the outer retinal layers, boarded by intact ELM and RPE layers. (c) En face OCT images on the level of the EZ demonstrating a regeneration of the EZ alterations over time in both eyes. Early images show a central hyporeflective oval zone surrounded by a distinct hyperreflective ring and again a faint, fuzzily bounded hyporeflective zone. Late images show a pronounced hyporeflective defect in the EZ, decreasing in size over follow-up. Note the inhomogeneous choroidal hypertransmission as an indirect sign of incomplete RPE and outer retina damage visible on days 11 and 46 in both eyes [10].

involved and light scattering) [14, 15]. With en face OCT, we could depict the total two-dimensional alterations of the EZ and carry out a quantitative analysis of the EZ reformation. All our patients showed significant reduction of EZ alteration.

Comparing solar maculopathy and laser injury, very similar findings were observed, except in one patient with a lamellar macular hole due to a laser injury, which was not seen in any of the solar maculopathy cases. This finding is most likely caused by the higher energy level in lasers compared to sun light: Local rise of temperature of the retina when sun gazing was calculated to be only about 2°, far below the 10° needed to cause thermal damage [16]. Solar maculopathy is most likely caused by photochemical damage, which involves cellular damage (ultimately resulting in cell death) by supercharged molecules. In laser light, energy can be far higher and therefore cause thermal (which involves direct corruption of the structure of proteins) or even disruptive damage [17, 3]. No qualitative difference could be seen in reformation of the EZ and subgroups were too small for statistical comparison.

Mechanism of the reformation of the EZ is unclear. There are multiple reports of total or partial EZ reformation in other retinal pathologies primarily involving photoreceptors such as in multiple evanescence white dot syndrome, acute macular neuropathy, and Vogt-Koyanagi-Harada disease [18–20]. Recent evaluations found that regeneration of only about 50% of photoreceptors might result in normal sensitivity to light [21]. However, reformation on the cellular

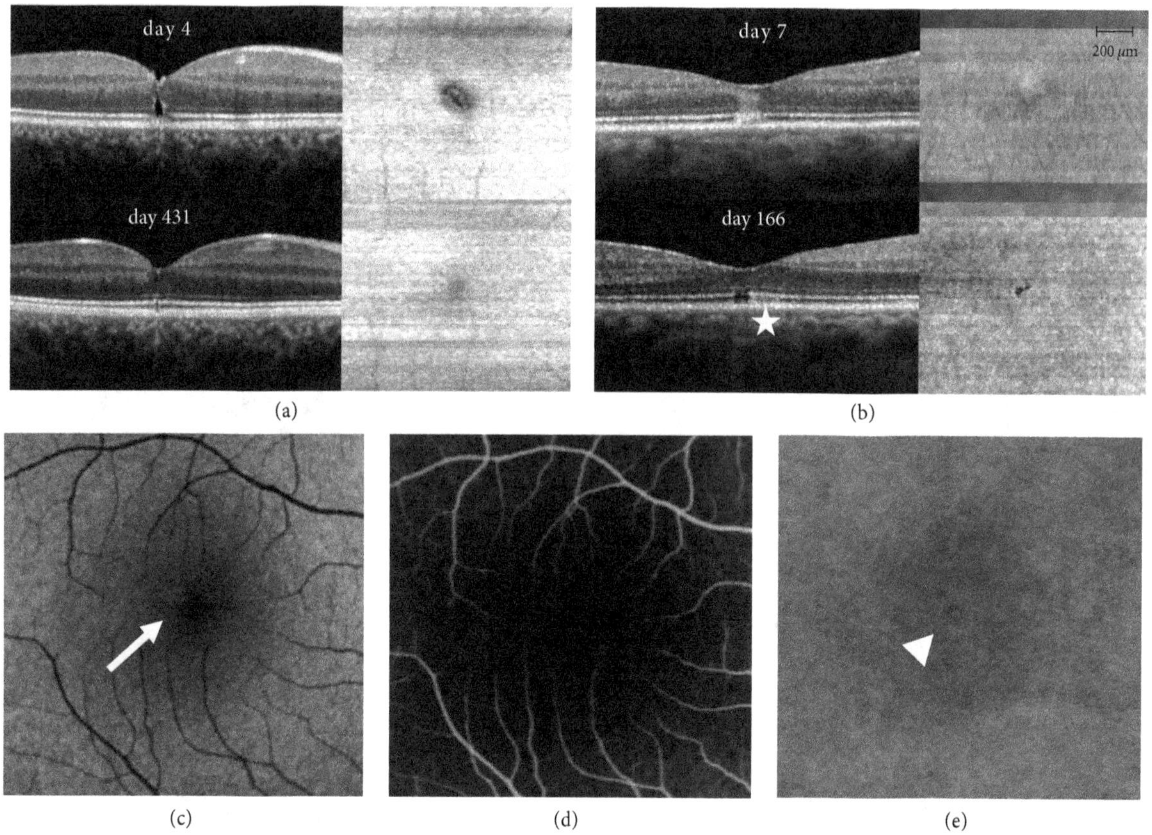

FIGURE 4: B-scan and en face OCT images of patient 2 and 3 (a and b) and multimodal imaging data including autofluorescence imaging (c), fluorescein (d) and indocyanine green (e) angiography of patient 2. (a) OCT B-scan on day 7 through the foveal center shows a lammelar hole reaching up to the outer nuclear layer; En face OCT shows an EZ alteration boarded by a hyperreflective ring; On day 166 (last follow-up) closure of the lamellar hole and near complete regeneration of the EZ. An inhomogeneous choroidal hypertransmission can be detected until the last follow-up (*star*). (b) B-scan OCT on day 4 through the foveal center demonstrates a typical hyperreflective band in the outer retina reaching from the RPE to the outer plexiform layer; there was no distinct hyporeflective zone and no thickening of the outer retinal layers. One month after the incident, B-scan showed a distinct hyporeflective defect in the ellipsoid zone (EZ), which persisted until last follow-up on day 431. En face OCT on day 4 shows a mild hyperreflective circle, partially surrounded by a scantly hyporeflective zone area; on day 431 a clearly demarcated EZ loss can be observed. (c) Autofluorescence (Heidelberg Spectralis HRA+OCT, excitation at 488nm, barrier filter wavelength of 500nm) showed a hyperautofluorescent zone at first presentation (seven days after the incidence) in the impact region (*arrow*). (d) Fluorescein angiography (ten minutes after injection) ten days after the incidence did not show any leakage or staining. (e) Indocyanine-green (ICG) angiography (ten minutes after injection) did show minimal irregular hyper- and hypocyanescence in the region of impact (*arrowhead*).

level is not well studied. Rabbits and mouse models show migration of photoreceptors from unaffected areas, thereby replacing the necrotic photoreceptors and building new functional synaptic contacts with unaffected overlying bipolar cells and light responsive retinal ganglion cell density recovers within 2 months [22, 23]. If similar cellular regeneration occurs in the human retina has yet to be investigated.

In our cases, most reformation of the EZ and recovery of visual acuity occurred within 2 months. BVA correlated with the extent of EZ alteration at any given time, but prediction of the visual outcome in a given injury at baseline is not possible. Clinical reports of laser injuries in children suggested a subdivision into "severe" injuries with poor visual outcome and "light" injuries with good visual outcome [24, 25]. Our cohort does support this subdivision, with only patient 4 presenting a severe injury (in both eyes) with only partial recovery and all others recovering to a BVA of 20/20 or better.

One major limitation of this study is that SD OCT can only visualize the EZ but neither the photoreceptors themselves nor their synaptic contacts; therefore, we can only describe the reformation of the EZ, which is in the end an artificial imaging effect solely existing on OCT, while the events on cellular level remain unknown. As in many other reports of solar maculopathies or laser injuries, the small number of patients limits the statistical significance of the results.

5. Conclusions

In our series of seven eyes, we demonstrated that there is reformation of the EZ on OCT in solar maculopathy as well as in laser injury to the central retina over time. Pattern of injury is very similar in both entities, where a laser injury may present additional risk of disruptive damage, in concordance with earlier publications. Further, we found a significant correlation of BVA and the extent of EZ loss at a given time.

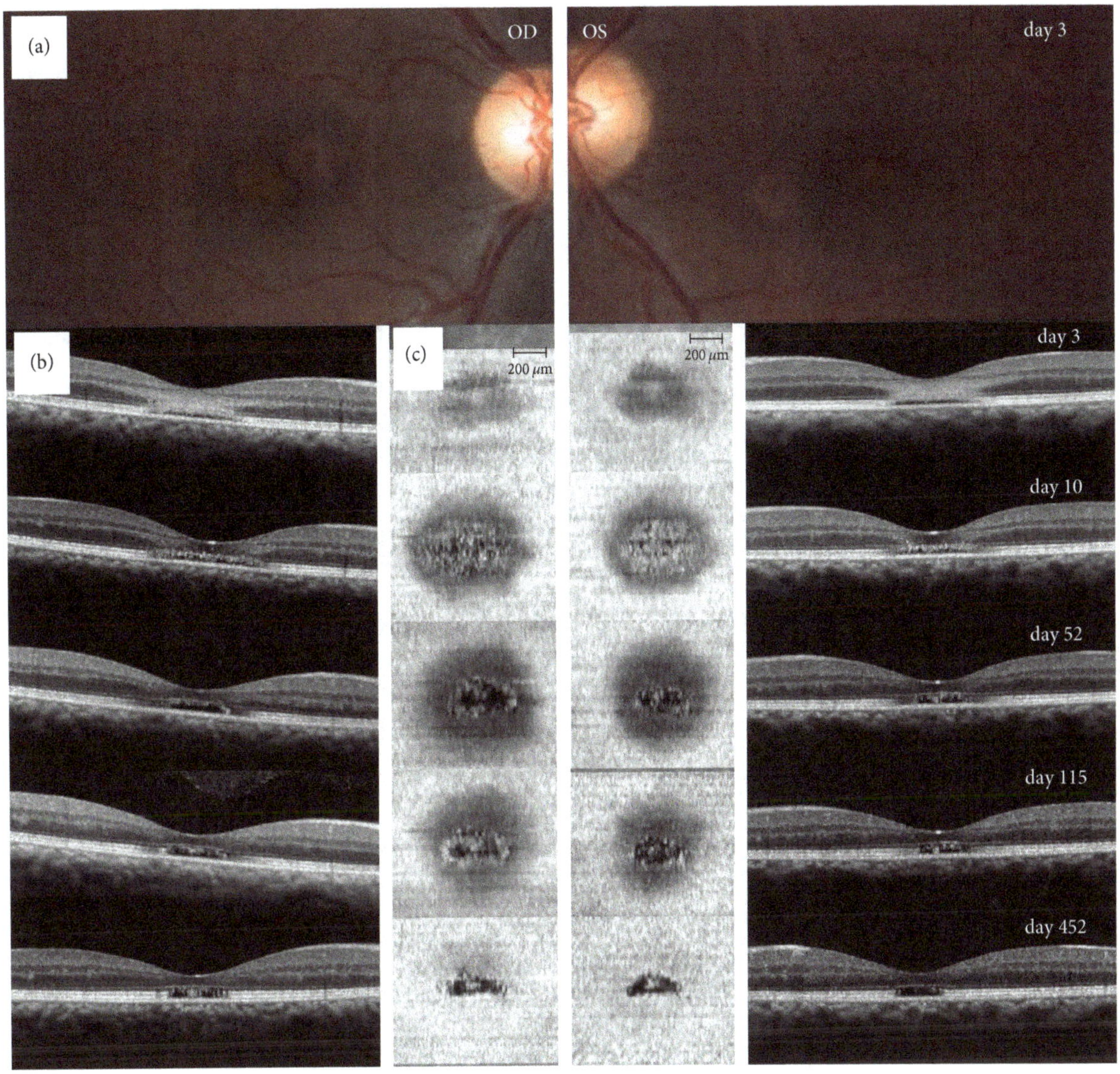

FIGURE 5: Fundus photography, B-scan, and en face OCT images of a patient with solar maculopathy. (a) Fundus photography on day 3 after the accident shows central pigment alterations in both eyes of patient 4. (b) B-scan OCT images through the fovea show disruption of the retinal pigment epithelium (RPE) and the ellipsoid zone (EZ) as well as a hyperreflective band reaching from the outer nuclear layer to the outer plexiform layer (whereas the external limiting membrane (ELM) seemed to be intact) in both eyes on day 3, diminishing in the follow-up images (days 10, 52 and 115), while presenting hyperreflective granular appearances at the level of the EZ. Last follow-up 452 days after the incidence showed a smaller, clearly delineated EZ alteration with persistent hyperreflective granular appearances boarded by intact ELM and RPE layers. (c) En face OCT at the level of the EZ on day 3 shows a hyporeflective defect surrounded by a hyperreflective ring in both eyes. On day 10, the hyporeflective defect expands to the region where the hyperreflective ring was seen and a central defect with granular appearances comes to light. Follow ups on days 52 and 115 show a regression of the granular appearing central defect. Last follow-up 452 days after the incidence shows a smaller, clearly delineated EZ loss suggesting a partial, centripetal regeneration of the EZ alteration over time in both eyes.

Disclosure

Primarily results were presented as an abstract at ARVO annual meeting 2017 in Baltimore under the title "Reformation of ellipsoid zone in en face OCT imaging in patients with solar maculopathy and laser injuries" (https://iovs.arvojournals.org/article.aspx?articleid=2638309).

Supplementary Materials

Figure 6: macular autofluorescence images of patient 4; day 3, day 10 and day 115 (Heidelberg Spectralis HRA+OCT, excitation at 488 nm, barrier filter wavelength of 500 nm). Images show extensive areas of hypoautofluorescence on day 3 and day 10 after the incident. Images on day 115 show normalization of autofluorescence. (*Supplementary Materials*)

References

[1] M. W. Hope-Ross, G. J. Mahon, T. A. Gardiner, and D. B. Archer, "Ultrastructural findings in solar retinopathy," *Eye*, vol. 7, no. 1, pp. 29–33, 1993.

[2] M. O. Tso and F. G. La Piana, "The human fovea after sungazing," *Transactions Section on Ophthalmology American Academy of Ophthalmology and Otolaryngology n.d.*, vol. 79, no. 6, 1975.

[3] J. J. Hunter, J. I. W. Morgan, W. H. Merigan, D. H. Sliney, J. R. Sparrow, and D. R. Williams, "The susceptibility of the retina to photochemical damage from visible light," *Progress in Retinal and Eye Research*, vol. 31, no. 1, pp. 28–42, 2012.

[4] G. Staurenghi, S. Sadda, U. Chakravarthy, and R. F. Spaide, "Proposed lexicon for anatomic landmarks in normal posterior segment spectral-domain optical coherence tomography," *Ophthalmology*, vol. 121, no. 8, pp. 1572–1578, 2014.

[5] A. Jain, R. U. Desai, R. A. Charalel, P. Quiram, L. Yannuzzi, and D. Sarraf, "Solar retinopathy: comparison of optical coherence tomography (OCT) and fluorescein angiography (FA)," *Retina*, vol. 29, no. 9, pp. 1340–1345, 2009.

[6] J. Mehlan, S. J. Linke, L. Wagenfeld, and J. Steinberg, "Unilateral solar maculopathy after gazing at solar eclipse," *Klinische Monatsblätter für Augenheilkunde*, vol. 233, no. 6, pp. 749–752, 2016.

[7] J. Comander, M. Gardiner, and J. Loewenstein, "High-resolution optical coherence tomography findings in solar maculopathy and the differential diagnosis of outer retinal holes," *American Journal of Ophthalmology*, vol. 152, no. 3, pp. 413–419.e6, 2011.

[8] C. Sánchez-Barahona, J. González-Martín-Moro, J. Zarallo-Gallardo, I. Lozano Escobar, and R. Cobo-Soriano, "Early changes in optic coherence tomography in a child with laser pointer maculopathy," *Archivos de la Sociedad Española de Oftalmología*, vol. 92, no. 1, pp. 33–36, 2017.

[9] S. M. Alsulaiman, A. A. Alrushood, J. Almasaud et al., "High-power handheld blue laser-induced maculopathy," *Ophthalmology*, vol. 121, no. 2, pp. 566–572.e1, 2014.

[10] S. R. Sadda, R. Guymer, F. G. Holz et al., "Consensus definition for atrophy associated with age-related macular degeneration on OCT," *Ophthalmology*, vol. 125, no. 4, pp. 537–548, 2018.

[11] K. V. Bhavsar, D. Wilson, R. Margolis et al., "Multimodal Imaging in Handheld Laser-Induced Maculopathy," *American Journal of Ophthalmology*, vol. 159, no. 2, pp. 227–231.e2, 2015.

[12] J. Wu, S. Seregard, and P. V. Algvere, "Photochemical damage of the retina," *Survey of Ophthalmology*, vol. 51, no. 5, pp. 461–481, 2006.

[13] R. M. DiCicco, B. A. Bell, C. Kaul et al., "Retinal regeneration following OCT-guided laser injury in zebrafish," *Investigative Opthalmology & Visual Science*, vol. 55, no. 10, p. 6281, 2014.

[14] G. Yiu, Z. Wang, C. Munevar et al., "Comparison of chorioretinal layers in rhesus macaques using spectral-domain optical coherence tomography and high-resolution histological sections," *Experimental Eye Research*, vol. 168, pp. 69–76, 2018.

[15] M. P. Rowe, J. M. Corless, N. Engheta, and E. N. Pugh, "Scanning interferometry of sunfish cones. I. Longitudinal variation in single-cone refractive index," *Journal of the Optical Society of America A*, vol. 13, no. 11, p. 2141, 1996.

[16] J. J. Vos, "A theory of retinal burns," *The Bulletin of Mathematical Biophysics*, vol. 24, no. 2, pp. 115–128, 1962.

[17] W. J. Ham, H. Mueller, R. Williams, and W. Geeraets, "Ocular hazard from viewing the sun unprotected and through various windows and filters," *Applied Optics*, vol. 12, no. 9, p. 2122, 1973.

[18] H. Hashimoto and S. Kishi, "Ultra-wide-field fundus autofluorescence in multiple evanescent white dot syndrome," *American Journal of Ophthalmology*, vol. 159, no. 4, pp. 698– 706, 2015.

[19] S. K. Vance, R. F. Spaide, K. B. Freund, R. Wiznia, and M. J. Cooney, "Outer retinal abnormalities in acute macular neuroretinopathy," *Retina*, vol. 31, pp. 441–5, 2011.

[20] S. S. Bae and F. Forooghian, "Optical coherence tomography-based quantification of photoreceptor injury and recovery in Vogt–Koyanagi–Harada Uveitis," *Ocular Immunology and Inflammation*, vol. 25, no. 3, pp. 338–343, 2017.

[21] J. C. Horton, A. B. Parker, J. V. Botelho, and J. L. Duncan, "Spontaneous regeneration of human photoreceptor outer segments," *Scientific Reports*, vol. 5, no. 1, 2015.

[22] Y. M. Paulus, A. Jain, R. F. Gariano et al., "Healing of retinal photocoagulation lesions," *Investigative Opthalmology & Visual Science*, vol. 49, no. 12, p. 5540, 2008.

[23] A. Sher, B. W. Jones, P. Huie et al., "Restoration of retinal structure and function after selective photocoagulation," *Journal of Neuroscience*, vol. 33, no. 16, pp. 6800–6808, 2013.

[24] N. Raoof, P. Bradley, M. Theodorou, A. T. Moore, and M. Michaelides, "The new pretender: a large UK case series of retinal injuries in children secondary to handheld lasers," *American Journal of Ophthalmology*, vol. 171, pp. 88–94, 2016.

[25] N. Raoof, J. O'Hagan, N. Pawlowska, and F. Quhill, ""Toy" laser macular burns in children: 12-month update," *Eye*, vol. 30, no. 3, pp. 492–496, 2016.

6

Hemianopia and Features of Bálint Syndrome following Occipital Lobe Hemorrhage: Identification and Patient Understanding Have Aided Functional Improvement Years after Onset

Nicola McDowell[1] **and Gordon N. Dutton**[2]

[1]*Institute of Education, Massey University, Albany Drive, Palmerston North 4474, New Zealand*
[2]*Department of Vision Sciences, Glasgow Caledonian University, Cowcaddens Road, Glasgow G4 0BA, UK*

Correspondence should be addressed to Nicola McDowell; nicolamcdowellnz@gmail.com

Academic Editor: Alexander A. Bialasiewicz

Introduction. Cerebral visual impairment (CVI) can present around birth or any time thereafter. Homonymous hemianopia is a common feature. The concept that functional improvement is unattainable augurs against active management. Dorsal stream dysfunction (or Bálint syndrome when severe) results from bilateral posterior parietal dysfunction but may go undetected, especially in children. *Case Presentation.* At 16 the patient suffered spontaneous left occipital lobe brain hemorrhage from a ruptured arteriovenous malformation. This was surgically excised. Short lived right upper limb intermittent jerking, with additional left sided weakness, ensued. Anomalous EEG recordings, with right-sided bias, arose from the posterior temporoparietal area. A right homonymous hemianopia was evident. During the ensuing 17 years she experienced multiple complex difficulties, until, at a lecture describing how to identify and support children with CVI, she realized she herself had many of the difficulties described. Visual assessment identified hemianopia and dorsal stream dysfunction. *Discussion.* Following identification, characterization, and explanation of the impact of her visual difficulties, she both gained greater awareness of her visual difficulties and their impact and developed a range of strategies leading to functional improvement of her visual field loss and amelioration of her dorsal stream dysfunction, with great improvement in quality of life.

1. Introduction

Cerebral visual impairment (CVI) can present around birth, often in relation to prematurity [1], hypoxic ischemic encephalopathy [2], and neonatal hypoglycemia [3], or it can be acquired at any time thereafter. Acquired causes include closed head injury, epilepsy, metabolic disorders, CNS infection [2], and brain neoplasia [4]. The most frequent manifestation of acquired CVI is homonymous hemianopia [5–7]. However, this common impairment often goes uncharacterized and untreated, owing to the belief that functional recovery from visual field loss is unattainable [6], despite recognition of the potential for persisting hemianopic blindsight, comprising the facility to respond predictably to visual stimuli in the hemianopic visual field, but without visual consciousness [6, 8, 9].

The identification of blindsight may facilitate visual rehabilitation in patients with homonymous hemianopia [10], founded on the hypothesis that residual nonconscious visual capacities can potentially be rendered conscious through training [6]. The requisite methodology has been shown to be beneficial in the case described by Arcaro and Thaler [11] of a patient who lost vision due to bilateral occipital infarction. Two years after the injury, the patient developed the Riddoch phenomenon enabling her to walk around obstacles and to mirror other's movements, despite reporting that she had no useful vision [11, 12]. The patient was encouraged and empowered to develop strategies to use motion and

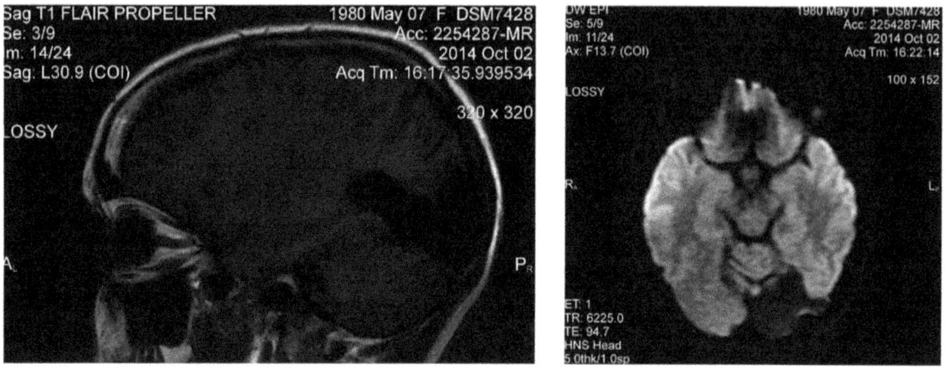

(a) Parasagittal view MRI image

(b) Axial view MRI image

Figure 1: (a) Parasagittal and (b) axial T2 weighted MRI images of the patient's brain after removal of her left occipital arteriovenous malformation.

self-motion to improve her visual abilities and her confidence to trust them. After an initial period of using these approaches to aid her vision, she became able to relinquish them as she learned to move freely through cluttered environments and achieve actions such as catching a moving ball [11].

Another well described CVI that results from cerebral injury in adults is Bálint syndrome [13]. This is caused by bilateral posterior parietal lobe dysfunction or injury [14]. It is characterized by three specific visual difficulties that impact on a person's visual access to the spatial characteristics of their surroundings. These comprise the following: simultanagnosia (an inability to see more than one or two objects at the same time; (described by Grüsser and Landis [4] as a 'disturbance of grasping the whole'), optic ataxia (impaired visual guidance of movement) [15] psychic paralysis, or apraxia of gaze (inability to volitionally direct visual gaze despite the requisite motor substrate) [13, 16]. Bálint syndrome has been infrequently reported in children, but recent case studies have highlighted that children can be significantly impacted by this triad of visual spatial difficulties [16].

Bálint syndrome-like features can occur in patients who have experienced bilateral posterior parietal lobe injury, but who are not as severely affected as those with Bálint syndrome in its most severe form [17]. This lesser, but yet still complex form of Bálint syndrome, is referred to as dorsal stream dysfunction and commonly occurs in children [18]. The dorsal visual stream runs within the superior longitudinal fasciculus from the occipital lobe to the posterior parietal cortex and is often referred to as the "vision for action" or the "where" pathway [19]. Difficulties due to dorsal stream dysfunction include the following:

(i) avoidance of crowded and cluttered environments or the increase of negative behaviors when in such places, such as tantrums and crying [20],

(ii) social withdrawal due to difficulty finding friends in groups of people [21],

(iii) avoidance of schoolwork due to difficulty copying information, difficulty simultaneously processing incoming visual and auditory information, and impaired ability to find numbers on a printed page and problems locating items, both on their work station and within the wider classroom environment [21, 22],

(iv) reluctance to move around both familiar and unfamiliar environments due to past embarrassing experiences of walking into objects and people and appearing clumsy [22],

(v) an unwillingness to participate in sporting activities due to issues with depth perception and eye-hand coordination [22],

(vi) memory difficulties, as visual information cannot be encoded in a robust and clear way [23].

We report a patient with combined hemianopia and dorsal stream dysfunction, for whom the insights gained from identification and explanation have changed her life for the better.

2. Case Presentation

A 16-year-old left handed girl suffered a spontaneous brain hemorrhage into her left occipital lobe. She lost consciousness and was resuscitated from respiratory arrest. Imaging showed left occipital and left frontoparietal subdural hematomata. Drug induced coma was implemented and maintained for eight days prior to left parietooccipital craniotomy and excision of the causative left occipital arteriovenous malformation (Figures 1(a) and 1(b)). At surgery small arterial feeders were evident 5cm from the midline. The hematoma cavity was evacuated. The arteriovenous malformation extended into the lateral horn of the left lateral ventricle and across the surface of the tentorium, draining into the transverse sinus. The medial aspect of the left occipital lobe was disconnected from the midline and the affected 4 x 4cm area was hinged up onto the draining vein. The vascular pedicles were coagulated and divided, and the vascular malformation was removed. Shortly following the surgery, the patient displayed intermittent jerking of the right upper limb, as well as marked weakness of the left side. EEG testing revealed irregular brain waves in

Table 1: Neuropsychology tests as reported (dates of assessments: A. 30.9.96, B. 16.1.1998).

Intelligence Wechsler Adult Intelligence Scale – Revised (WAIS -R)
(Pre-accident: High average range)
A. Not done
B. Superior range of functioning

Reading Wide Range Achievement – Third Ed (WRAT-3) and SCOLP spot the Word subtest
A. Low average (reading single words out loud)
B. Slight improvement into the average range (reading single words)

Confrontation naming Boston Naming Test
A. Low average range
B. Average range*

Speed of information processing SCOLP speed of compression subtest
A. 10th centile
B. Improvement into the average range*

Attentional and psychomotor skills WAIS-R Digit Symbol subtest and Trial Marking Test
A. Speed of visual motor responding and visual scanning low average
B. Slight improvement into the average range*

Verbal memory abilities California verbal learning test
A. Intact abilities in learning new verbal material preserved abilities in reading recently learned verbal material from long-term memory
B. 'No change' reported

Visuospatial skills and visual memory abilities Rey complex figure test
A. "Misplacement of detail"
B. "Copied the design in piecemeal fashion as she was unable to see the entire figure at a glance"

Executive and problem-solving abilities Trail making test
A. Slow speed of information processing
B. Now has no problems alternating her attention between number and letter concepts under time pressure

Cognitive flexibility and problem-solving skills Wisconsin card sorting test (for conceptual flexibility, hypothesis formation, testing abilities, skills in using feedback to modify problem-solving)
A. Above average range
B. Above average range

*'Inconsistent with WAIS-R test results'
The items underlined are indicative of persistent difficulties with visual information processing.

the posterior temporal and parietal regions with a right-sided bias. Both the jerking and the weakness resolved over 4 days. A right-sided homonymous hemianopia became evident. On discharge, the patient and her parents were informed of a possibility of spontaneous recovery of the hemianopia, but this was deemed unlikely. Her neuropsychological tests showed focal visual dysfunction, suggestive of difficulties in visual search (Table 1), but their origin was not identified at the time. For the following 17 years, the patient experienced challenges with many aspects of her life, including her mobility, her ability to access learning material at school, her social interactions, specific daily living activities including finding items on a supermarket shelf or clothes in her wardrobe, and the control of emotion. In 2013, at a conference presentation on identifying and supporting children with CVI, the patient recognized the difficulties described as being identical to her own. The patient introduced herself to the presenter and explained this.

Visual assessment confirmed persisting right hemianopia. No evidence of visual impairment in the sighted visual field [24] was elicited. A body turn to the right (without a head turn) slightly extended the field of vision to the right, suggestive of an additional element of right inattention. Nevertheless, repeated small discreet finger movements made by the examiner in multiple locations within the hemianopic field were correctly intuited on more than 70% of occasions, consistent with blindsight. Uncorrected visual acuities and stereopsis were in the normal range. Structured history taking for evidence of perceptual visual impairment [25] revealed great difficulty finding an item from within clutter or within a pattern and great difficulty copying, consistent with simultanagnostic vision. Standard eye movement examination was normal, with normal convergence, pursuits, and saccades to command (e.g., 'look right'), but instruction to look at specific items nominated by the examiner resulted in anarchic visual search movements until the specified item was eventually found. This feature is consistent with apraxia of gaze, a phenomenon known to accompany simultanagnostic vision [17]. When asked to look at a large group of people, the patient could only identify the presence of one person. Careful observation of eye movements during such search consistently showed them to be sparse and apparently random. In an outdoor café she was asked to count the number of support poles for the sun-shading roof. She randomly found and identified 3 out of 11, with the same lack of visual search strategy.

The accuracy of the patient's visual guidance of reach was evaluated. Careful observation of the in-flight gap between the fingers, and their orientation while reaching for discreet targets in the intact visual field showed consistent features of a gap much wider than necessary, with inaccuracy of orientation [19]. These features are consistent with a degree of accompanying optic ataxia.

The patient was given a detailed tutorial concerning the nature of her vision and strategies that she could employ to make best use of her vision.

3. Discussion

Receiving an in-depth explanation for the unexplained challenges that she had lived with for 17 years had an immediate impact on the patient's feelings of self-worth and overall well-being. Just the knowledge that she had been living with a significant visual impairment that had only recently been identified helped her to understand that it was this impairment that impacted on many aspects of her daily life, as opposed to her feeling 'useless' and unable to achieve simple activities, such as the grocery shopping for her family.

As each specific visual difficulty was assessed and thoroughly explained to her, she found herself able to connect her anomalies of visual function, to the specific challenges she experienced. For example, the reason she did not like spending time in crowded and cluttered environments (supermarkets and shopping malls) was not only due to her hemianopia, but also because of a combination of her simultanagnostic visual dysfunction and hemianopia together. Also, the reason she often got frightened by people suddenly 'looming' in front of her, when walking in a busy environment, was because of a combination of the hemianopia and her impaired visually guided movement making it difficult for her to judge how far away people actually were. But probably the most important concept that she learnt about her CVI was that she had the potential to improve her visual functioning through personal endeavor.

As with patient MC, described by Arcaro and Thaler [11], the patient was surprised that she had been able to accurately respond to stimuli in her right visual field, even though she felt she could not 'see' any image. Although she had previously been aware that at times she was able to detect movement in her right visual field, the concept of blindsight had never been explained to her. Therefore, her new recognition that she had the potential to improve her awareness of movement within her right visual field, to begin to look and see, was empowering [26]. As with MC, the patient was encouraged to develop strategies to use motion and self-motion to improve her visual abilities and her confidence to trust them [11]. Although at first she used the motion of head nodding to experiment with detecting visual stimuli on her right in her home environment, it was not a strategy she used when out and about. However, not long after receiving her CVI diagnosis following the conference presentation, she began to become more aware of movements in her right visual field. When this occurred, she made a conscious effort to try and interpret what she was seeing, instead of ignoring it, as she had in the past. She soon found that the more conscious awareness she gave to understanding what she was seeing, the more she became able to interpret her visual responses to the movements on her right. This is in line with studies focusing on increasing the detection and awareness of stimuli within the blind hemifield, which have shown that with repeated stimulation, the incidence of reported awareness also increases [27] and may well relate to the type of increased saccadic amplitudes resulting from more structured training in visual search, recently shown to be effective in extending the functional field of vision in children with hemianopia [28].

Each day she challenged herself to interpret movement she was detecting on her right side. Her approaches included attempting to detect any movement the driver on her right was making while she was sitting in the left hand passenger seat, looking straight ahead; walking on the left hand side of the path when out for her daily walks and trying to establish the exact moment, runners, other walkers, or cyclists passing her on her right hand side (while wearing headphones and listening to music so she could not hear them); and choosing a place to sit in her lounge that meant that the doorway was on her right and trying to detect any movement through the door while looking straight ahead at the television while ensuring she acknowledged and described everything she saw when detecting stimuli on her right side.

These approaches are in line with visual field training techniques described by Pollock and Hazelton [29] where patients are trained to detect stimuli that are repeatedly presented in their blind hemifield, to help increase their overall sensitivity to them by helping the brain to enhance visual awareness. Within the first year of implementing these strategies, the patient was beginning to be aware of more stimuli in her right visual field. After two years of her continuous visual self-training regime, she was surprising even herself on the occasions that she detected and correctly identified that the family (black) cat was on her right side or that someone was walking past her from behind. Her most exciting detection was when she looked up from reading her book to respond to an air hostess at the exact moment she appeared on her right side. With the continued self-training, over time she also began to detect more and more stimuli that were unrelated to her training regime, for instance, detecting changes in a familiar environment, such as furniture being moved.

During the six years following her diagnosis, visual field testing was performed by her optometrist using the Humphrey FDT Viewfinder (Figure 2). The first was undertaken in 2013 and showed little change from the plots of 1996 following her brain hemorrhage. Successive testing, however, revealed progressive improvement in the right visual field of both eyes. This remarkable functional improvement supports the hypothesis that it is potentially possible for neuroplastic brain change to occur through focusing on the belief and expectation that things can change, while striving to gain greater conscious visual awareness, perhaps through

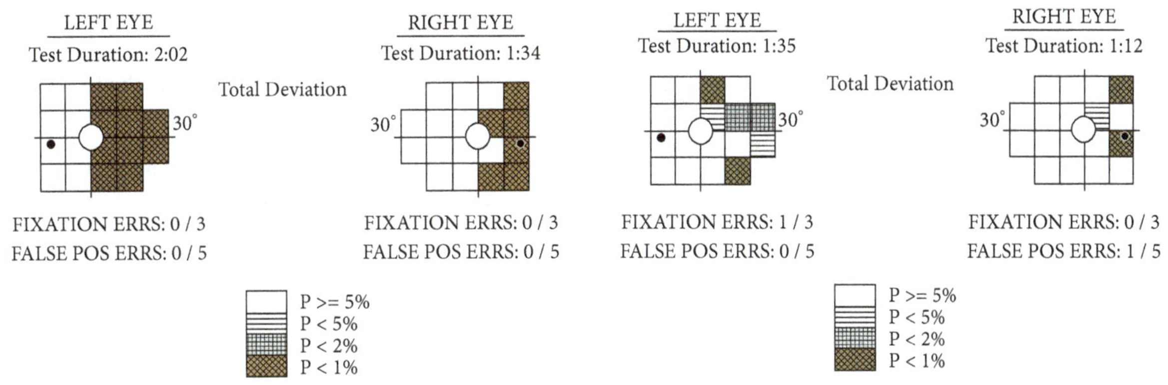

Visual field test 02/19/2013 Visual field test 06/22/2018

FIGURE 2: It comprises images of two visual field plots on a Humphrey FDT Viewfinder, demonstrating improvement in visual fields. The first image is from 02/19/13 and the second is from 06/22/18.

modulating processes in the brain that control and facilitate change [30].

As well as focusing on functionally improving her visual field, the patient also concentrated on improving her overall visual function. An important aspect of this was to firstly develop an in-depth understanding of her Bálint-like symptoms / dorsal stream difficulties of simultanagnostic visual dysfunction, optic ataxia, and apraxia of gaze and how they impacted on her in everyday life. This meant focusing on each specific issue separately, followed by the combined impact of living with a significant visual spatial impairment. Once the patient understood the nuances of her impaired unconscious visual functions, she was able to compare her current experiences of the visual world to how she had previously seen the world prior to her brain hemorrhage. With this unique insight, she was able to develop strategies to help improve her visual functioning in challenging activities and environments.

As a dorsal stream dysfunction largely affects nonconscious visual functions [19], the patient used the analogous approach to the one she used for developing her Riddoch phenomenon and focused on becoming more conscious of what was occurring when she was experiencing difficulties as a result of her simultanagnostic vision, optic ataxia, and apraxia of gaze. To strive to develop effective conscious viewing, she followed the concept outlined by Doidge [31] of using conscious actions to overcome unconscious processes, which requires a focused meditative level of concentration. This process has been used successfully for a man suffering from Parkinsonian symptoms, also described by Doidge [31] as using a form of conscious walking, whereby he trained himself to overcome many of his symptoms, by forcing himself to focus on the specific actions of walking and not letting his body adopt compensatory movements as a result of his Parkinson's disease.

At first, she adopted a different form of conscious viewing for each of her visual difficulties. For instance, for her simultanagnostic vision, she developed a strategy that she termed as 'wagon wheel visual fixation.' This strategy required the patient to consciously recognize when her gaze had wandered from what she was looking at in a crowded or complex environment, to enable her to build up the complete visual scene over time. For this strategy to be effective, she found the first step was to establish an anchor point (an obvious and appealing visual target in the middle of the chosen environment). She then trained herself to consciously recognize whenever her gaze had moved from this anchor point and work hard to force her gaze back to it. This process was repeated over and over again, applying a wagon wheel approach to consciously chosen eye movement, until the whole scene had been mapped out.

To aid her mobility in relation to her optic ataxia, especially in busy environments, she again adopted a process of conscious viewing and worked hard to focus her attention on processing and interpreting the visual information in her surroundings. For this, as she was moving, she focused her visual attention upon the space ahead of her that she would be moving in to. She then repeatedly glanced at the different elements in her travel pathway to make sure she had an enhanced opportunity to accurately map the environment around her. To ensure that this process was effective, she had to mentally block out all other sensory distractions, so that she could focus solely on processing the visual information.

Both of these techniques were difficult to implement and although she could immediately see the potential benefits of each strategy, they both had to be repeatedly practiced in the environments that required such strategies, before she was confident with her ability to implement them. However, while experimenting with these strategies, the patient also realized that she could only use them when she was feeling calm and relaxed. If anxious or stressed in any way, especially in a complex environment, she found them difficult to implement. Although she had developed a very good understanding of what types of environments were difficult for her (supermarkets, busy restaurants, shopping malls, and crowded parks), this knowledge alone was insufficient to help her cope in such locations. She then came to realize that along with her unconscious visual behaviors, she was also experiencing unconscious emotional reactions, including anxiety, panic, and high levels of stress as a result of the dorsal stream dysfunction [32].

The difficulty in implementing strategies requiring forced conscious actions necessitating intense cognitive functioning is in line with the awareness that when a person's sympathetic nervous system causes a fight or flight response in their primitive brain, their ability to think logically and coherently is absent [33]. The patient, therefore, realized that to be able to implement the specific visual strategies she had developed, she needed to identify techniques to keep herself calm, to allow any chance of overcoming both her visual difficulties and her behaviors due to her emotional reactions. To help reduce her constant high levels of anxiety when in complex environments, the patient began daily mindfulness practice, which has been shown to be useful in preventing feelings of anxiety and stress by helping a person to concentrate on their breathing and to not focus on negative or disruptive thoughts or feelings [34]. To aid in her practice, she used an online mindfulness based intervention program, as this has been proven to be effective in treating a variety of mental health conditions in adults, including anxiety and stress [35–38]. Although there is currently no literature concerning the use of cognitive based therapies such as mindfulness to support children and adults with CVI, they have been shown to be effective in helping children with High Functioning Autism Spectrum Disorder (HFASD) and anxiety disorders [39]. The concept of focusing on her breathing also helped reinforce the strategy of focusing on an anchor point when implementing the wagon wheel visual fixation process. Over time, focusing on an anchor point became easier to achieve, which supports the concept that regular mindfulness practice changes the brain patterns that cause day to day anxiety and stress [34].

With regular practice of both the mindfulness exercises to reduce environment based anxiety and her specific visual strategies of wagon wheel visual fixation and conscious viewing, the patient started to notice that the uncomfortable compensatory behaviors she had developed on account of her visual difficulties started to diminish. For instance, she stopped withdrawing from social activities and interactions and instead started engaging in activities such as going out for dinner with friends once more. She also started feeling more confident in her mobility, even in crowded environments, and felt more comfortable travelling independently in these environments. She found it easier to control her emotions and greatly reduced the number of occasions where she experienced high levels of anxiety and stress around her visual difficulties. It also helped to improve her overall well-being and confidence and helped to render normal daily activities, such as taking her children to the playground less fatiguing and more enjoyable.

Most significantly, she also noticed that her visual functioning had greatly improved and that she was less handicapped by her simultanagnostic vision, optic ataxia, and apraxia of gaze. She could now cope in busy, crowded environments for longer periods of time. She did not feel as clumsy and was not frightened by people looming in front of her. She also found it easier to spot objects in the distance that were pointed out to her, and she felt confident in her ability to handle any situation and environment that she found herself in.

4. Conclusions

What this case highlights is that for patients who do not have other cognitive disorders (such as memory or frontal disorders), it is possible to overcome some of the most disabling effects of a homonymous hemianopia and dorsal stream dysfunction. This is despite the fact that both these conditions can greatly impact on the quality of life for those affected, both physically and mentally [27, 29, 32]. However, for this to happen, the patient needs to firstly, whenever possible, fully understand the nature of their visual difficulties and how they impact on their day-to-day living. This requires timely and accurate diagnosis of not only the overarching condition of CVI, but also the specific visual difficulties of simultanagnostic vision, optic ataxia, and apraxia of gaze. In regard to their hemianopia, patients also need to be introduced to the concept of blindsight and the Riddoch phenomenon, so that if they do experience subconscious or conscious perception of movement in their blind visual fields, they are aware that this could aid their rehabilitation. Secondly, the patient also needs to be empowered through this understanding and the awareness that they have the ability to possibly functionally improve their impairments, through utilizing the resilience and plasticity of the brain to be able to reorganize itself after brain damage [27, 29, 40]. This case study also gives weight to the hypothesis that along with passive bottom up processes that can influence the cortical reorganization, neuroplastic brain change can occur through simply the belief and expectation that things can change [30], if the patient has the desire to implement strategies to bring about such change.

Consent

The patient has read the manuscript and consents to its publication.

References

[1] L. Jacobson, O. Flodmark, and L. Martin, "Visual field defects in prematurely born patients with white matter damage of immaturity: a multiple-case study," *Acta Ophthalmologica Scandinavica*, vol. 84, no. 3, pp. 357–362, 2006.

[2] G. N. Dutton, *Visual Impairment in Children Due to Damage to the Brain*, M. Bax, Ed., Mac Keith Press, London, UK, 2010.

[3] C. Macintyre-Béon, D. Young, G. N. Dutton et al., "Cerebral visual dysfunction in prematurely born children attending mainstream school," *Documenta Ophthalmologica*, vol. 127, no. 2, pp. 89–102, 2013.

[4] O.-J. Grüsser and T. Landis, *Visual Agnosias and Other Disturbances of Visual Perception and Cognition*, Macmillan, Basingstoke, UK, 1991.

[5] X. Zhang, S. Kedar, M. J. Lynn, N. J. Newman, and V. Biousse, "Natural history of homonymous hemianopia," *Neurology*, vol. 66, no. 6, pp. 901–905, 2006.

[6] C. Perez and S. Chokron, "Rehabilitation of homonymous hemianopia: insight into blindsight," *Frontiers in Integrative Neuroscience*, vol. 8, no. 82, 2014.

[7] G. Holmes, "Disturbances of vision by cerebral lesions," *British Journal of Ophthalmology*, vol. 2, no. 7, pp. 353–384, 1918.

[8] S. Chokron, C. Perez, M. Obadia, I. Gaudry, L. Laloum, and O. Gout, "From blindsight to sight: cognitive rehabilitation of visual field defects," *Restorative Neurology and Neuroscience*, vol. 26, no. 4-5, pp. 305–320, 2008.

[9] L. Weiskrantz, J. L. Barbur, and A. Sahraie, "Parameters affecting conscious versus unconscious visual discrimination with damage to the visual cortex (V1)," *Proceedings of the National Acadamy of Sciences of the United States of America*, vol. 92, no. 13, pp. 6122–6126, 1995.

[10] T. Ro and R. Rafal, "Visual restoration in cortical blindness: insights from natural and TMS-induced blindsight," *Neuropsychological Rehabilitation*, vol. 16, no. 4, pp. 377–396, 2006.

[11] M. J. Arcaro, L. Thaler, D. J. Quinlan et al., "Psychophysical and neuroimaging responses to moving stimuli in a patient with the Riddoch phenomenon due to bilateral visual cortex lesions," *Neuropsychologia*, 2018.

[12] G. N. Dutton, "Cognitive vision, its disorders and differential diagnosis in adults and children: Knowing where and what things are," *Eye*, vol. 17, no. 3, pp. 289–304, 2003.

[13] R. Bálint, "Seelenlähmung des 'Schauens' optische ataxie räumliche störung der aufmerksamkeit," *Monatsschr Psychiatr Neurol*, vol. 25, no. 1, pp. 51–81, 1909.

[14] M. Lehmann, J. Barnes, G. R. Ridgway et al., "Basic visual function and cortical thickness patterns in posterior cortical atrophy," *Cerebral Cortex*, vol. 21, no. 9, pp. 2122–2132, 2011.

[15] M. A. Goodale, "Separate visual systems for perception and action: a framework for understanding cortical visual impairment," *Developmental Medicine & Child Neurology*, vol. 55, no. 4, pp. 9–12, 2013.

[16] S. S. Philip, S. E. Mani, and G. N. Dutton, "Pediatric balint's syndrome variant: a possible diagnosis in children," *Case Reports in Ophthalmological Medicine*, vol. 2016, Article ID 3806056, 5 pages, 2016.

[17] M. N. Maia da Silva, R. S. Millington, H. Bridge, M. James-Galton, and G. T. Plant, "Visual dysfunction in posterior cortical atrophy," *Frontiers in Neurology*, vol. 8, 2017.

[18] C. Williams, K. Northstone, R. Sabates, L. Feinstein, A. Emond, and G. N. Dutton, "Visual perceptual difficulties and underachievement at school in a large community-based sample of children," *PLoS ONE*, vol. 6, e14772, no. 3, 2011.

[19] M. A. Goodale and A. D. Milner, *Sight Unseen: An Exploration of Conscious and Unconscious Vision*, Oxford University Press, Oxford, United Kingdom, 2nd Edition edition, 2013.

[20] F. C. Lam, F. Lovett, and G. N. Dutton, "Cerebral visual impairment in children: a longitudinal case study of functional outcomes beyond the visual acuities," *Journal of Visual Impairment & Blindness*, vol. 104, no. 10, pp. 625–635, 2010.

[21] S. S. Philip and G. N. Dutton, "Identifying and characterising cerebral visual impairment in children: a review," *Clinical and Experimental Optometry*, vol. 97, no. 3, pp. 196–208, 2014.

[22] L. Hyvärinen, R. Walthes, C. Freitag, and V. Petz, "Profile of visual functioning as a bridge between education and medicine in the assessment of impaired vision," *Strabismus*, vol. 20, no. 2, pp. 63–68, 2012.

[23] E. Fazzi, S. Bova, A. Giovenzana, S. Signorini, C. Uggetti, and P. Bianchi, "Cognitive visual dysfunctions in preterm children with periventricular leukomalacia," *Developmental Medicine & Child Neurology*, vol. 51, no. 12, pp. 974–981, 2009.

[24] C. Cavézian, C. Perez, C. Peyrin et al., "Hemisphere-dependent ipsilesional deficits in hemianopia: sightblindness in the 'intact' visual field," *Cortex*, vol. 69, pp. 166–174, 2015.

[25] G. N. Dutton, "Assessment of functional vision: history taking for children with CVI," in *Vision and the Brain: Understanding Cerebral Visual Impairment in Children*, A. Lueck and G. N. Dutton, Eds., pp. 261–277, AFB Press, New York, NY, 2015.

[26] J. Zihl and R. Werth, "Contributions to the study of "blindsight"-II. the role of specific practice for saccadic localization in patients with postgeniculate visual field defects," *Neuropsychologia*, vol. 22, no. 1, pp. 13–22, 1984.

[27] A. Sahraie, C. T. Trevethan, M.-J. Macleod, L. Weiskrantz, and A. R. Hunt, "The continuum of detection and awareness of visual stimuli within the blindfield: from blindsight to the sighted-sight," *Investigative Ophthalmology & Visual Science*, vol. 54, no. 5, pp. 3579–3585, 2013.

[28] I. V. Ivanov, S. Kuester, M. MacKeben et al., "Effects of visual search training in children with hemianopia," *PLoS ONE*, vol. 13, no. 7, 2018.

[29] A. Pollock, C. Hazelton, C. A. Henderson et al., "Interventions for visual field defects in patients with stroke," *Cochrane Database of Systematic Reviews*, vol. 5, CD008388, no. 10, 2011.

[30] M. Merzenich, *Soft-Wired: How the New Science of Brain Plasticity Can Change Your Life*, Parnassus Publishing, LLC, San Francisco, USA, 2013.

[31] N. Doidge, *The Brain's Way of Healing: Remarkable Discoveries and Recoveries from the Frontiers of Neuroplasticity*, Scribe Publications, Brunswick, Scoresby, Australia, 2015.

[32] R. Freeman, "Psychiatric Considerations in Cortical Visual Impairment," in *Visual Impairment in Children due to Damage to the Brain*, G. N. Dutton and M. Bax, Eds., Mac Keith Press, London, UK, 2010.

[33] D. Goleman, *Emotional Intelligence*, New York Bantam Books, New York, USA, 1995.

[34] M. Williams and D. Penman, *Mindfulness: A Practical Guide to Finding Peace in a Frantic World*, Hachette Digital, 2011.

[35] E. Bohlmeijer, R. Prenger, E. Taal, and P. Cuijpers, "The effects of mindfulness-based stress reduction therapy on mental health of adults with a chronic medical disease: a meta-analysis," *Journal of Psychosomatic Research*, vol. 68, no. 6, pp. 539–544, 2010.

[36] A. Chiesa and A. Serretti, "Mindfulness-based stress reduction for stress management in healthy people: a review and meta-analysis," *The Journal of Alternative and Complementary Medicine*, vol. 15, no. 5, pp. 593–600, 2009.

[37] N. W. Bailey, J. Nguyen, E. Bialylew et al., "Effect on Well-Being from an Online Mindfulness Intervention: "Mindful in May"," *Mindfulness*, vol. 9, no. 5, pp. 1637–1647, 2018.

[38] M. P. J. Spijkerman, W. T. M. Pots, and E. T. Bohlmeijer, "Effectiveness of online mindfulness-based interventions in improving mental health: a review and meta-analysis of randomised controlled trials," *Clinical Psychology Review*, vol. 45, pp. 102–114, 2016.

[39] C. Perry-Parrish, N. Copeland-Linder, L. Webb, and E. M. Sibinga, "Mindfulness-based approaches for children and youth," *Current Problems in Pediatric and Adolescent Health Care*, vol. 46, no. 6, pp. 172–178, 2016.

[40] A. Brodtmann, A. Puce, D. Darby, and G. Donnan, "Extrastriate visual cortex reorganizes despite sequential bilateral occipital stroke: Implications for vision recovery," *Frontiers in Human Neuroscience*, vol. 9, 2015.

7

Evaluation of the Effect of Repeated Intravitreal Bevacizumab Injections on the Macular Microvasculature of a Diabetic Patient Using Optical Coherence Tomography Angiography

Ayman G. Elnahry, Ahmed A. Abdel-Kader, Karim A. Raafat, and Khaled Elrakhawy

Department of Ophthalmology, Faculty of Medicine, Cairo University, Cairo, Egypt

Correspondence should be addressed to Ayman G. Elnahry; ayman_elnahri@hotmail.com

Academic Editor: Stephen G. Schwartz

A 53-year-old female patient with center-involving diabetic macular edema affecting the left eye was imaged using optical coherence tomography angiography (OCTA) in both eyes. She underwent three monthly intravitreal bevacizumab injections in the left eye only and OCTA was repeated in both eyes one month following the last injection and showed decreased vascular density (VD) in the treated left eye but not in the untreated right eye compared to baseline. No further injections were required in either eye, and OCTA was done in both eyes 4 months following the last injection which showed improved VD of the left eye with stable VD in the right. Three monthly intravitreal bevacizumab injections were then required in both eyes; then OCTA was repeated following the last injection and revealed decreased VD in both eyes compared to previous scan. OCTA could be a useful tool for detecting VD changes following bevacizumab injections in diabetics.

1. Introduction

Diabetic macular edema (DME) is a major cause of vision loss worldwide that is partly mediated by excess vascular endothelial growth factor (VEGF) production by hypoxic and damaged retinal tissues. Several agents, including bevacizumab, aimed at targeting and blocking VEGF molecules, have been developed, and have proven useful in the treatment of DME [1, 2]. Because the action of these agents, however, is not long lasting, treatment may be required for extended periods which raises the concern for long term effects of these agents such as worsening of macular perfusion through increasing capillary nonperfusion and vasoconstriction [2, 3].

Studies evaluating macular perfusion following intravitreal anti-VEGF injections have mainly relied on fluorescein angiography (FA) [4]. Optical coherence tomography angiography (OCTA) is a new noninvasive modality capable of imaging the different retinal capillary layers of the macula in greater detail compared to conventional FA. Unlike FA, it does not need dye injection and uses several technologies, including the split-spectrum amplitude decorrelation angiography (SSADA) algorithm, to image blood flow in the retinal and choroidal blood vessels [5]. Previously, we and others have shown that OCTA can detect areas of capillary nonperfusion not appreciated on fluorescein angiography [6, 7].

We evaluated the effect of repeated intravitreal bevacizumab injections on the capillary density of the maculae of a diabetic patient using OCTA.

2. Case Report

A 53-year-old female presented with gradually progressive diminution of vision in her left eye for 2 months. She had a history of diabetes mellitus for 20 years for which she is taking insulin. Her most recent HbA1C was 7.5%. She had no history of hypertension or renal problems. She had no past ocular history. Examination revealed a corrected distance visual acuity (CDVA) of 20/40 in her right eye and 20/100 in the left. Anterior segment examination showed nuclear sclerosis in both eyes. Posterior segment examination revealed intraretinal hemorrhages in all 4 quadrants indicating severe

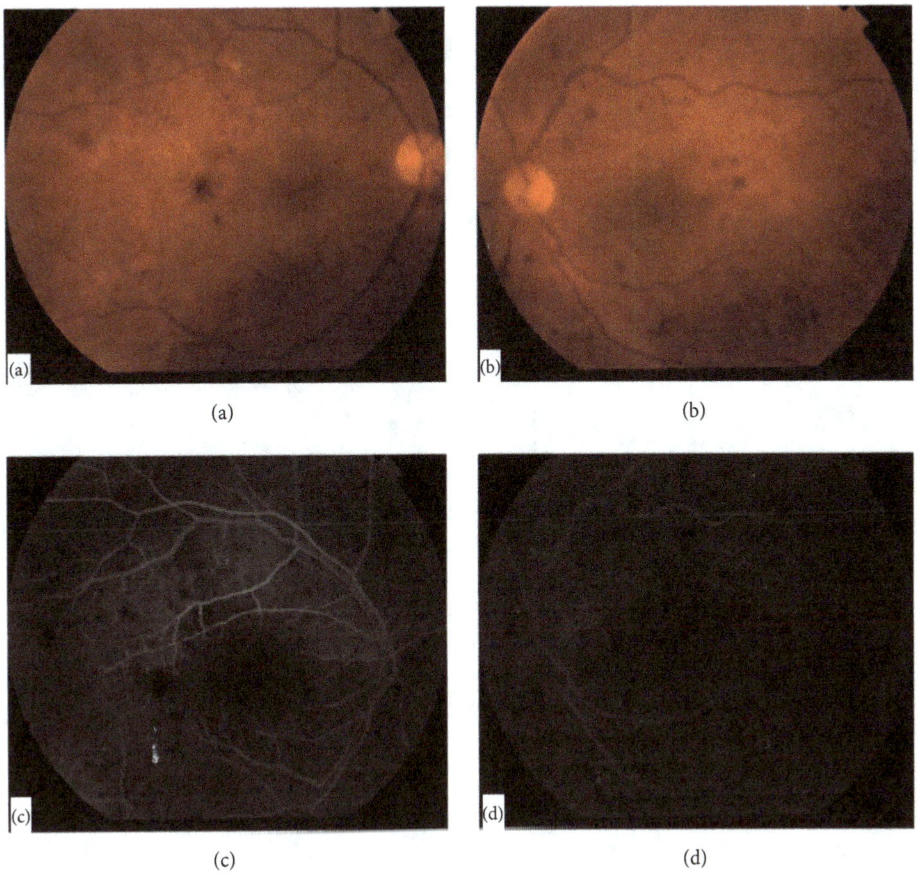

FIGURE 1: Fundus photography and fluorescein angiography of both eyes. Fundus photography showed retinal hemorrhages affecting the posterior pole in both eyes with clinically significant macular edema in the left eye (a and b). Fluorescein angiography revealed microaneurysms and areas of blocked fluorescence due to retinal hemorrhages in both eyes with leakage of fluorescein in the left macula (c and d).

nonproliferative diabetic retinopathy in both eyes with clinically significant macular edema in the left eye confirmed by fluorescein angiography (Figure 1). Spectral domain optical coherence tomography (OCT) of the macula was done and revealed multiple cystic spaces, mild subfoveal neurosensory detachment, and diffuse retinal thickening with a central subfield macular thickness of 332 μm in the left eye (Figure 2(a)). The right eye showed only few cystic spaces with minimal thickening. OCTA (Optovue, Inc., Fremont, CA, USA) was done in both eyes and showed areas of capillary nonperfusion in the superficial capillary plexus (SCP) of the maculae of both eyes (Figures 3(a) and 3(e)). Three monthly intravitreal bevacizumab injections were done to treat the macular edema in the left eye. One month following the last intravitreal injection, CDVA improved to 20/60 in the left eye and was stable in the right eye. OCT showed improvement of the macular edema in the left eye (Figure 2(b)). OCTA was performed in both eyes and showed decreased vascular density of the SCP of the left eye compared to pretreatment OCTA while a mild increase was noted in the vascular density of the SCP of the untreated right eye (Figures 3(b) and 3(f)). The patient was then followed up without requiring further intravitreal injections and 4 months following the last intravitreal injection OCTA was repeated in both eyes and showed improvement of the vascular density of the SCP of the left eye with unchanged SCP in the right eye (Figures 3(c) and 3(g)). CDVA was 20/60 in the right eye and 20/100 in the left. Clinical examination revealed retinal neovascularization in the right eye with clinically significant macular edema in both eyes. OCT showed increased center-involving macular edema in both eyes with recurrent neurosensory detachment in the left eye (Figure 2(c)). Three monthly intravitreal bevacizumab injections were then done for treatment of proliferative diabetic retinopathy in the right eye and the macular edema in both eyes. One month following the last intravitreal injection, CDVA was 20/40 in the right eye and 20/60 in the left, OCT showed decreased macular thickness in both eyes (Figure 2(d)), and OCTA revealed decreased vascular density of the SCP of both eyes (Figures 3(d) and 3(h)). Changes in the deep capillary plexus closely followed those in the SCP at all stages.

3. Discussion

According to the World Health Organization criteria on drugs and adverse drug reactions, a certain association is

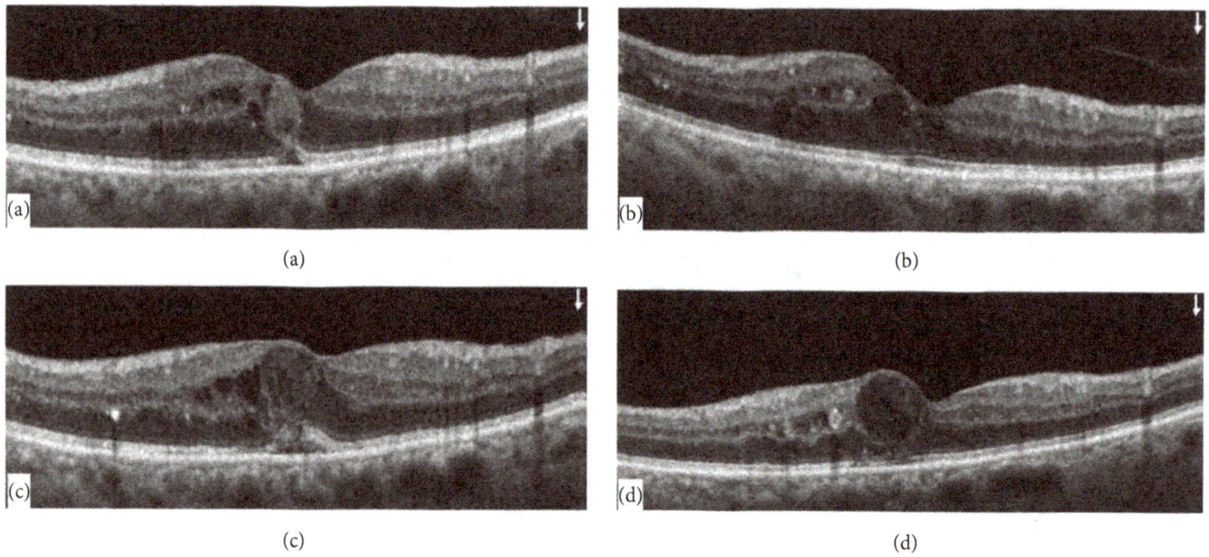

Figure 2: Structural OCT of the left macula. (a) At presentation, there were multiple intraretinal cystic spaces with mild subfoveal neurosensory detachment and diffuse retinal thickening. (b) Following 3 monthly intravitreal bevacizumab injections, there was improvement of the retinal edema and neurosensory detachment. (c) Follow-up 4 months following the last injection showed increased intraretinal cystic spaces and retinal thickness with recurrence of neurosensory detachment. (d) Following another 3 intravitreal injections, there was improvement of the neurosensory detachment and retinal thickness.

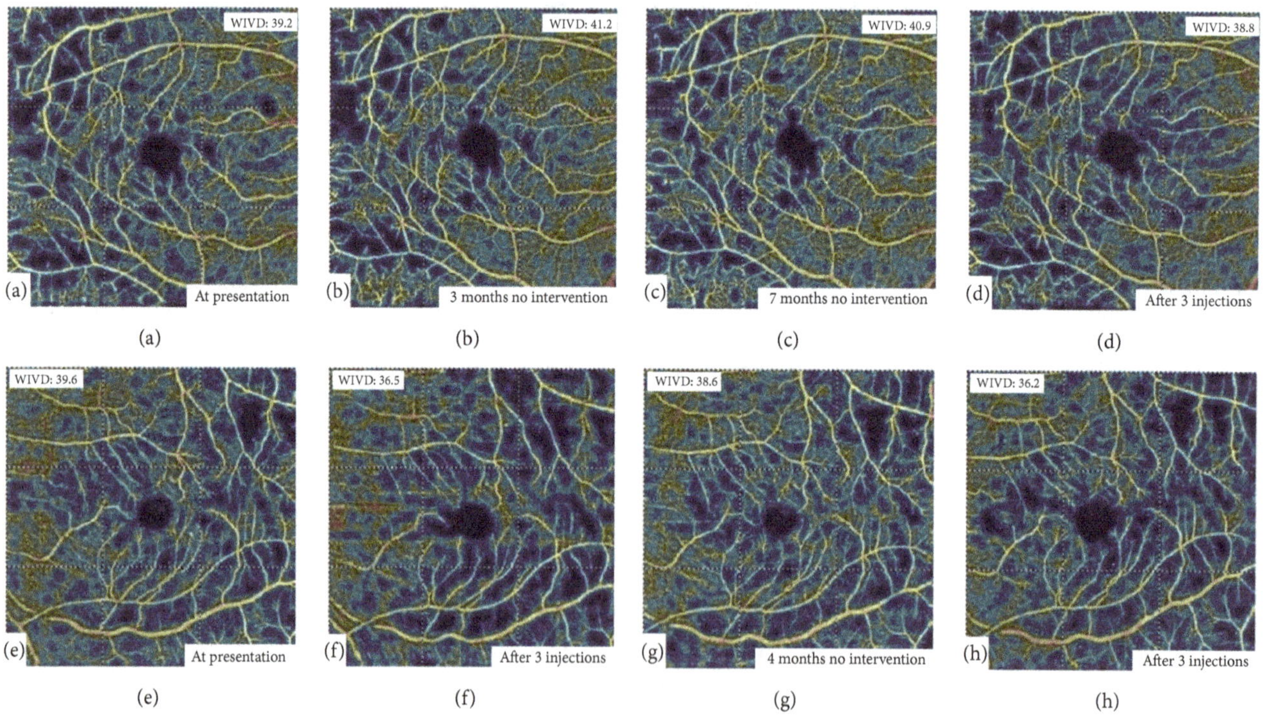

Figure 3: OCTA of the SCP of the right (top row) and left (bottom row) maculae. At presentation, there were areas of capillary nonperfusion detected in the SCP of both eyes especially temporally (a and e). Following three months of no intervention in the right eye and three monthly intravitreal injections in the left eye, there was increased vascular density (VD) in the right eye (b) and decreased VD in the left (f). After four months of no interventions in either eye, there was no change in the VD in the right eye (c) and increased VD in the left (g). Finally, following three monthly intravitreal injections in both eyes, there was decreased VD in both eyes (d and h). Scan quality was 6/10 or higher in all images and there were no significant segmentation errors detected. Whole image vascular density (WIVD), as measured by the built-in machine software, is shown at each visit.

present between the drug and the adverse event, including an abnormal laboratory test, if the event occurs in a plausible time relationship to drug administration and could not be explained by any other factor. The response to withdrawal of the drug, known as dechallenge, should be plausible, and the event must be definitive pharmacologically and using a satisfactory rechallenge procedure if necessary [8]. These criteria were all fulfilled in the presented case.

In a previous study assessing the effect of bevacizumab injections on the macular perfusion in diabetic patients without severe macular ischemia, there was no worsening of macular ischemia following 3 intravitreal injections given at 6 weeks' interval. This study, however, relied on FA for this assessment and assessed mainly parameters related to the foveal avascular zone which may not be fully representative of the whole macular perfusion [2, 4]. In another study evaluating the visual outcomes of bevacizumab injections in patients with DME with and without macular ischemia defined by FA, there was a negative effect from macular ischemia on the visual outcome of injections [9]. This may indicate further worsening of macular perfusion by VEGF inhibition in these cases [3, 9]. OCTA has been shown to be more sensitive in detecting areas of capillary nonperfusion when compared to FA and could therefore be more suited for assessing the status of the macular perfusion before and after anti-VEGF injections in diabetic patients [6, 7]. Because areas of capillary nonperfusion are more prevalent in diabetic patients in the SCP than the deep plexus as imaged by OCTA, with less projection artifacts, we focused our analysis on the SCP [7].

The increased areas of capillary nonperfusion detected by OCTA following bevacizumab injections could also be the result of slowing of blood flow in these capillaries rather than due to complete capillary obliteration. This would explain the apparent perfusion of these capillaries when imaged by FA but not OCTA, a phenomenon often observed with some microaneurysms detected by FA but not OCTA and suggested to be due to inability of the SSADA algorithm to detect retinal capillary flow less than 0.3 mm per second [7]. Indeed, intravitreal bevacizumab injections have been shown to reduce the mean blood flow velocities in the central retinal, posterior ciliary, and ophthalmic arteries of patients with wet age-related macular degeneration 4 weeks following a single intravitreal injection [10], an effect that may be more exaggerated in diabetic patients.

Lastly, there is a remote possibility that the increase and decrease in the capillary density observed with OCTA in this case may be a part of the natural history of diabetic retinopathy. This, however, is unlikely given that the capillary density decreased only when intravitreal bevacizumab injections were given but otherwise improved or was stable in the absence of injections in either eye.

This case, therefore, highlights the urgent need for further studies to evaluate the effect of repeated intravitreal bevacizumab injections, and other anti-VEGF agents, on the macular microvasculature of diabetic patients using the new flow-detecting OCTA imaging modality.

References

[1] D. R. Lally, C. P. Shah, and J. S. Heier, "Vascular endothelial growth factor and diabetic macular edema," *Survey of Ophthalmology*, vol. 61, no. 6, pp. 759–768, 2016.

[2] M. Michaelides, A. Kaines, R. D. Hamilton et al., "A prospective randomized trial of intravitreal bevacizumab or laser therapy in the management of diabetic macular edema (BOLT study) 12-month data: report 2," *Ophthalmology*, vol. 117, no. 6, pp. 1078–1086, 2010.

[3] K. Manousaridis and J. Talks, "Macular ischaemia: a contraindication for anti-VEGF treatment in retinal vascular disease?" *British Journal of Ophthalmology*, vol. 96, no. 2, pp. 179–184, 2012.

[4] M. Michaelides, S. Fraser-Bell, R. Hamilton et al., "Macular perfusion determined by fundus fluorescein angiography at the 4-month time point in a prospective randomized trial of intravitreal bevacizumab or laser therapy in the management of diabetic macular edema (bolt study): Report 1," *Retina*, vol. 30, no. 5, pp. 781–786, 2010.

[5] R. F. Spaide, J. M. Klancnik Jr., and M. J. Cooney, "Retinal vascular layers imaged by fluorescein angiography and optical coherence tomography angiography," *JAMA Ophthalmology*, vol. 33, no. 1, pp. 45–50, 2015.

[6] A. G. Elnahry, F. K. Hassan, and A. A. Abdel-Kader, "Bevacizumab for the treatment of intraretinal cystic spaces in a patient with gyrate atrophy of the choroid and retina," *Ophthalmic Genetics*, vol. 39, no. 6, pp. 759–762, 2018.

[7] A. Couturier, V. Mané, S. Bonnin et al., "Capillary plexus anomalies in diabetic retinopathy on optical coherence tomography angiography," *Retina*, vol. 35, no. 11, pp. 2384–2391, 2015.

[8] F. W. Fraunfelder and A. B. Richards, "Diplopia, blepharoptosis, and ophthalmoplegia and 3-Hydroxy-3-Methyl-Glutaryl-CoA reductase inhibitor use," *Ophthalmology*, vol. 115, no. 12, pp. 2282–2285, 2008.

[9] E. J. Chung, M. I. Roh, O. W. Kwon, and H. J. Koh, "Effects of macular ischemia on the outcome of intravitreal bevacizumab therapy for diabetic macular edema," *Retina*, vol. 28, no. 7, pp. 957–963, 2008.

[10] P. Bonnin, J.-A. C. Pournaras, Z. Lazrak et al., "Ultrasound assessment of short-term ocular vascular effects of intravitreal injection of bevacizumab (Avastin®) in neovascular age-related macular degeneration," *Acta Ophthalmologica*, vol. 88, no. 6, pp. 641–645, 2010.

8

Corneal Opacity Induced by Antiglaucoma Agents Other than Brimonidine Tartrate

Yuka Kasuya, Ichiya Sano, Shinji Makino, and Hidetoshi Kawashima

Department of Ophthalmology, Jichi Medical University, Shimotsuke, Tochigi, Japan

Correspondence should be addressed to Shinji Makino; makichan@jichi.ac.jp

Academic Editor: Cristiano Giusti

The aim of this study is to report a patient with corneal opacity that developed after the use of topical antiglaucoma medications other than brimonidine tartrate (BT). An 85-year-old woman presented with corneal opacity and neovascularization in both eyes. A diagnosis of glaucoma was made 20 years previously, and antiglaucoma agents were prescribed (latanoprost, tafluprost, timolol maleate, travoprost, bimatoprost, ripasudil hydrochloride hydrate, and brinzolamide/timolol maleate) for both eyes. Ocular examination revealed semicircular fan-shaped corneal sterile infiltration with neovascularization. Anterior-segment optical coherence tomography (OCT) showed marked corneal opacity and thickened corneal stroma. The topical drugs were discontinued and replaced with 0.1% betamethasone eye drops. Two weeks after topical drugs were discontinued and replaced with betamethasone, the corneal sterile infiltration markedly improved, although the corneal opacity remained across the stromal layer. In addition, corneal opacity, intermixed with separate transparent sections, was observed as a striped shape. OCT showed an improvement of the thickened corneal stroma. Six weeks after the initial visit, the remaining corneal opacity could be seen as a mixture of opaque and nonopaque areas in stripes. The corneal stromal thickness decreased almost back to the normal range, while the area of the corneal opacity remained unchanged. *In vivo* laser confocal microscopy showed hyperreflective materials with needle-like structures in the corneal stroma. The corneal opacity showed several similarities to the previous reports of the cases treated with BT. Therefore, clinicians should be mindful of a possible development of corneal opacity in patients treated with antiglaucoma medications other than BT.

1. Introduction

Brimonidine tartrate (BT) ophthalmic solution, a topical $\alpha 2$-adrenoreceptor agonist, has been used for glaucoma therapy, and reports of adverse side effects include allergic conjunctivitis, blepharitis, and conjunctival hyperemia [1]. However, corneal side effects are uncommon [2]. In 2017, Maruyama et al. [3] reported two cases of peripheral corneal opacity that developed after treatment with BT. To date, four reports including eight cases have been described in Japan [3–6]. In this study, we report a case of bilateral corneal stromal opacity, which showed several similarities to previous cases treated with BT that presumably developed after treatment with topical antiglaucoma medications other than BT.

2. Case Presentation

An 85-year-old woman presented with corneal opacity and neovascularization in both eyes. She was diagnosed as having primary open-angle glaucoma 20 years previously and had been treated with seven different ocular hypotensive agents (latanoprost, tafluprost, timolol maleate, travoprost, bimatoprost, ripasudil hydrochloride hydrate, and brinzolamide/timolol maleate) for both eyes (OU). In detail, she was initially treated with latanoprost eye drops (Xalatan; Pfizer Inc., New York, USA), with timolol maleate (Timoptol, Santen Pharmaceutical Co. Ltd., Osaka, Japan) being added to her treatment regimen in 2005. In April 2013, her treatment was switched from latanoprost to tafluprost (Tapros, Santen

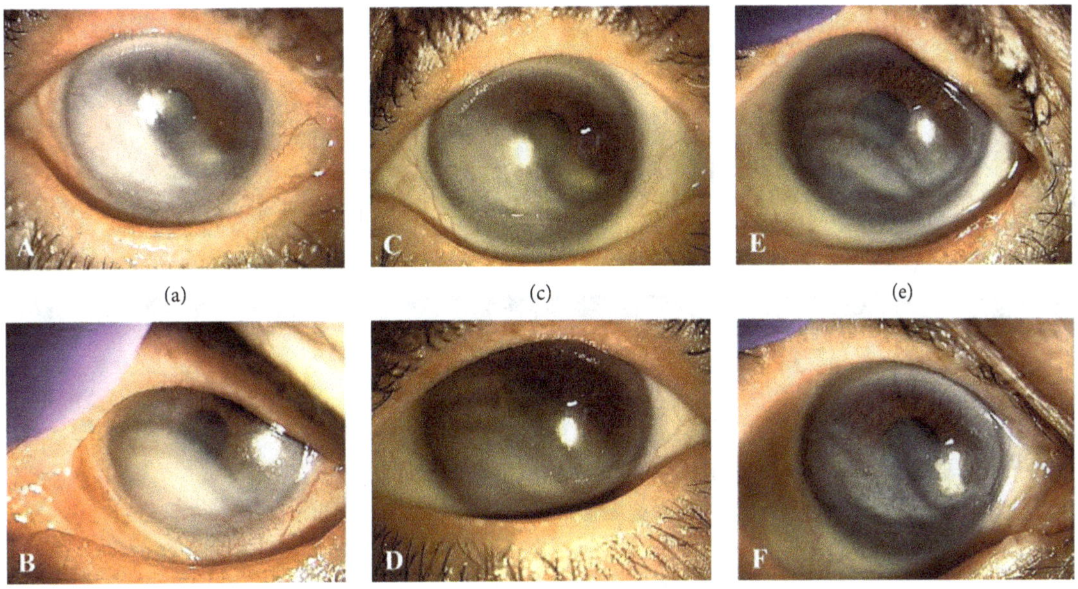

(a) (c) (e)

(b) (d) (f)

Figure 1: Corneal findings in the right (a, c, and e) and left (b, d, and f) eyes. (a, b) Slit-lamp examination shows corneal sterile infiltration and neovascularization in the temporal-lower side of the right eye and in the nasal-lower side of the left eye at the initial visit. (c, d) Two weeks after the initial visit (after topical agents were discontinued and replaced with betamethasone), slit-lamp examination showed a marked regression of the corneal vascularization and decreased corneal opacity bilaterally, while the area of the corneal opacity remained unchanged. (e, f) Six weeks after the initial visit, corneal opacity, intermixed with separate transparent sections, was clearly seen bilaterally, while the area of the corneal opacity remained unchanged.

Pharmaceutical Co. Ltd., Osaka, Japan). In May 2014, her treatment was switched from timolol maleate to brinzolamide/timolol maleate (Azorga Combination Ophthalmic Suspension, Novartis, Basel, Switzerland). In April 2015, her treatment was switched from tafluprost to travoprost (Travatan Z Ophthalmic Solution 0.004%, Novartis, Basel, Switzerland) and then to bimatoprost (Lumigan, Senju Pharmaceutical Co. Ltd., Osaka, Japan) in November 2017. Furthermore, ripasudil hydrochloride hydrate (Glanatec ophthalmic solution 0.4%, Kowa Co. Ltd., Nagoya, Japan) was added to her treatment regimen for both eyes since October 2016. Thus far, she was being treated with three kinds of eye drops (brinzolamide/timolol maleate, ripasudil hydrochloride hydrate, and bimatoprost) at the time of the consultation. She has had no history of BT use. Corneal opacity was observed since December 2018 at the referral eye clinic. She had no remarkable ophthalmological, medical, allergic histories and rosacea.

At the initial presentation, the best-corrected visual acuities (BCVAs) were 0.3 in her right eye (OD) and 0.15 in her left eye (OS) in decimal; the intraocular pressures (IOPs) were 11 mmHg OD and 15 mmHg OS. Bilateral gonioscopy showed open iridocorneal angles, and fundoscopy showed typical glaucomatous changes in the optic nerve heads OU. Ocular examination revealed follicular conjunctivitis and blepharitis OU and corneal sterile infiltration with neovascularization in the temporal lower side OD and in the nasal lower side OS (Figures 1(a) and 1(b)). Anterior-segment optical coherence tomography (OCT) showed a marked corneal opacity and thickened corneal stroma OU (Figures 2(a) and 2(b)). Although she had no history of BT use, she was diagnosed with stromal opacity with deep corneal vascularization possibly associated with certain topical medications. Therefore, we discontinued all three ocular hypotensive agents and initiated treatment with 0.1% betamethasone sodium phosphate (Sanbetason ophthalmic and otorhinologic solution 0.1%, Santen Pharmaceutical Co. Ltd., Osaka, Japan) four times daily OU. Two weeks after the discontinuation of topical drugs and administration of betamethasone, both the blepharitis and corneal sterile infiltration markedly improved (Figures 1(c) and 1(d)). In addition, corneal opacity, intermixed with separate transparent sections, was observed as a striped shape. OCT showed an improvement in the thickened corneal stroma (Figures 2(c) and 2(d)). The BCVAs were 0.5 OD and 0.2 OS, and the IOP was 15 mmHg OU. Six weeks after the initial visit, corneal opacity, intermixed with separate transparent sections, was clearly seen bilaterally (Figures 1(e) and 1(f)). Corneal stromal thickness improved almost normally, while the area of the corneal opacity remained unchanged (Figures 2(e) and 2(f)). The BCVAs were 0.7 OD and 0.6 OS, and the IOP was 16 mmHg OU. *In vivo* laser confocal microscopy (IVCM; Heidelberg Retina Tomograph II Rostock Cornea Module) showed hyperreflective materials with needle-like structures in the corneal stroma (Figures 3(a)–3(f)). The progression of corneal thinning and definite lipid deposition was not detected during the 18-month follow-up period.

3. Discussion

In this study, we report a case of bilateral corneal stromal opacity that resembles previous cases that were treated with

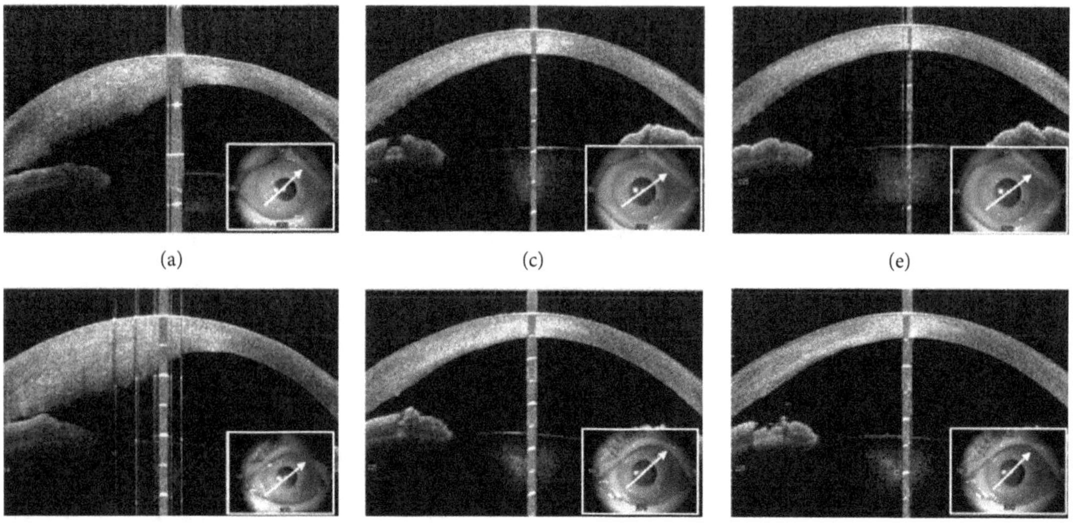

(a) (c) (e)

(b) (d) (f)

FIGURE 2: Anterior-segment optical coherence tomography (OCT) images in the right (a, c, and e) and left (b, d, and f) eyes. (a, b) Anterior OCT images showing opacity deep in the marked thickening corneal stroma in both eyes at the initial visit. (c, d) Two weeks after the initial visit (after topical agents were discontinued and replaced with betamethasone), an improvement of the thickened corneal stroma was observed. (e, f) Six weeks after the initial visit, corneal stromal thickness improved almost back to normal.

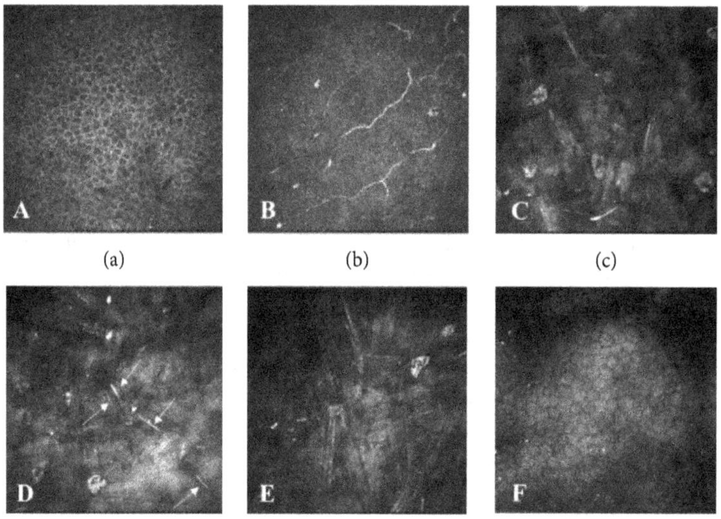

(a) (b) (c)

(d) (e) (f)

FIGURE 3: *In vivo* confocal microscopic (IVCM) images (a–f): (a) the basal epithelium (12 μm depth), (b) subbasal nerve plexus (129 μm depth), (c) anterior stroma (206 μm depth), (d) mid stroma (235 μm depth), (e) posterior stroma (266 μm depth), and (F) endothelium (483 μm depth). IVCM showed hyperreflective materials with needle-like structures in the corneal stroma (d arrows). Each image represents a $400 \times 400\,\mu m^2$ area.

BT and that presumably developed after the use of topical antiglaucoma medications other than BT.

BT has been associated with ocular side effects including conjunctival injection, allergic conjunctivitis, and blepharitis; however, corneal side effects are uncommon [1, 2]. To date, four reports including eight cases with severe corneal disorder have been reported in Japan [3–6]. According to these reports, the clinical features of BT-induced corneal opacity were as follows. First, peripheral corneal sterile infiltration was observed, especially below the cornea, and was semicircular or fan-shaped with blepharitis. Second, corneal lesions were present deep in the corneal stroma with vascular invasion. Third, corneal disorder developed several years after the induction of topical BT. Fourth, the use of topical steroid and discontinuance of topical BT led to improved clinical symptoms. Last, the remaining corneal opacity could be seen as a mixture of opaque and nonopaque areas in stripes.

According to previous cases that were treated with BT, corneal opacity might be due to an allergic reaction, interaction between BT and other antiglaucoma medications, effects of preservatives such as benzalkonium chloride and sodium chlorite, and racial differences. However, the exact mechanism for corneal opacity remains unknown.

Additionally, lipid keratopathy can result from corneal sterile infiltration with neovascularization and can be secondary to stromal corneal herpes, other corneal diseases, trauma, contact lens wear, or systemic diseases [7–10]. In cases of lipid keratopathy, crystalline- or needle-like structures have been observed by IVCM [10]. These findings are consistent with the histopathological description, which states that the opacity of the cornea was caused by deposition of cholesterol in the corneal stroma [7]. IVCM findings in our case of corneal opacity that developed after treatment with topical antiglaucoma agents indicate the mechanisms behind; i.e., long-term use of multiple topical antiglaucoma agents led to the corneal sterile infiltration with neovascularization. As a result, serum lipid components accumulated in the corneal stroma as observed in cases of lipid keratopathy. From this point of view, IVCM can be a useful examination for the diagnosis of this rare corneal disorder in future cases.

We present a case of bilateral corneal stromal opacity, which showed several similarities to previous cases that were treated with BT and that presumably developed after treatment with topical antiglaucoma medications other than BT. The present case indicates that clinicians should therefore be mindful of a possible development of corneal opacity in patients treated with antiglaucoma medications other than BT. A further accumulation of reports may be needed.

References

[1] G. Manni, M. Centofanti, M. Sacchetti et al., "Demographic and clinical factors associated with development of brimonidine tartrate 0.2%-induced ocular allergy," *Journal of Glaucoma*, vol. 13, no. 2, pp. 163–167, 2004.

[2] A. A. Shah, Y. Modi, B. Thomas, S. R. Wellik, and A. Galor, "Brimonidine allergy presenting as vernal-like keratoconjunctivitis,," *Journal of Glaucoma*, vol. 24, no. 1, pp. 89–91, 2015.

[3] Y. Maruyama, Y. Ikeda, N. Yokoi et al., "Severe corneal disorders developed after brimonidine tartrate ophthalmic solution use," *Cornea*, vol. 36, no. 12, pp. 1567–1569, 2017.

[4] A. Tsujinaka, Y. Takai, Y. Inoue, and M. Tanito, "A case of bilateral deep stromal corneal opacity and vascularization after use of multiple antiglaucoma medications including brimonidine tartrate ophthalmic solution," *Acta Ophthalmologica*, vol. 97, no. 6, pp. e948–e949, 2019.

[5] Y. Manabe, A. Sawada, and K. Mochizuki, "Corneal sterile infiltration induced by topical use of ocular hypotensive agent," *European Journal of Ophthalmology*, p. 112067211985008, 2019, [Epub ahead of print].

[6] A. Yorifuji, Y. Hosotani, M. Okamoto, Y. Kasumoto, and F. Gomi, "Three cases of corneal disorders developed after brimonidine tartrate ophthalmic solution use," *Ganka*, vol. 61, no. 13, pp. 1527–1533, 2019.

[7] K. U. Loeffler and P. Seifert, "Unusual idiopathic lipid keratopathy: a newly recognized entity?," *Archives of Ophthalmology*, vol. 123, no. 10, pp. 1435–1438, 2005.

[8] J. Levy, D. Benharroch, and T. Lifshitz, "Bilateral severe progressive idiopathic lipid keratopathy," *International Ophthalmology*, vol. 26, no. 4-5, pp. 181–184, 2005.

[9] J. Y. Oh, M. K. Kim, and W. R. Wee, "Subconjunctival and intracorneal bevacizumab injection for corneal neovascularization in lipid keratopathy," *Cornea*, vol. 28, no. 9, pp. 1070–1073, 2009.

[10] Y. Pang, Q. Zhang, and Y. A. Bao, "A CARE-compliant article: ipsilateral progressive idiopathic lipid keratopathy: a case report," *Medicine (Baltimore)*, vol. 98, no. 35, p. e16589, 2019.

9

Idiopathic Isolated Acquired Steroid Dependent SO Palsy: A Rare Case Report

Isha Agarwal, Mayuresh Naik, and HarinderSingh Sethi

Department of Ophthalmology, V.M.M.C. & Safdarjung Hospital, Ring Road, Ansari Nagar, New Delhi 110029, India

Correspondence should be addressed to Mayuresh Naik; mayureshpnaik@gmail.com

Academic Editor: Ruth Huna-Baron

15-year-old boy presented with sudden onset, stable, nonprogressive painless diplopia (greatest in right gaze and inferior field of view) and hyperdeviation of left eye for a year. On ophthalmic examination, the patient had uncrossed diplopia with tilt and separation maximum in dextrodepression. On Park's three step test, left eye hypertropia increased on right gaze and left tilt suggestive of left superior oblique (SO) palsy. On prism bar cover test (PBCT), deviation was more than 25 PD base-down over the left eye for both distance and near in all gazes. MRI head and orbit revealed a normal study while the myasthenia and inflammatory work-up was unremarkable. A provisional diagnosis of "Idiopathic Acquired Left Superior Oblique Palsy" was made and the patient was given trial of oral steroids at 1 mg/kg body weight. At 6 weeks, patient's diplopia resolved and PBCT neutralised at 6PD. Oral steroids were gradually tapered off by 10 mg per week with weekly follow-up. Upon decreasing the dose of prednisolone to 5 mg, intermittent diplopia and 18 PD left hypertropia reappeared. When patient was again restarted on oral steroids at 1 mg/kg body weight, diplopia-hypertropia disappeared at 10 mg OD prednisolone only to reappear at 5 mg OD dosage, leading to the final diagnosis of a "Steroid Dependent Isolated Superior Oblique Palsy". Presently, the patient is maintained on a daily dose of 10 mg oral prednisolone.

1. Case Report

A 15-year-old boy presented with sudden onset painless diplopia and hyperdeviation of left eye for almost a year, which was stable, painless, and nonprogressive. The binocular diplopia persisted both for near and for distance and was greatest in right gaze and inferior field of view.

There was no history of any associated vision loss, pain, trauma, febrile illness, or any other systemic illness. There was neither any history of weakness after prolonged work or in the evenings nor any past history of strabismus or squinting for far.

There was no history of any weakness, of decreased sensations in body part, of tremors or jerks, of sudden severe pain, of neck stiffness, or of loss of consciousness at the onset of the symptoms. There were no associated neurological symptoms including no other cranial nerve abnormalities. The patient's past medical history and birth history were uneventful. Also there was no history of similar complains among family members.

General physical examination and systemic review were unremarkable.

On ophthalmic examination, the Best Corrected Visual Acuity (BCVA) in both the eyes was 6/6 Snellen's for distance and J6 Jaeger's for near. The patient had a compensatory head posture with the chin at level, face turned towards the right side, and a head tilt to right. Extra ocular movements were full and free in both the eyes with inferior oblique over action in left eye (Figure 1). On diplopia charting, patient had uncrossed diplopia with tilt and separation maximum in dextrodepression. Park-Bielschowski's three step test suggested a left superior oblique (SO) palsy. On prism bar cover test (PBCT) with prism over the left eye, the deviation was more than 25 PD base-down for both distance and near in all cardinal gazes. Hess charting corroborated the clinical findings. Forced duction test (FDT) and force generation testing (exaggerated FDT) were carried out in an ICU setting and revealed neither any restriction of movement nor laxity of muscles in any gaze.

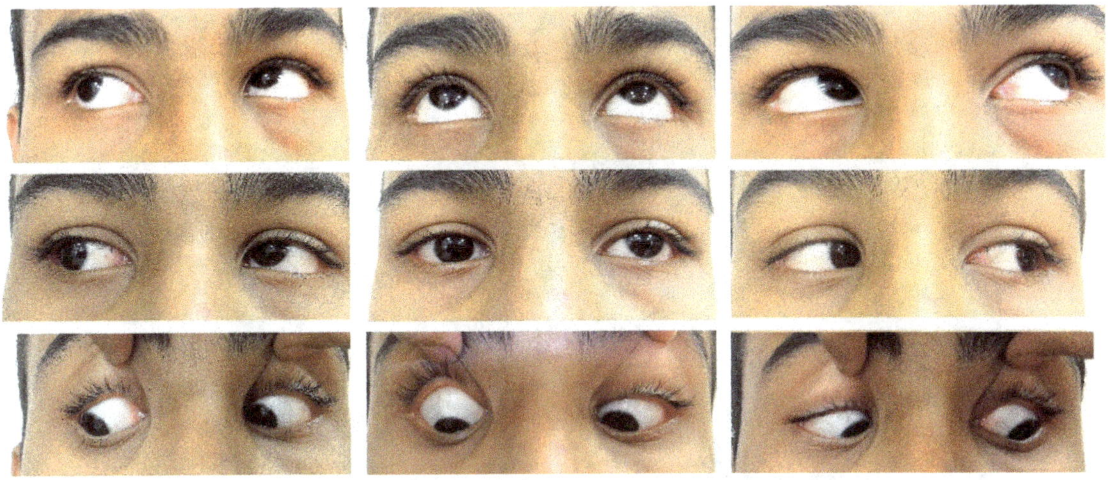

FIGURE 1: Clinical photograph of 9 cardinal gazes at presentation.

Revisiting old photographs did not reveal any plagiocephaly or facial asymmetry, thus negating a congenital deviation. Hematological investigations also did not reveal any anaemia, thyroid dysfunction, or any other abnormality.

Ultrasound (USG)-B scan of both the eyes was unremarkable. Gadolinium enhanced MRI of head and orbit was normal, neither any inflammatory lesions in the orbit or the cavernous sinus nor any demyelinating plaques in the periventricular areas (Figures 2 and 3). Anti-AchR and anti-MUSK antibodies were negative and single fiber electromyography (SF-EMG) was within normal limits, thus ruling out the possibility of ocular myasthenia. Blood count and thyroid functions were normal. An inflammatory work-up revealed normal ESR and CRP and negative RF, ANA, cANCA, and pCNCA. A provisional diagnosis of "Idiopathic Acquired Superior Oblique Palsy" was made.

The patient was given a trial of oral steroids, i.e., Prednisolone 1 mg/kg body weight. After 2 weeks, the patient was symptomatically better, now with only intermittent diplopia in inferior gaze and decrease in the upward deviation of left eye according to patient's father. PBCT for both near and distance (with prism over the left eye) neutralised the hypertropia with 18 PD base-down over left eye. 4 weeks after starting the oral steroids, the patient's diplopia resolved the left hyperdeviation measured 6PD. After 6 weeks of treatment, the patient remained free of diplopia-hypertropia. Oral steroids were gradually tapered off by 10 mg per week and weekly follow-up was done (Figure 4). Upon decreasing the dose of prednisolone to 5mg per day, the intermittent diplopia and 18PD left hypertropia reappeared. Oral steroids were restarted at 1 mg/kg body weight and in 2 weeks the diplopia had resolved again and the left hypertropia decreased to 6PD. When the steroid dose was again gradually tapered, intermittent diplopia and 16PD hypertropia reappeared upon reducing the dose to 5 mg per day.

The oral steroid dose was increased back to 10 mg per day and after a week the diplopia disappeared and PBCT neutralised at 6PD base-down in front of left eye.

This unique sequence of events, i.e., disappearance of diplopia-hypertropia at 10 mg OD prednisolone and reappearance at 5 mg OD dosage, led to the final diagnosis of a "Steroid Dependent Isolated Acquired Superior Oblique Palsy". Presently the patient is maintained on a daily dose of 10 mg oral prednisolone.

2. Discussion

The trochlear nerve, also known as the fourth cranial nerve, arises from the trochlear nucleus, situated on the dorsal aspect of the midbrain below the inferior colliculus just lateral to the frenulum veli [1, 2]. It is the only cranial nerve that arises from the dorsal aspect of the brain resulting in the longest intracranial course of any cranial nerve and has the fewest axons of all the cranial nerves, making it slender and vulnerable to trauma. It is the only decussated cranial nerve apart from optic nerve, thus innervating the contralateral superior oblique muscle. Nuclear lesions cause contralateral SO palsy and peripheral lesions cause ipsilateral SO palsy [3].

The most common etiology of isolated 4th nerve palsy is congenital, contributing to around 39.5% of the cases, closely followed by traumatic (34%), idiopathic (23.2%), and neurologic (2.9%) paralyses [4, 5].

Congenital fourth nerve palsy often remains compensated and unrecognized during childhood due to large vertical fusional vergence amplitudes and can manifest later either spontaneously or after a minor trauma [1].

Trauma commonly leads to bilateral fourth nerve palsy due to injury to the decussating nerve fibers at the anterior medullary velum. Other etiologies of acquired causes of 4th nerve palsy include compressive lesions (aneurysms and tumors), demyelination, ocular myasthenia, diabetic neuropathy, and herpes zoster. Around 20% cases are idiopathic [6–8]. 4th nerve palsy of microvascular etiology is usually seen in older patients with vascular risk factors.

Several syndromes (superior orbital fissure syndrome, orbital apex syndrome, and cavernous sinus syndrome) cause

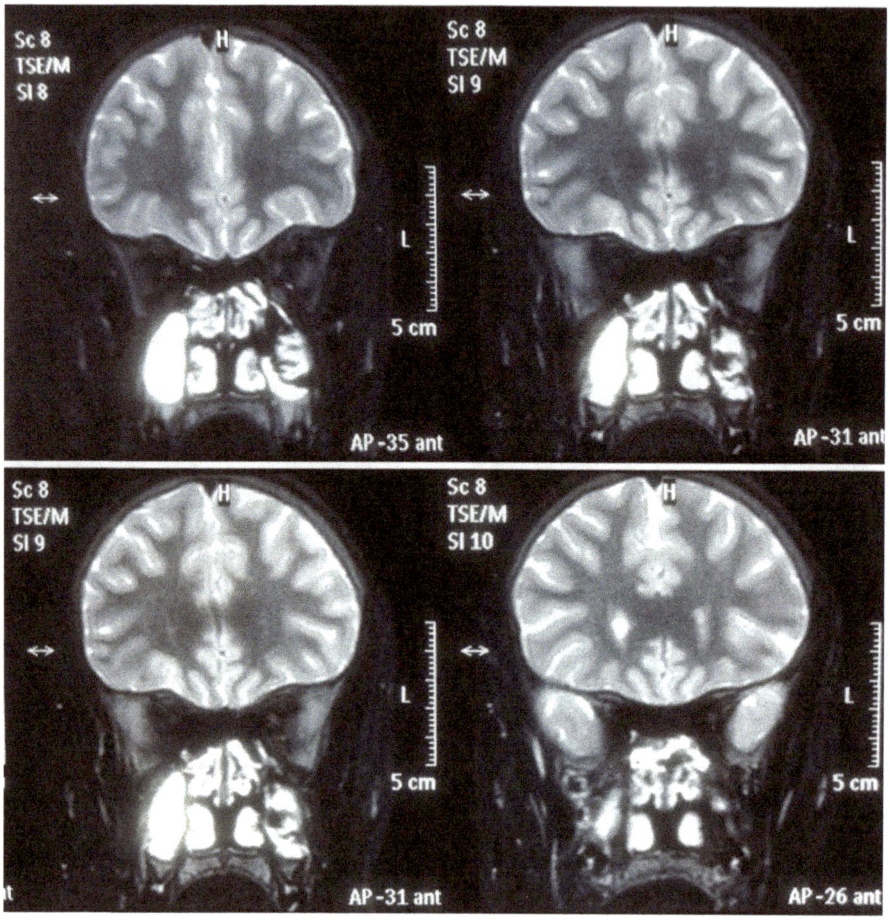

Figure 2: MRI head and orbit coronal section at the level of the midorbit and apex showing absence of any granulomatous lesions nor any extraocular muscle thickening (ruling out myositis or orbital pseudotumor).

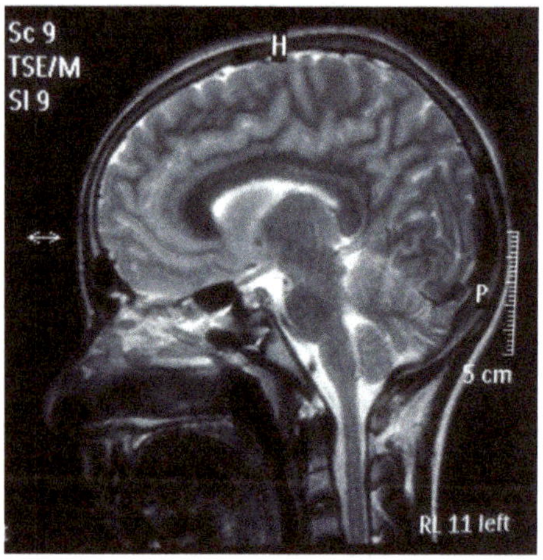

Figure 3: MRI head and orbit at the level of the midorbit and apex showing absence of any granulomatous lesions nor any extraocular muscle thickening (ruling out myositis or orbital pseudotumor).

trochlear nerve palsy associated with variable involvement of cranial nerves 2nd through 6th. However, our patient presented with isolated 4th nerve palsy.

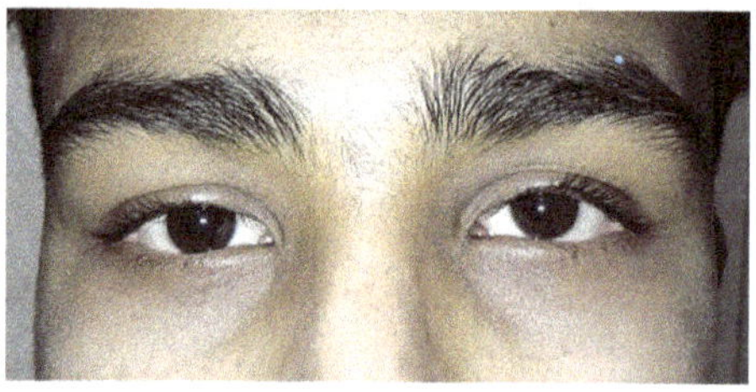

Figure 4: Clinical photograph of patient after 4 weeks of 1 mg/kg oral steroid.

For an isolated nonprogressive 4th nerve palsy, neuroimaging is not required routinely; however imaging is recommended if there is any neurologic deficit, in acute traumatic cases and in patients with unclear etiology [9, 10]. The recently established guideline for the cost-effective evaluation of patients with SO palsy suggests that isolated congenital or old traumatic cases may not require neuroimaging [11]. In most cases of 4th nerve palsy, detailed evaluation with an elaborate history and thorough clinical examination and high index of suspicion reveal the etiology. According to a recent study, neuroimaging is now recommended in all patients presenting with acute onset isolated ocular motor cranial nerve palsy [10, 12–15].

Pain is an important indicator of etiology. Painful SO palsy occurs in traumatic cases, neurological syndromes, extraocular muscle (EOM) myositis, nonspecific idiopathic orbital inflammatory disorders (NSIOID), Graves ophthalmopathy, and cysticercosis with microscopic leaks. Painless SO palsy more commonly occurs in congenital cases, myasthenia, chronic progressive ophthalmoplegia CPEO, demyelination, and nuclear palsies.

In our patient, there was no improvement in vertical diplopia or hypertropia over a year and further investigations did not reveal any abnormality. Since there was conspicuous absence of pain throughout the duration of the diplopia, a differential diagnosis of ocular myasthenia, demyelinating lesion (?multiple sclerosis), and central inflammatory lesion (vasculitis) was considered. Gadolinium enhanced MRI imaging of the head and orbit was done looking for any inflammatory or demyelinating lesion, both of which were absent. AntiAChR and antiMuSK antibodies were negative. Extensive inflammatory work-up was unremarkable so that other autoimmune diseases were ruled out. Thereafter a trial of oral steroids [10] was administered, to which the patient responded very well. However to our surprise, upon withdrawal of steroids after a tapering regime, the diplopia and hypertropia recurred. Taking into account the systemic side effects of long term oral steroids, steroid sparing immunosuppressive agents are considered for the patient.

To the best of our knowledge after a thorough review of literature, such a clinical presentation has not been reported previously and this is the first instance of a "Steroid Dependent Isolated Acquired Superior Oblique Palsy".

Authors' Contributions

All the authors were involved in the concept and design of the study, data acquisition, data analysis and interpretation, drafting manuscript, technical support, and final review of the manuscript.

References

[1] J. C. Sargent, "Nuclear and infranuclear ocular motility disorders," in *Walsh and Hoyt's Clinical neuroophthalmology*, N. R. Miller and N. J. Newman, Eds., pp. 969–1040, Lippincott Williams and Wilkins, Maryland, Md, USA, 2005.

[2] N. J. Newman, "Third, fourth and sixth-nerve lesions and the cavernous sinus," in *Principles and Practice of Ophthalmology*, D. M. Albert and F. A. Jackobiec, Eds., vol. 3, pp. 4071–4100, WB Saunders, Pennsylvania, Pa, USA, 2008.

[3] E. M. Helveston, J. S. Mora, and S. N. Lipsky, "Surgical treatment of superior oblique palsy," *Transactions of the American Ophthalmological Society*, vol. 94, pp. 315–328, 1996.

[4] G. K. Von Noorden, E. Murray, and S. Y. Wong, "Superior oblique paralysis: a review of 270 cases," *JAMA Ophtalmology*, vol. 104, no. 12, pp. 1771–1776, 1986.

[5] H. K. Yang, J. H. Kim, and J.-M. Hwang, "Congenital superior oblique palsy and trochlear nerve absence: A clinical and radiological study," *Ophthalmology*, vol. 119, no. 1, pp. 170–177, 2012.

[6] J. A. Rush and R. R. Younge, "Paralysis of cranial nerves III, IV, and VI. Cause and prognosis in 1,000 cases," *JAMA Ophtalmology*, vol. 99, no. 1, pp. 76–79, 1981.

[7] B. W. Richards, F. R. Jones Jr., and B. R. Younge, "Causes and prognosis in 4,278 cases of paralysis of the oculomotor, trochlear, and abducens cranial nerves," *American Journal of Ophthalmology*, vol. 113, no. 5, pp. 489–496, 1992.

[8] J. M. Holmes, S. Mutyala, T. L. Maus, R. Grill, D. O. Hodge, and D. T. Gray, "Pediatric third, fourth, and sixth nerve palsies: A population-based study," *American Journal of Ophthalmology*, vol. 127, no. 4, pp. 388–392, 1999.

[9] J. Kanski and B. Bowling, *Strabismus*, chapter 19, article 827, 8th edition, 2011.

[10] D. Ray, A. Gupta, V. Sachdeva, and R. Kekunnaya, "Superior oblique palsy: epidemiology and clinical spectrum from a tertiary eye care center in South India," *Asia-Pacific Journal of Ophthalmology*, vol. 3, no. 3, pp. 158–163, 2014.

[11] A. G. Lee, L. A. Haymann, H. A. Beaver et al., "A guide to the evaluation of fourth nerve cranial nerve paralysis," *Srabismus*, vol. 6, article 191, 1998.

[12] K. L. Chou, S. L. Galetta, G. T. Liu et al., "Acute ocular motor mononeuropathies: prospective study of the roles of neuroimaging and clinical assessment," *Journal of the Neurological Sciences*, vol. 219, no. 1-2, pp. 35–39, 2004.

[13] M. A. Tamhankar and N. J. Volpe, "Management of acute cranial nerve 3, 4 and 6 palsies: role of neuroimaging," *Current Opinion in Ophthalmology*, vol. 26, no. 6, pp. 464–468, 2015.

[14] A. P. Murchison, M. E. Gilbert, and P. J. Savino, "Neuroimaging and acute ocular motor mononeuropathies: a prospective study," *JAMA Ophtalmology*, vol. 129, no. 3, pp. 301–305, 2011.

[15] N. J. Volpe and A. G. Lee, "Do patients with neurologically isolated ocular motor cranial nerve palsies require prompt neuroimaging?" *Journal of Neuro-Ophthalmology*, vol. 34, no. 3, pp. 301–305, 2014.

10

Closantel Retinal Toxicity: Case Report and Literature Review

Sepideh Ghods, Elias Khalili Pour, Hamid Riazi-Esfahani, Hooshang Faghihi, and Bahman Inanloo

Retina Ward, Farabi Eye Hospital, Tehran University of Medical Sciences, Tehran, Iran

Correspondence should be addressed to Bahman Inanloo; inanloobahman96@gmail.com

Academic Editor: Takaaki Hayashi

A 57-year-old shepherd was referred with a 2-week history of decreased visual acuity in both eyes. Optical coherence tomography (OCT) (Heidelberg Engineering GmbH, Heidelberg, Germany) revealed diffuse outer nuclear layer hyperreflectivity and indistinguishable external limiting membrane and ellipsoid zone. The patient announced to us that he took two 500 mg of closantel tablets (15.15 mg/kg) three days before the initiation of visual problems for sore throat as an antibiotic. Electroretinography displayed severely attenuated responses in both eyes. We decided to admit the patient with the presumed diagnosis of closantel retinal toxicity and treated him with intravenous methylprednisolone 1 g per day and intravenous erythropoietin 10000 IU twice a day, and reevaluation of the patient proved no change in his visual acuity on the third day of admission. Closantel is a veterinary drug with serious side effects in the human retina and central nervous system even in previously reported doses. Public awareness and appropriate drug labeling about its side effects could prevent accidental toxicity. OCT is a noninvasive and rapid diagnostic modality that should be done in suspected toxic retinopathy.

1. Case Presentation

A 57-year-old shepherd was referred to the retina clinic of Farabi Eye Hospital complaining about 2-week sudden vision loss in both eyes. He weighed about 66 kg. His visual acuity was count fingers at 50 cm and 1 m for the right and left eye, respectively. His past medical history was unremarkable, and he denied any recent self-medication. On slit-lamp examination, the anterior segment was normal except for mild symmetric nuclear sclerosis and middilated and poorly reacting pupils. The fundus exam showed a small area of myelinated axons on the right optic nerve head and very mild peripapillary whitening and nerve fiber layer swelling more prominent in the right eye (Figure 1(a)). Fundus autofluorescence and infrared reflectance (Heidelberg Engineering GmbH, Heidelberg, Germany) images were normal (Figure 1(b)). Optical coherence tomography (OCT) (Heidelberg Engineering GmbH, Heidelberg, Germany) revealed diffuse outer nuclear layer hyperreflectivity and indistinguishable external limiting membrane and ellipsoid zone (Figure 1(c)). Systemic laboratory tests and brain MRI were performed before his referral. Laboratory documents were unremarkable except for the liver enzyme test twice the normal range. T2-weighted brain MRI without gadolinium showed multiple bright foci at peri- and paraventricular, centrum semiovale, and junctional areas (not showed) that were diagnosed as a microvascular disease by a radiologist.

Based on our previous experience on closantel retinal toxicity and its typical OCT features, we returned to the patient's history and asked about inadvertent veterinary drug use. The patient announced to us that he took two 500 mg of closantel (15.15/kg) tablets 3 days before the initiation of visual problems for sore throat as an antibiotic. Electroretinography displayed severely attenuated responses in both eyes (Figure 1(d)). As we came across some plasma exchange beneficial reports in literature [1], we referred the patient to toxicologists but they were reluctant for performing the procedure, as there was a low chance of recovery. Consequently, we decided to admit the patient and treated him with intravenous methylprednisolone 1 g per day and intravenous

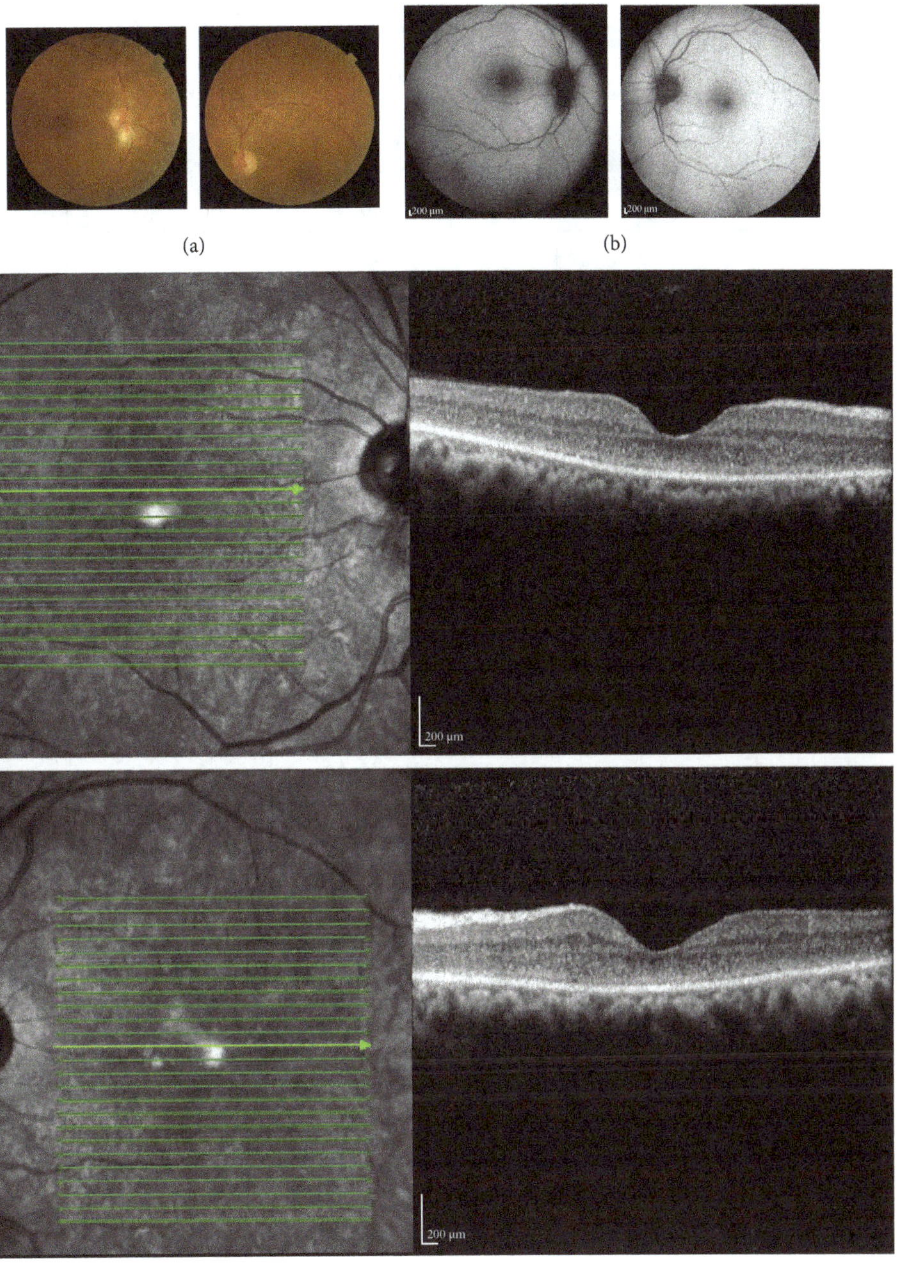

(a) (b)

(c)

Figure 1: Continued.

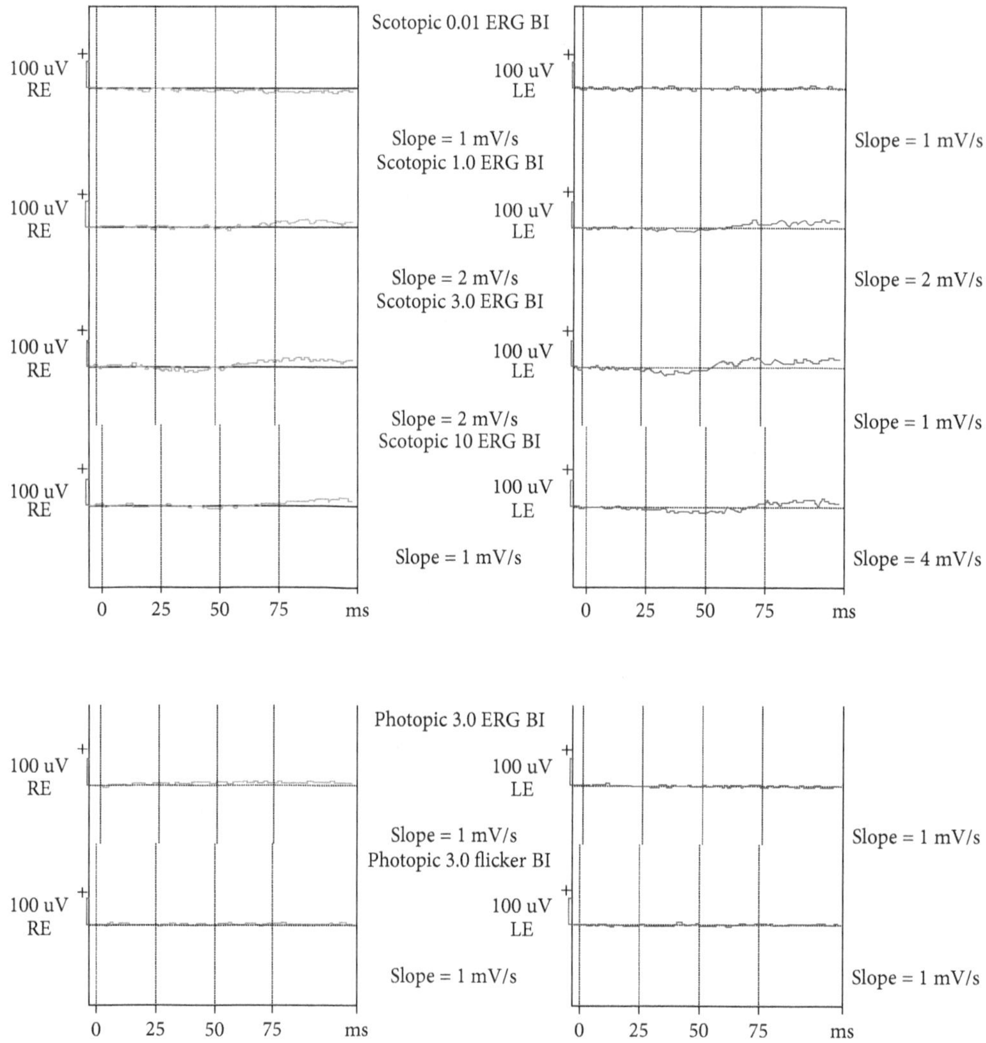

(d)

Figure 1: (a) The fundus photograph of both eyes shows a small area of myelinated axons on the inferior margin of the right optic nerve head and very mild peripapillary whitening and nerve fiber layer swelling more prominent in the right eye. (b) Fundus autofluorescence images show a hypoautofluorescent area corresponding to the small area of myelinated axons on the inferior margin of the right optic nerve head and the normal appearance of the left eye. (c) Macular optical coherence tomography (OCT) revealed diffuse outer nuclear layer hyperreflectivity and indistinguishable external limiting membrane and ellipsoid. (d) Electroretinography displayed severely attenuated responses in both eyes.

erythropoietin 10000 IU twice a day and reevaluation of the patient proved no change in his visual acuity on the third day of admission.

2. Discussion

Closantel is an old veterinary antihelmetic drug used broadly for the treatment of Fasciola and Haemonchus infestation [2]. It is a halogenated salicylanilide that acts on the energy metabolism pathway by blocking oxidative phosphorylation [3]. There are several reports of the toxic effect of closantel on the central nervous system, optic nerve, and retinal tissues in animals [3–5]. However, reports in humans are limited and mainly was associated with visual manifestations. Therefore, closantel is contraindicated in humans and should be used with caution in milk-producing animals. It has been claimed that a low dose of closantel is safe in humans [6], but our case clarified that it could be devastating in doses as low as 1000 mg.

Previous studies on the animal brain and ocular tissues explained pathologic changes. Gill et al. showed severe edema in the myelinated intracranial optic nerve and optic tract and small scattered foci of myelinic edema in the brain stem and cerebellar peduncles of goats and sheep. They observed retrograde axonal degeneration because of myelinic edema and its compressive effect at the intracanalicular portion of the optic nerve [5]. Studies on retinal tissues demonstrated acute and severe outer retinal cells, particularly photoreceptor necrosis [2].

In 1993, ‘t Hoen and Hodgkin published a series of blindness in 11 women following mistaken treatment for gynecological problems [7]. Badran et al. reported 3 cases of severe visual impairment following accidental closantel ingestion

[8]. There is another paper from Morocco about blindness in a 5-year-old girl after 8 days of closantel ingestion with partial visual recovery that occurred after medical treatment by vitamin K, vitamin B12, and glucocorticoid [9]. Koziolek et al. reported a case of visual loss after 3 days of closantel intake. They performed plasma exchange 4 days after the last dose, and the patient experienced significant visual recovery [1]. Previous studies in animals showed that closantel reaches its peak plasma level after 8-48 hours of oral administration and its half-life in plasma was 2-3 weeks. As closantel has a high serum protein binding capacity and low metabolism rate, plasma exchange in the early phase after ingestion can effectively remove it from circulation [1, 10]. Tabatabaei et al. treated a case of blindness due to closantel toxicity with intravenous steroid and erythropoietin which did not affect visual prognosis [11]. Recently, Khalili and Zareei reported a complete recovery of vision and electroretinography parameters of a patient with retinal closantel toxicity by single intravenous injection of methylprednisolone acetate 250 mg. Unlike our patient, their case was referred early and steroid therapy commenced on the 5th day after intoxication [12]. Since there was 2 weeks of delay in referral and diagnosis of our patients, toxicology specialists refuse to do plasma exchange. Administration of high doses of intravenous methylprednisolone and erythropoietin was also ineffective, so we consider these medical management options futile in closantel toxicity.

In our patient, OCT revealed diffuse outer nuclear layer hyperreflectivity and indistinguishable external limiting membrane and ellipsoid zone. Tabatabaei et al. reported very similar findings of OCT in a closantel toxicity case [11]. OCT image is an inexpensive, widely available, and easy to interpret modality. We believe OCT could be a key diagnostic imaging for early detection of closantel toxicity. Additionally, ERG showed severely reduced and flat responses in both photopic and scotopic conditions, which indicates severe photoreceptor loss.

Para- and periventricular bright spots on brain MRI in our patient might be due to the toxic effect of closantel on central neural tissues of the visual pathway. Visual evoked responses could show reduced response in this situation, but because severe retinal impairment would affect VER, we did not accomplish this modality. A mild increase in serum liver enzymes has also been reported after higher doses of closantel, but this was observed in our case with far lower doses of the drug.

In a recent study, Asoklis et al. assessed late ocular changes in 5 patients with inadvertent use of at least three tablets of 500 mg closantel. Visual acuity changes were partly reversible, but visual-field defects deteriorated with time, and changes in the fundus, like retinal thinning, were seen. They concluded that closantel has a long-term detrimental impact on the retina, with no discernible recovery after 22 years [13].

3. Conclusion

Closantel is a veterinary drug with serious side effects in the human retina and central nervous system even in previously reported doses. Public awareness and appropriate drug labeling about its side effects could prevent accidental toxicity. OCT is a noninvasive and rapid diagnostic modality that should be done in suspected toxic retinopathy. Since early treatment by plasma exchange could remove the drug from circulation and lessen its damages, timely diagnosis is very mandatory.

References

[1] M. J. Koziolek, D. Patschan, H. Desel, M. Wallbach, and J. Callizo, "Closantel poisoning treated with plasma exchange," *JAMA Ophthalmol.*, vol. 133, no. 6, pp. 718–720, 2015.

[2] J. A. Bacon, R. G. Ulrich, J. P. Davis et al., "Comparative in vitro effects of closantel and selected beta-ketoamide anthelmintics on a gastrointestinal nematode and vertebrate liver cells," *Journal of Veterinary Pharmacology and Therapeutics*, vol. 21, no. 3, pp. 190–198, 1998.

[3] J. J. van der Lugt and I. Venter, "Myelin vacuolation, optic neuropathy and retinal degeneration after closantel overdosage in sheep and in a goat," *Journal of Comparative Pathology*, vol. 136, no. 2-3, pp. 87–95, 2007.

[4] A. S. Borges, L. C. Mendes, A. L. de Andrade, G. F. Machado, and J. R. Peiro, "Optic neuropathy in sheep associated with overdosage of closantel," *Veterinary and Human Toxicology*, vol. 41, no. 6, pp. 378–380, 1999.

[5] P. A. Gill, R. W. Cook, J. G. Boulton, W. R. Kelly, B. Vanselow, and L. A. Reddacliff, "Optic neuropathy and retinopathy in closantel toxicosis of sheep and goats," *Australian Veterinary Journal*, vol. 77, no. 4, pp. 259–261, 1999.

[6] Organization WH and on Food Additives JFEC, Food, of the United Nations AO, *Evaluation of Certain Veterinary Drug Residues in Food: Eighty-Fifth Report of the Joint FAO/WHO Expert Committee on Food Additives*, World Health Organization, 2018.

[7] E. T. Hoen, C. Hodgkin, and D. Milkevicius, "Harmful human use of donated veterinary drug," *Lancet*, vol. 342, no. 8866, pp. 308-309, 1993.

[8] N. Badrane, A. Abbada, H. Chaoui et al., "XXXIII International Congress of the European Association of Poisons Centres and Clinical Toxicologists (EAPCCT) 28–31 May 2013, Copenhagen, Denmark," *Clinical Toxicology*, vol. 51, no. 4, pp. 252–378, 2013.

[9] L. Essabar, T. Meskini, S. Ettair, N. Erreimi, and N. Mouane, "Harmful use of veterinary drugs: blindness following closantel poisoning in a 5-year-old girl," *Asia Pacific Journal of Medical Toxicology*, vol. 3, no. 4, pp. 173–175, 2014.

[10] M. Michiels, W. Meuldermans, and J. Heykants, "The metabolism and fate of closantel (Flukiver) in sheep and cattle," *Drug Metabolism Reviews*, vol. 18, no. 2-3, pp. 235–251, 1987.

[11] S. A. Tabatabaei, M. Soleimani, M. R. Mansouri et al., "Closantel; a veterinary drug with potential severe morbidity in humans," *BMC Ophthalmology*, vol. 16, no. 1, p. 207, 2016.

[12] M. R. Khalili and A. Zareei, "Case report: restored vision after ocular closantel intoxication and blindness," *BMC Ophthalmology*, vol. 21, no. 1, p. 158, 2021.

[13] R. Asoklis, A. Cimbalas, A. Augyte, E. Jasinskiene, and R. Strupaite, "Late ocular changes after closantel poisoning in five women," *Eye (London, England)*, vol. 32, no. 12, pp. 1800–1802, 2018.

11

Conjunctival Pigmentation at the Sclerotomy Site following 23 G Vitrectomy with Silicone Oil Injection

Nazimul Hussain[1,2]

[1]*Department of Ophthalmology, Mediclinic Parkview Hospital, Dubai, UAE*
[2]*Department of Ophthalmology, Al Zahra Hospital, Sharjah, UAE*

Correspondence should be addressed to Nazimul Hussain; nazimul.hussain@gmail.com

Academic Editor: Stephen G. Schwartz

54-year-old gentleman undergoing 23 Gauge vitrectomy with silicone oil injection developing conjunctival pigmentation at one of the entry sites of trocar and cannula 1 week postoperative. The conjunctival tissue was biopsied at the time of silicone oil removal and correlated histopathological. Biopsy of the conjunctival tissue showed intracellular and stromal melanin pigments. This report highlights conjunctival pigmentation in suture less entry site and silicone oil as intraocular tamponade than earlier published reports of with or without intraocular gas tamponade.

1. Introduction

Conjunctival pigmentation can occur following traumatic scleral tear repair or following microincisional vitreous surgery [1–3]. Such pigmentations can also be congenital or acquired following melanoma, drug induced, or other systemic illnesses [4–7].

We present a case of conspicuous conjunctival pigmentation following 23 G suture vitrectomy with silicone oil injection in one of the entry sites.

2. Case Report

A 54-year-old gentleman presented to the retina clinic with complaints of sudden diminution of vision in the left eye noticed in the past 1 week. There is no significant past ocular or systemic history of illness. On examination, his distant visual acuity was uncorrected 6/6 in the right eye and counting fingers 2 meters in the left eye. Best corrected near vision was N6 in the right eye and < N36 in the left eye. Intraocular pressure was 14 mm Hg in the right eye and 11 mm Hg in the left eye. Anterior segment examination was unremarkable including the conjunctiva in both eyes except the lens showed early cortical changes in both eyes. Dilated fundus examination showed clear ocular media with attached retina and multiple lattice degeneration in the peripheral retina in the right eye. Left eye showed clear ocular media, temporal hemiretina detachment involving the macula, and peripheral lattice degeneration with retinal holes (Figure 1). Based on clinical examination, he was diagnosed as lattice degeneration in the right eye and rhegmatogenous retinal detachment in the left eye.

After informed consent and discussion, he underwent barrage laser photocoagulation around the lattice degeneration in the right eye and 23 G vitrectomy, silicone oil injection, and endolaser in the left eye uneventfully. On the first postoperative day, anterior segment examination showed flat lids, mild congested conjunctiva, clear cornea, deep and quiet anterior chamber, mild dilated pupil, and cortical cataract changes in the left eye. Intraocular pressure was 15 mm Hg in the left eye. Fundus examination of the left eye showed clear media, attached retina, fresh laser marks in the periphery, and silicone oil in the vitreous cavity. An impression of stable status and reattached retina was made. On 1-week postoperative follow up, his retina status was stable, but anterior segment examination showed conjunctival pigmentation in the superotemporal quadrant at the site of trocar cannula entry. 3 months postoperative, his best

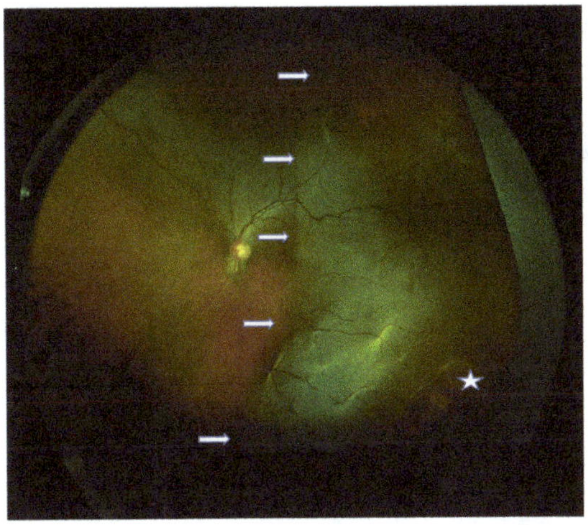

FIGURE 1: Wide-field fundus photo of left eye showing the temporal retinal detachment involving partially the macula (arrow) and lattice degeneration with retinal hole (Asterisk).

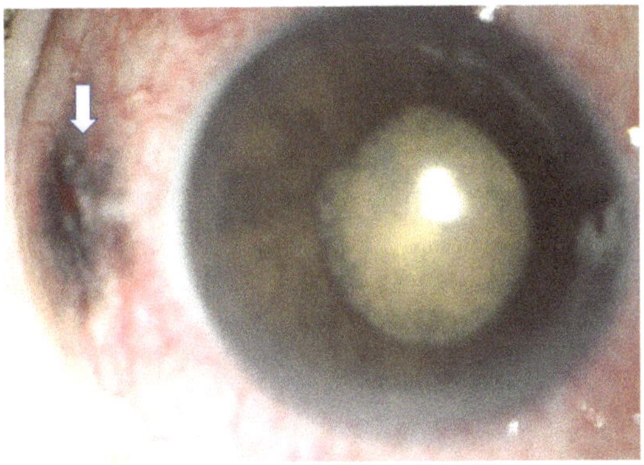

FIGURE 2: Showing conjunctival bluish black pigmentation of the conjunctiva (Arrow) in the superotemporal quadrant in the left eye.

corrected visual acuity was 6/18 in the left eye. Anterior segment examination in left eye showed conjunctival pigmentation in the superotemporal quadrant (Figure 2) and quiet conjunctiva, clear cornea, deep and quiet anterior chamber, and round and reacting pupil; lens showed early posterior subcapsular cataract with cortical cataract, and intraocular pressure was 16 mm Hg. Fundus examination showed mild hazy media, silicone oil in the vitreous cavity, attached retina, and peripheral laser scars in the left eye. An impression of secondary postsurgical conjunctival pigmentation, cataract, and reattached retina with silicone oil in the left eye was made. He then underwent conjunctival biopsy and silicone oil removal in the left eye.

Intraoperatively, the area of conjunctival pigmentation demonstrated extensive scarring with entrapped minute silicone oil bubbles within the subconjunctival scar. Dispersed light pigmentation was also seen on the scleral surface (Figures 3(a)–3(d)). The dissected conjunctival tissue was sent for Histopathological examination. Gross examination showed a wedge of conjunctival tissue measuring 0.3 cm. Microscopic examination showed intracellular and stromal infiltration of dark pigments seen in the stroma and intracellular (Figure 4). The Masson-Fontana special stain was positive for melanin pigments (Figure 5).

3 months post silicone oil removal, the patient underwent phacoemulsification with intraocular lens implantation in the left eye, and his visual acuity achieved 6/9, N6 in the left eye.

Informed consent and using patient data for research purposes was taken, and institutional review board permission was taken for research and publication of the case.

3. Discussion

Acquired conjunctival melanosis is seen secondary to many conditions including drug-induced, trauma or systemic disorders [3]. Smiddy et al. [3] have narrated a 34-year-old gentleman undergoing pars plana vitrectomy with fluid gas exchange for retinal detachment developing conjunctival pigmentation in the inferotemporal quadrant 6 weeks later. The pupil colour was brown, and he was Caucasian male. The surgery was performed with 20G instruments, and conjunctival pigmentation was attributed to cryotherapy applied before vitrectomy. They proposed that this could be due to reactivation of preexisting quiescent melanocytes, and the pigment distribution appears exogenous. They concluded that the source of melanin is probably from ruptured uveal and RPE cells treated by cryotherapy prior to vitrectomy.

Park et al. [2] have shown in their series of patients who underwent 23 G microincision vitreous surgery (MIVS) with fluid gas exchange and endolaser developing conjunctival pigmentation at the entry sites in 4.3% (8/185 patients) of patients. Interestingly, Park et al. have closed the entry sites at the end of surgery with a single releasable 8-0 polyamide suture. All patients showed conjunctival pigmentation within 7 days of surgery. Conjunctival pigmentation was observed in inferotemporal and superotemporal as well as superonasal entry sites. It was also observed that in eyes which had C3F8 tamponade, the surface area of pigmentation was larger than those eyes which did not have tamponade. The etiology of the cases was mostly proliferative diabetic retinopathy and one eye with rhegmatogenous retinal detachment. Multivariate logistic regression analysis confirmed that C3F8 tamponade (OR 9.4; 95% CI, 1.9-44.5; $P = 0.005$) was associated with conjunctival pigmentation after 23G MIVS in the study. However, performing complete vitrectomy as a responsible factor cannot be ruled out. It may increase the possibility of pigment exterior pigment fall out.

Our case showed conjunctival pigmentation in the superotemporal quadrant near to the entry site at 1 week. A 23G MIVS trocar cannula was used, and no sutures were applied at the end of the procedure. Histopathology and special stain for melanin have shown that the melanin pigments were both in the stroma and intracellular suggesting non-preexisting pigments. Besides, as shown in Figure 3, minute silicone oil bubbles enmeshed in the subconjunctival scar along with pigmentation suggest its origin from the uveal tissue at the entry site. However, silicone oil infiltration was not seen in the biopsied conjunctival tissue. Possible slow gradual leakage of in the

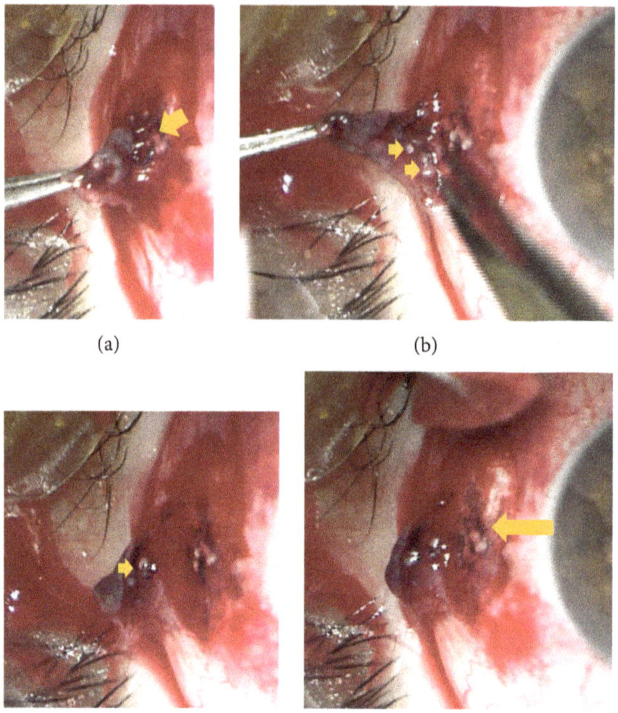

(a) (b)

(c) (d)

FIGURE 3: (a) Showing subconjunctival scarring (arrow), (b, c) subconjunctival silicone oil bubbles, and (d) dispersed pigmentation on the scleral surface .

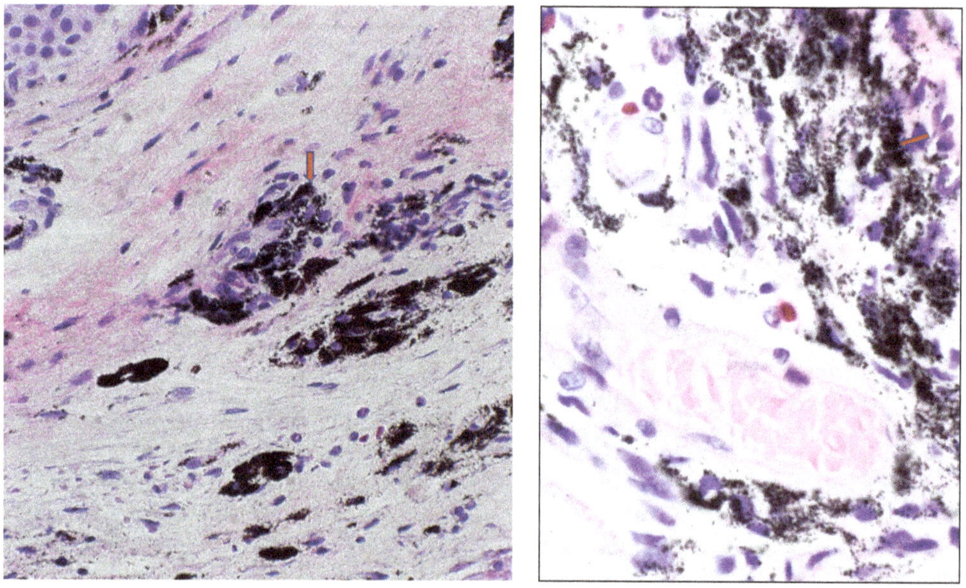

(a) (b)

FIGURE 4: (a) Showing light microscopy and (b) higher magnification with intracellular pigments and stromal pigments (arrow).

initial time of healing of the wound has resulted in silicone oil bubbles and visibility of conjunctival pigmentation at 1 week.

Several studies [8–11] have shown that the migration of silicone oil bubbles in the subconjunctival tissue initiates chronic inflammatory process evident by presence of histiocytes and multinucleated lymphocytes. This suggests granulomatous inflammatory reaction to silicone oil. This chronic inflammatory process causes scar, and subconjunctival trapped silicone oil droplets. In our case, silicone oil droplets were seen in the subconjunctival tissue entrapped in the scar tissue.

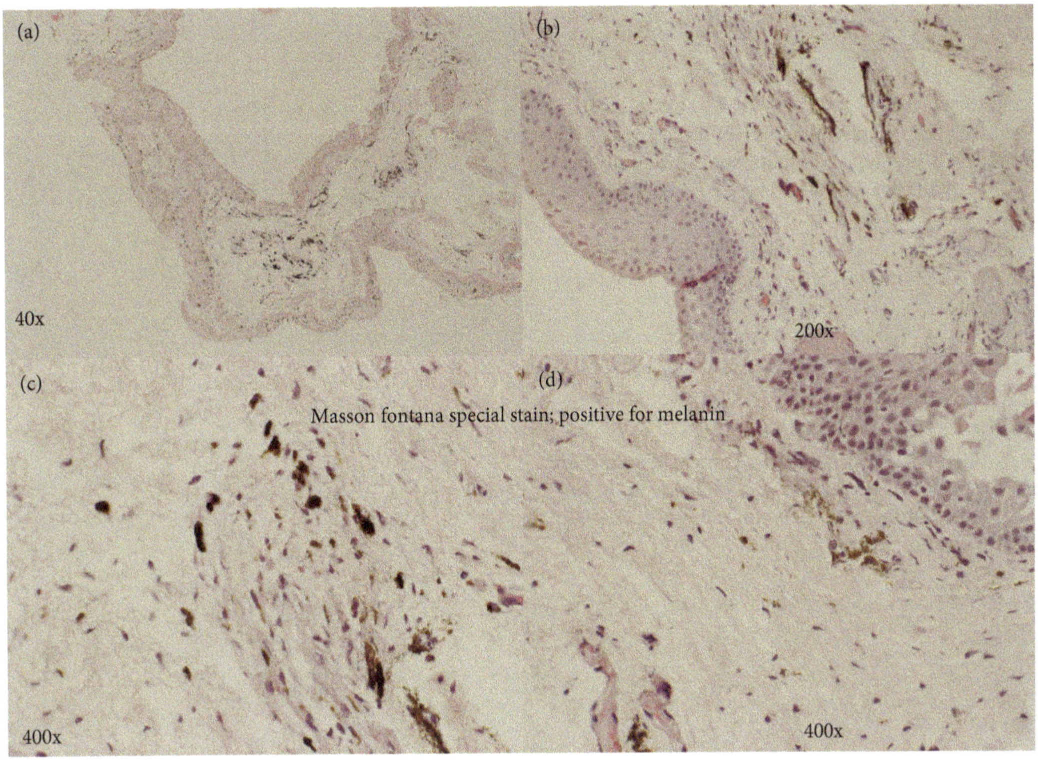

Figure 5: The Masson-Fontana special stain showing positive for melanin pigments.

Uveal pigment migration mostly happens in the initial period of minimal leakage along with silicone oil migration from entry site as evident in intracellular and intrastromal melanin pigments on histology. Chronic inflammation causes the subconjunctival scarring and heals the leaking entry site.

The highlight of the present case in contrast to the published reports is the use of silicone oil tamponade and not suturing the entry sites in 23G MIVS. The patient has brown eyes and middle eastern ethnicity.

In conclusion, the present case suggests that postoperative acquired conjunctival melanosis can occur in a patient undergoing 23G MIVS, and the possible use of sutures at the entry site can reduce the incidence lower than 4.3% as published earlier. Use of finer gauge MIVS like 27G can reduce such occurrence, but checking for leakage at the entry site seems mandatory especially in brown eyes.

Consent

Consent from patient to use for research is obtained at the time consulting the patient as information will be used for clinical study or research with confidentiality maintained.

Authors' Contributions

NH prepared, conceptualize, and reviewed the manuscript.

Acknowledgments

I am thankful to Dr. Hamzeh Tarabichi MD, department of Pathology, Al Zahra Hospital, Sharjah, UAE for histopathology collaboration.

References

[1] M. T. Benson, I. Rennie, and J. Talbot, "External ocular pigmentation secondary to perforating eye injury," *British Journal of Ophthalmology*, vol. 74, no. 4, pp. 251–253, 1990.

[2] D. H. Park, J. P. Shin, and S. Y. Kim, "Conjunctival pigmentation after 23-gauge microincisional vitrectomy surgery," *Eye*, vol. 25, no. 11, pp. 1465–1470, 2011.

[3] W. E. Smiddy, J. H. Yeo, R. G. Michels, and W. R. Green, "Conjunctival pigmentation following pars plana vitrectomy," *Retina*, vol. 7, no. 1, pp. 38–40, 1987.

[4] G. S. Negretti, K. A. Roelofs, B. Damato, M. Sagoo, S. Parvizi, and V. M. L. Cohen, "The natural history of conjunctival naevi in children and adolescents," *Eye*, vol. 35, no. 9, pp. 2579–2584, 2021.

[5] T. T. Khan and U. P. Reddy, "Conjunctival pigmentation following minocycline therapy," *Ophthalmic Plastic & Reconstructive Surgery*, vol. 32, no. 6, pp. e129–e130, 2016.

[6] D. M. Brothers and A. A. Hidayat, "Conjunctival pigmentation associated with tetracycline medication," *Ophthalmology*, vol. 88, no. 12, pp. 1212–1215, 1981.

[7] G. Feuntes-Paez, M. C. Mendez, J. Montanez, J. M. Herreras, M. A. Saornil, and M. Calonge, "Conjunctival pigmentation

in Stevens Johnson syndrome," *Comprehensive Therapy*, vol. 33, no. 2, pp. 99–103, 2007.

[8] A. Algethami, S. A. Schellini, S. M. Elkhamary, M. A. Talea, and V. A. Semidey, "Orbital and periorbital migration of silicone oil associated with emphysema development after retinal detachment repair - Case report and literature review," *American journal of ophthalmology case reports*, vol. 25, article 101376, 2022.

[9] M. Corbett and S. Wood, "OP-9 Subconjunctival silicone oil - presentation, histology and surgical management," *BMJ open ophthalmology*, vol. 7, Supplement 1, 2022.

[10] C. P. Azarcon, H. E. Grossniklaus, and J. R. Wells, "Foreign body giant cell reaction to silicone oil presenting as a salmon-patch conjunctival lesion," *American Journal of Ophthalmology Case Reports*, vol. 27, article 101676, 2022.

[11] J. Biswas, P. S. Bhende, L. Gopal, S. Parikh, and S. S. Badrinath, "Subconjunctival cysts following silicone oil injection: a clinicopathological study of five cases," *Indian Journal of Ophthalmology*, vol. 47, no. 3, pp. 177–180, 1999.

12

Optical Coherence Tomography Angiography Evolution of Choroidal Neovascular Membrane in Choroidal Rupture Managed by Intravitreal Bevacizumab

Massimo Lorusso,[1] Luisa Micelli Ferrari,[2]
Eleni Nikolopoulou,[1] and Tommaso Micelli Ferrari[1]

[1]Department of Ophthalmology, Ente Ecclesiastico "F. Miulli" Hospital, Acquaviva delle Fonti, Bari, Italy
[2]Department of Ophthalmology, "G. Moscati" Hospital, Taranto, Italy

Correspondence should be addressed to Eleni Nikolopoulou; elenigisotti@gmail.com

Academic Editor: Winfried M. Amoaku

Purpose. To describe a case of a 25-year-old man with choroidal neovascularization (CNV) secondary to traumatic choroidal rupture treated with intravitreal bevacizumab and to evaluate the vascular structure of the area near the traumatic choroidal rupture. *Methods.* The patient underwent complete ophthalmologic evaluation, including best-corrected visual acuity (BCVA), intraocular pressure, anterior segment and funds examination, and optical coherence tomography angiography (OCTA) at baseline and on each follow-up visit. Fluorescein angiography (FA) was performed at baseline. Intravitreal bevacizumab was administered at the time of choroidal neovascular membrane diagnosis. *Results.* At baseline, ophthalmoscopic examination of the left eye revealed four subretinal macular hemorrhages and two choroidal ruptures located temporally to the fovea. On OCT angiograms, the choroidal rupture appeared as a hypointense break in choriocapillaris plexus. At 4-week follow-up, the OCTA disclosed a well circumscribed lesion characterized by numerous and fine anastomotic vessels. Patient received intravitreal injection of bevacizumab. At 6-week post injection, OCTA documented regression of the neovascular complex. *Conclusion.* Choroidal neovascularization is a common complication associated with traumatic choroidal rupture and OCTA may represent a complementary diagnostic technique to evaluate the vascular structure of the area near the traumatic choroidal rupture.

1. Introduction

Choroidal rupture is a break in the choroid, Bruch membrane, retinal pigment epithelium (RPE) that results from blunt ocular trauma. In most cases choroidal ruptures are secondary to indirect trauma, non-penetrating closed-globe blunt trauma [1]. After blunt trauma, the ocular globe undergoes mechanical compression and then sudden hyperextension. The sclera and the retina can resist this insult because of their elasticity but Bruch's membrane breaks because it does not have enough tensile strength. Small capillaries in the choriocapillaris and deep choroidal vessels are damaged leading to sub-RPE hemorrhages.

Choroidal neovascularization (CNV) is a common complication associated with traumatic choroidal rupture [2]. Bevacizumab, a humanized monoclonal antibody to vascular endothelial growth factor, has been given as an intravitreal injection to treat choroidal neovascularization (CNV) secondary to CR [3]. We used a non-invasive imaging modality, optical coherence tomography angiography (OCTA), to detect and follow the progression of the CNV in a patient with traumatic choroidal rupture.

2. Case Report

A healthy 25-year-old man presented with recent visual acuity reduction in the left eye (LE) after a blunt ocular trauma he received the day before. Complete ophthalmologic evaluation showed best-corrected visual acuity (BCVA) of 20/20 in the RE and of 20/25 in the LE. Slit-lamp biomicroscopy examination of the anterior segment of the LE showed conjunctival hyperemia and normal pupillary reflex to light. The anterior

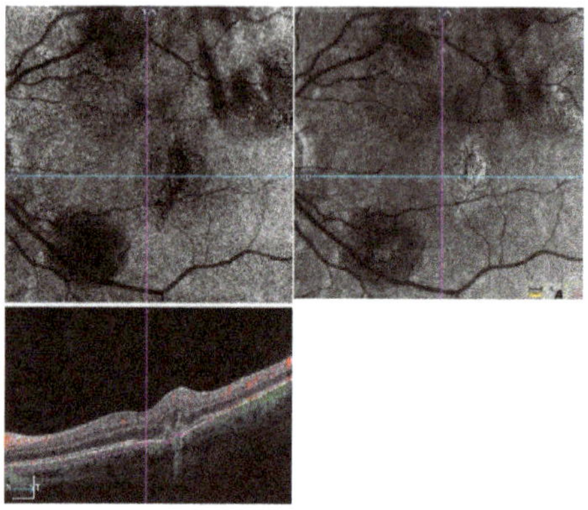

FIGURE 1: **Baseline examination of choroidal rupture.** OCTA shows a hyporeflective line corresponding to retinal pigment epithelium (RPE)-choriocapillaris defects near to the foveal area. B-scan reveals a disruption of the RPE-Bruch membrane and a hyperreflective intraretinal area associated with backscattering effect was also present.

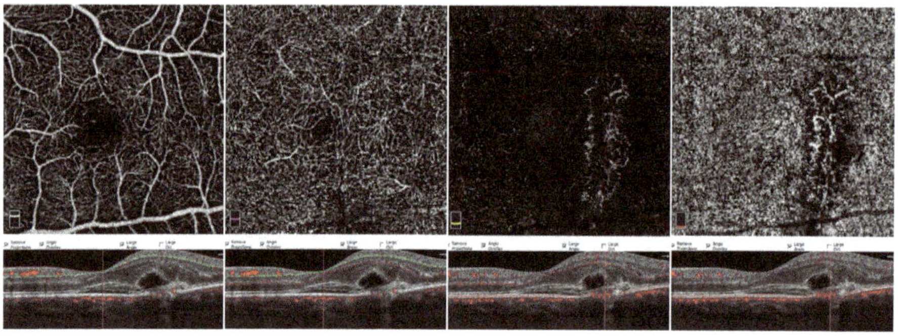

FIGURE 2: **Optical coherence tomography angiography (OCTA): enface angiograms at 4-week visit.** Angiograms of outer retina (A) and choriocapillaris (B) demonstrate the presence of a well circumscribed lesion with a clear hyperintense signal and characterized by numerous anastomotic vessels. Neovascular lesion extends along the primary RPE-Bruch membrane defect. OCT B-scan shows subretinal fluid.

segment of the RE was normal. Intraocular pressure was 17 mmHg in both eyes. Ophthalmoscopic examination of the LE revealed commotio retinae in the inferior quadrants, four subretinal macular hemorrhages, and two choroidal ruptures located temporally to the fovea. Fundus examination of the RE was unremarkable. The patient underwent imaging with fluorescein angiography (FA), spectral domain optical coherence tomography (SD-OCT), and optical coherence tomography angiography (OCT-A). On FA, choroidal ruptures (CR) were hyperfluorescent in the mid and late phases due to staining. Hemorrhages appeared as round hypofluorescent areas. SD-OCT scans revealed disruption of the retinal pigment epithelium (RPE)-Bruch membrane (BM) complex associated with back-scattering effect. OCTA allows a depth resolved visualization of retinal and choriocapillaris microvasculature. On OCT angiograms, the choroidal rupture appeared as a hypointense break in choriocapillaris plexus (Figure 1). At 4-week follow-up, FA was repeated and revealed leakage in the perifoveal area in correspondence of the CR. SD-OCT showed an hyperreflective lesion involving the ellipsoid zone (EZ) and outer nuclear layer such as hyporeflective subretinal fluid present next to the choroidal rupture. In the OCT-A enface scan, taken above the retinal pigment epithelium, a well circumscribed lesion with a clear hyperintense signal was observed. Lesion was characterized by numerous and fine anastomotic vessels with a well-shaped peripheral arcade (Figure 2). Superficial and deep retinal vasculature were spared. Diagnosis of choroidal neovascular membrane (CNV) secondary to choroidal rupture was done. After a written consent was signed by the patient, an off-label intravitreal injection of Bevacizumab (1.25 mg/0.05 ml) was administered in his LE. At 6-week post injection, visual acuity has improved to 20/20. OCTA documented the closure of CNV (Figure 3). C-scans of the outer retina and choriocapillaris did not show any hyperintense signal. SD-OCT revealed RPE wound healing process as lesion covered by a less hyperreflective layer of RPE. This layer was less hyperreflective than normal RPE.

3. Discussion

Choroidal ruptures are breaks in the retinal pigment epithelium, Bruch's membrane, and choroid that occur in 5% of blunt ocular trauma [4]. CR may be complicated with haemorrhagic or serous macular detachment, optic disc pallor, and choroidal neovascularization [1]. The formation of CNV must consider the distance of the CR from the fovea and the length of the break [2].

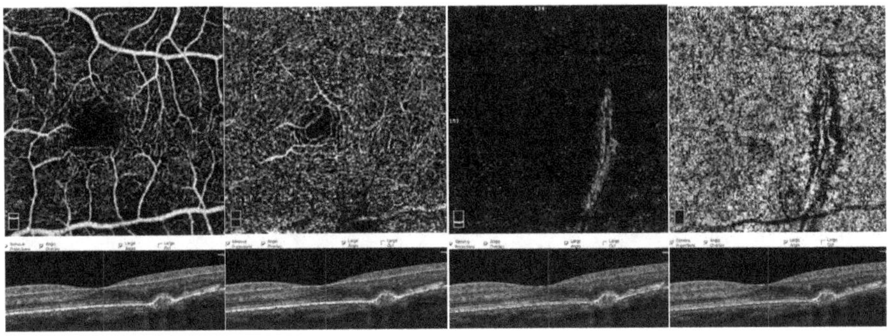

FIGURE 3: **Optical coherence tomography angiography (OCTA): enface angiograms at 6-week visit.** OCTA reveals shrinkage of the choriocapillaris defect; enface scan of outer retina and choriocapillaris show no hyperintense flow signal. OCT B-scan demonstrates partial healing of the RPE wound, covered by a less reflective RPE and a reduction of hyperreflective intraretinal material; no subretinal fluid is evident.

In this report, we used OCT-A, a new imaging tool, to investigate the choroidal and retinal vasculature in a patient with traumatic choroidal rupture. OCT-A is a recent, non-invasive imaging technology, able to visualize the microvasculature without any dye injection [5]. OCT-A shows an in vivo three-dimensional vasculature of the retina and choroid and performs a segmentation in different layers. We used OCT-A initially to evaluate and describe the vascular structure of the area near the traumatic choroidal rupture. Monitoring the patient with OCT-A, we observed the presence of CNV and its regression after anti-VEGF therapy.

Choroidal neovascularization is a well-known complication of traumatic choroidal rupture. Most of the post-traumatic membranes are sub- or juxta-foveal [6]. The more abundant blood supply from the choroidal vasculature and the more intense healing response may be linked to the increased propensity to CNV in the fovea [7]. Many growth factors, including those of the VEGF family, are involved in wound healing process. A local higher level of elastin-derived peptides released from the rupture of Bruch membrane could induce VEGF upregulation [8]. Anti-VEGF therapy is recognized as gold standard treatment of post-traumatic CNV [9].

In clinical practice, OCT-A represents a new non-invasive method that provides important information about vascular flow in macular area and represents an early diagnostic tool for CNV detection that can also be used to follow its progression over time.

To our knowledge, for the first time, we used OCT angiography to early detect and follow the evolution of CNV, one of the common complications of choroidal rupture. OCT-A is a fast, non-invasive imaging tool that can be used for an early diagnosis of disease. This imaging technology might provide relevant information about microvascular response to anti-VEGF therapy and wound healing process without use of exogenous dye. Further studies are needed to establish the value of OCT-A in early diagnosis of CNV in blunt ocular trauma with choroidal rupture and to assess the role in the follow-up of the lesion.

Additional Points

Summary. The authors report a case of a 25-year-old man with choroidal neovascularization (CNV) secondary to traumatic choroidal rupture. OCT angiography was used to evaluate the vascular structure of the area near the traumatic choroidal rupture at baseline visit and during follow-up.

References

[1] L. C. Glazer, D. P. Han, and M. S. Gottlieb, "Choroidal rupture and optic atrophy," *British Journal of Ophthalmology*, vol. 77, no. 1, pp. 33–35, 1993.

[2] M. Secrétan, M. Sickenberg, L. Zografos, and B. Piguet, "Morphometric characteristics of traumatic choroidal ruptures associated with neovascularization," *Retina*, vol. 18, no. 1, pp. 62–66, 1998.

[3] B. Chanana, R. V. Azad, and N. Kumar, "Intravitreal bevacizumab for subfoveal choroidal neovascularization secondary to traumatic choroidal rupture," *Eye*, vol. 23, no. 11, pp. 2125-2126, 2009.

[4] C. M. Wood and J. Richardson, "Chorioretinal neovascular membranes complicating contusional eye injuries with indirect choroidal ruptures," *British Journal of Ophthalmology*, vol. 74, no. 2, pp. 93–96, 1990.

[5] Y. Huang, Q. Zhang, M. R. Thorell et al., "Swept-source OCT angiography of the retinal vasculature using intensity differentiation-based optical microangiography algorithms," *Ophthalmic Surgery, Lasers and Imaging Retina*, vol. 45, no. 5, pp. 382–389, 2014.

[6] J. Y. Shin, B. Chung, Y. H. Na, J. Lee, H. Chung, and S. H. Byeon, "Retinal pigment epithelium wound healing after traumatic choroidal rupture," *Acta Ophthalmologica*, vol. 95, no. 7, pp. e582–e586, 2017.

[7] S. A. Mousa, W. Lorelli, and P. A. Campochiaro, "Role of hypoxia and extracellular matrix-integrin binding in the modulation of angiogenic growth factors secretion by retinal pigmented epithelial cells," *Journal of Cellular Biochemistry*, vol. 74, no. 1, pp. 135–143, 1999.

[8] H. Wang, Y. Ninomiya, I. K. Sugino, and M. A. Zarbin, "Retinal pigment epithelium wound healing in human Bruch's mem-

brane explants," *Investigative Ophthalmology & Visual Science*, vol. 44, no. 5, pp. 2199–2210, 2003.

[9] U. De Benedetto, M. Battaglia Parodi, K. A. Knutsson et al., "Intravitreal bevacizumab for extrafoveal choroidal neovascularization after ocular trauma," *Journal of Ocular Pharmacology and Therapeutics*, vol. 28, no. 5, pp. 550–552, 2012.

13

Acquired Immunodeficiency Syndrome Presented as Atypical Ocular Toxoplasmosis

Elias Khalili Pour,[1] Hamid Riazi-Esfahani,[1] Nazanin Ebrahimiadib,[1] Violet Zaker Esteghamati,[2] and Mohammad Zarei[1]

[1]*Eye Research Center, Farabi Eye Hospital, Tehran University of Medical Sciences, Tehran, Iran*
[2]*Imam Khomeini General Hospital, School of Medicine, Tehran University of Medical Sciences, Tehran, Iran*

Correspondence should be addressed to Mohammad Zarei; mzareiran81@gmail.com

Academic Editor: Kamal Kishore

Background. The aim is to report an atypical presentation of ocular toxoplasmosis which led to the diagnosis of Acquired Immunodeficiency Syndrome (AIDS). *Case Report.* The 38-year-old woman was referred with metamorphopsia and reduced vision in the right eye over the past 3 weeks. Slit-lamp examination revealed granulomatous keratic precipitates (KPs), 2+ cells in the anterior chamber, and posterior synechiae. Fundus examination was remarkable for a white patch surrounding a scar, inferonasal to the optic disc with fibrous bands emanating from the lesion, and the retina around this region was detached with considerable extension towards the periphery, while no breaks could be appreciated. She mentioned anorexia and losing 10 kg in the past three months, and signs of anemia like paleness of face skin, bed nails, and bilateral angular cheilitis were observed on systemic evaluation. The results of the patient's complete blood count revealed anemia and leukopenia and CD4 lymphocytes: 79 cells/μL. Enzyme-linked immunosorbent assays (ELISA) for HIV antibodies came back positive which was later confirmed with the Western blot test. Brain magnetic resonance imaging (MRI) showed multiple ring-enhancing lesions in both cerebral cortices. The patient underwent antitoxoplasmosis and anti-HIV treatment and serous retinal detachment completely resolved. *Conclusion.* This report highlights the fact that sometimes, the eyes are the site of the first presentation of a systemic life-threatening condition and emphasizes the role of ophthalmologists in such cases. In cases of atypical presentation, appropriate laboratory tests and CNS imaging should be requested. Systemic treatment with antitoxoplasmosis regimens and highly active antiretroviral therapy (HAART) is mandatory in AIDS patients with ocular toxoplasmosis.

1. Background

Since the 1950s, ocular toxoplasmosis has been reported as the most common cause of infectious uveitis worldwide. *Toxoplasma gondii* is a ubiquitous obligate intracellular microorganism, which is estimated to affect one-third of the world's population [1–3].

Active ocular toxoplasmosis is characterized by a necrotizing retinochoroiditis lesions accompanied by localized or diffuse vitritis. In immunocompetent patients, lesions are usually self-limited and resolve within two months. Atypical forms of ocular toxoplasmosis such as diffuse outer retinitis, which can mimic acute retinal necrosis (ARN), punctuate outer retinal toxoplasmosis, occlusive retinal vasculitis, neuroretinitis, scleritis, and exudative retinal detachment, have been reported [4]. Atypical lesions may occur bilaterally and have been reported in the immunocompromised, neonates, and elderly patients [5].

This parasite can be fatal in immunocompromised individuals, such as HIV/AIDS patients especially those with CD4 T lymphocyte cell counts less than 200 cells/μL. In such a setting, reactivation of opportunistic organisms like *Toxoplasma gondii* can occur with multiorgan involvement, especially central nervous system (CNS), and with much lower incidence, ocular involvement [5–7].

The central nervous system, as the most common site of Toxoplasma reactivation, can be involved in about 30% of patients with AIDS, especially in those who are

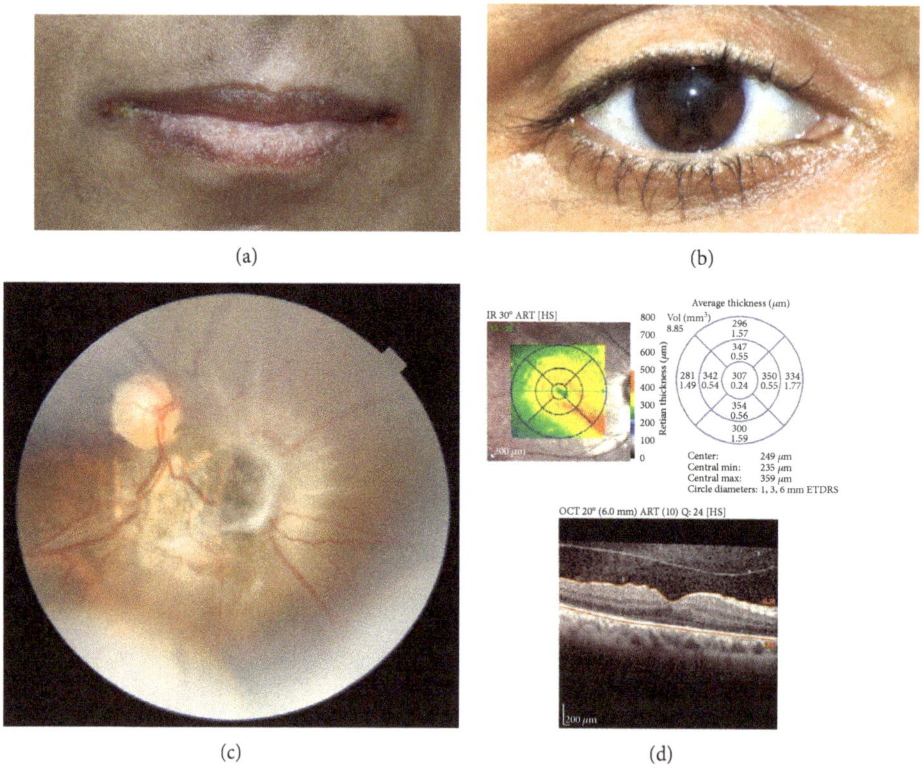

FIGURE 1: Clinical features of the patient at the time of presentation. Bilateral angular cheilitis (a), posterior synechiae, and keyhole-shaped pupil (b), In the right eye inferonasal to the optic disc, an annular white patch centered with a pigmented scar is seen. White subretinal bands are extending from the lesion. The size of the lesion is about three-disc diameter, and the adjacent retina is detached (c). Macular optical coherence tomography of the right eye demonstrates evidence of vitritis, detached posterior hyaloid, and a fine epiretinal membrane nasal to the fovea (d).

treatment-naive and Toxoplasma seropositive with CD4 < 100 cells/μL [8–11].

Here, we report an atypical presentation of ocular toxoplasmosis with a serous retinal detachment which led to the diagnosis of AIDS. The serous retinal detachment resolved with antitoxoplasmosis treatments and HAART.

2. Case Report

The 38-year-old woman was referred to the retina department of Farabi Eye Hospital with metamorphopsia and reduced vision in the right eye over the past 3 weeks. At the time of the presentation, she mentioned anorexia and losing 10 kg in the past three months, and signs of anemia like paleness of face skin, bed nails, and bilateral angular cheilitis were observed (Figure 1(a)). Uncorrected visual acuity in the right eye was counting fingers at two meters. Posterior synechia (PS) and pigment deposit over the anterior crystalline lens capsule precluded precise refraction in this eye. Slit-lamp examination revealed granulomatous keratic precipitates (KPs) distributed in Arlt's triangle, 2+ cells in the anterior chamber, and a relatively broad-based PS causing a keyhole appearance in the pupil (Figure 1(b)). The crystalline lens was clear and 2+ cells were present in the anterior vitreous. Fundus examination was remarkable for a white patch surrounding a scar, inferonasal to the optic disc with three-disc diameter size. Some fibrous bands were emanating from the lesion, and the retina around this region was detached with considerable extension towards the superior, nasal, and inferior periphery, while no breaks could be appreciated (Figure 1(c)). The vision in the left eye was 20/20, and ophthalmic examination was unremarkable in this eye.

Spectral-domain optical coherence tomography (SD-OCT) (Spectralis Heidelburg Germany) disclosed evidence of vitritis, a detached posterior hyaloid face, and a fine epiretinal membrane (ERM) nasal to the fovea in the right eye (Figure 1(d)).

She denied using any medications or having other illnesses. Considering systemic symptoms and signs and due to involuntary weight loss, the patient underwent a comprehensive infectious, neoplastic, and rheumatologic workup. The results of the patient's complete blood count (CBC) are summarized in Table 1. Based on the ocular findings, additional tests were ordered for *Toxoplasma gondii* antibodies which revealed the presence of IgG antibodies (18 IU/mL; reference range: positive ≥ 12 IU/mL, suspicious 10-11 9 IU/mL, negative ≤ 9 IU/mL) while IgMs were absent (0.1 IU/mL; reference range: positive ≥ 0.65 IU/mL, suspicious 0.55-0.64 IU/mL, negative ≤ 0.55 IU/mL).

Imaging studies including chest-X-ray, abdominal sonography, and age-related neoplastic workup including mammography, Pap smear, and colonoscopy were unremarkable except for nonspecific polyps in the patient's large intestine.

Table 1: The results of the patient's CBC-diff.

Blood component		Reference range
White blood cells	3400	4500-11,000/mm^3
Red blood cells	4.19	Male: 4.3-5.9 million/mm^3 Female: 3.5-5.5 million/mm^3
Hemoglobin	8.1	Male: 13.5-17.5 g/dL Female: 12.0-16.0 g/dL
Hematocrit	26.8	Male: 41%-53% Female: 36%-46%
Mean corpuscular volume	64.0	80-100 μm^3
Mean corpuscular hemoglobin	19.3	25.4-34.6 pg/cell
Mean corpuscular hemoglobin concentration	30.2	31%-36% Hb/cell
Platelets	236000	150,000-400,000/mm^3
Neutrophil	61.7	40-60%
Lymphocytes	27.9	20-40%
Monocytes	7.8	4-8%
Eosinophil	2.6	1-3%
Basophil	0	0-1%
CD4 lymphocytes	79 cells/μL	500-1400 cells/μL

Enzyme-linked immunosorbent assays (ELISA) for HIV antibodies came back positive which was later confirmed with the Western blot test.

Once the diagnosis of toxoplasmic retinochoroiditis in an immunosuppressed patient was established, treatment with trimethoprim/sulfamethoxazole (TMP/SMX) 160/800 mg twice daily was commenced. Brain magnetic resonance imaging (MRI) showed multiple ring-enhancing lesions in both cerebral cortices (Figure 2). Meanwhile, three weeks after initial ophthalmic presentations, the patient developed a right hemiparesis. Due to the numerous lesions in the patient's motor cortex in the left and right lobes, the diagnosis of toxoplasmic encephalitis was made for the patient.

Highly active antiretroviral therapy (HAART) was added to her antitoxoplasmosis treatment four weeks after initial presentation and the dose of trimethoprim/sulfamethoxazole (TMP/SMX) increased to 160/800 mg/three times a day and azithromycin 250 mg/daily was added to the antitoxoplasmic regimen. The systemic steroid was not added to the patient's treatment regimen due to concerns about the patient's immunosuppression. Two months after initial presentation, vitreous inflammation decreased substantially, subretinal fluid gradually resolved, and the uncorrected visual acuity improved to 20/100 (Figure 3). Yellow subretinal hard exudates appeared in the perifoveal area with complete reattachment of the retina in three months. Two months after starting HAART, the patient's hemiparesis improved significantly during this time.

3. Discussion

The presence of cells in the anterior chamber and vitreous cavity, large Kps, PS, and a patch of retinitis adjacent to a pigmented retinochoroidal scar are clinical clues to the diagnosis of toxoplasmic retinochoroiditis. According to the fundus examination, weight loss, anemia, and leukopenia of the patient, internal medicine and infectious disease service consultation were requested. The patient's neuroimaging and the appearance of typical ring-enhanced lesions besides positive HIV test and diminished CD4+ cells suggested a possible diagnosis of toxoplasmosis in the patient, and therefore, no intraocular fluid PCR test requested for the patient. Positive Toxoplasma IgG antibody along with negative IgM indicates infection with the organism at some time [2, 12, 13]. According to a meta-analysis conducted by Borna et al., for estimating the level of immunity to toxoplasmosis in reproductive ages in Iran, the overall estimation for the prevalence of antitoxoplasma total antibody was 39.9% (95% CI: 26.1-53.7) [14].

However, this case shows some ocular and systemic features that are not commonly expected in the typical case of toxoplasmic retinochoroiditis. In this case, pursuing these atypical features led us to the diagnosis of AIDS.

The first red flag was the presence of an extensive retinal detachment with tractional bands surrounding the central scar and no responsible break which could be suggestive of tractional and/or exudative retinal detachment in our case. Although tractional, exudative, and rhegmatogenous retinal detachments can occur in ocular toxoplasmosis, such reports are limited; the reported prevalence of retinal detachment in acquired toxoplasmosis varies between 2.5 and 11 percent which is mostly of tractional or rhegmatogenous type [13, 15–17].

There are several reports on the management of retinal detachment in the setting of ocular toxoplasmosis. Among the 193 patients with ocular toxoplasmosis, Kianersi et al. reported five patients with RD: three rhegmatogenous and two tractional. All five patients underwent vitrectomy or scleral buckling surgery. It is well known that severe intraocular inflammation can lead to tractional retinal detachment. With the progression of traction, a retinal hole and subsequent rhegmatogenous detachment may develop. Another possible mechanism of hole formation is the occurrence of full-thickness necrosis in the retinitis patch [17].

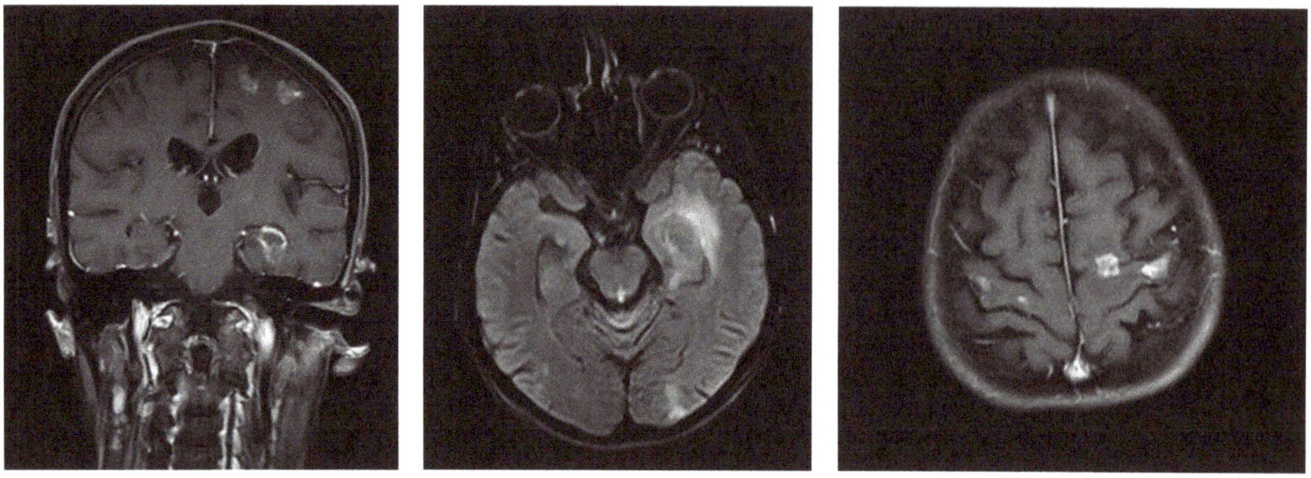

(a) (b) (c)

FIGURE 2: Magnetic resonance imaging (MRI): T1 with contrast in coronal (a) and axial planes (b, c): multiple ring-enhancing lesions in the left and right cerebral cortices.

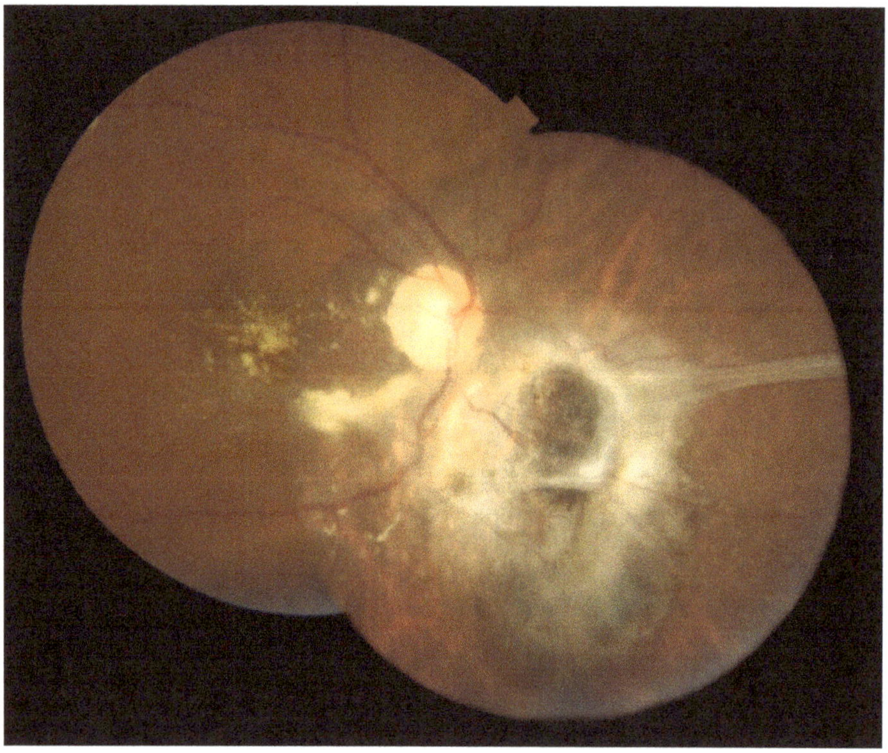

FIGURE 3: Montage fundus photography of the patient's right eye three months after initiation of antitoxoplasmosis treatment and HAART shows complete retinal reattachment. A retinal fold extends from the lesion to the nasal periphery. Subretinal exudates are seen in the inferior area of the disc and around the macula.

In another study, Al-Zahrani et al. reported a 24-year-old man with exudative RD secondary to reactivation of a toxoplasmosis lesion, which was successfully managed with antitoxoplasmosis treatment [15].

In a study by Faridi et al., on thirty-five eyes of 28 patients with ocular toxoplasmosis and sufficient follow-up, they identified 4 eyes (11 percent) with secondary RD, which was either rhegmatogenous, tractional, or a combination of the two. All eyes with retinal detachment underwent surgical repair of which 50% developed recurrent RDs (two of 4 patients). They concluded that handling ocular toxoplasmosis and related RDs may necessitate several measures, including surgical management, systemic therapy, and intravitreal injections. Formation of new breaks or PVR-related complications may necessitate multiple surgeries in cases with recurrent RD [16]. Our case represents the exudative detachment with no distinct retinal break. Observation of a retinal fold may advocate the presence of a tractional component in this case. The resolution of RD following an antitoxoplasmic regimen and HAART and without surgical intervention may suggest that decision upon surgery should not be rushed in such patients, and a period of close follow-up visits for ocular examination combined with appropriate systemic treatment may be warranted.

Angular cheilitis and significant weight loss are not expected to occur in typical ocular toxoplasmosis. The presence of angular cheilitis calls for investigating the possibility of anemia and its underlying etiology. In our case, CBC revealed hypochromic microcytic anemia suggestive of iron-deficiency anemia and leukopenia which necessitates a thorough investigation for immunodeficiency.

Increased energy expenditure happens in the setting of opportunistic infections. Weight loss in patients with HIV is associated with poor prognosis, increased risk of disease progression, and opportunistic pathology [18].

In a study by Neves et al. on 37 immunocompetent patients with acute acquired toxoplasmosis, the frequency of systemic manifestations was inspected. Weight loss, anemia, and leukopenia were seen in 62.2%, 10.8%, and 16.2% of patients, respectively [12]. Although our patient was not a case of acquired toxoplasmosis and the results of the study by Neves et al. could not be generalized to reactivated congenital toxoplasmosis, another similar study could investigate the possibility of anemia, leukopenia, and weight loss in this group of patients.

The possibility of toxoplasmic encephalitis should be investigated in every patient with HIV and retinochoroidal toxoplasmosis [19, 20]. The study of choice for this purpose is brain MRI with contrast that can illustrate characteristic enhancing ring lesions. While not pathognomonic, the presence of several brain abscesses is the most characteristic feature of *T. gondii* infection in AIDS patients. Autopsy usually shows a global involvement of both hemispheres, though the basal ganglia and the corticomedullary junction are the most common sites of involvement [9–11].

This report highlights the fact that sometimes the eyes are the site of the first presentation of a systemic life-threatening condition and emphasizes the role of ophthalmologists in such cases. Judicious ocular and systemic evaluation of patients with ocular toxoplasmosis are of utmost importance. In cases of atypical presentation, appropriate laboratory tests and CNS imaging should be requested. Systemic treatment with antitoxoplasmosis regimens and HAART is mandatory in AIDS patients with ocular toxoplasmosis. Treatment options for retinal detachment in this setting should be meticulously approached.

References

[1] S. Abgrall, C. Rabaud, and D. Costagliola, "Incidence and risk factors for toxoplasmic encephalitis in human immunodeficiency virus-infected patients before and during the highly active antiretroviral therapy era," *Clinical Infectious Diseases*, vol. 33, no. 10, pp. 1747–1755, 2001.

[2] G. N. Holland, "Ocular toxoplasmosis: a global reassessment. Part I: epidemiology and course of disease," *American Journal of Ophthalmology*, vol. 136, no. 6, pp. 973–988, 2003.

[3] C. S. Subauste, D. Ajzenberg, and A. Kijlstra, "Review of the series "Disease of the year 2011: toxoplasmosis" pathophysiology of toxoplasmosis," *Ocular Immunology and Inflammation*, vol. 19, no. 5, pp. 297–306, 2011.

[4] J. R. Smith and E. T. J. Cunningham, "Atypical presentations of ocular toxoplasmosis," *Current Opinion in Ophthalmology*, vol. 13, no. 6, pp. 387–392, 2002.

[5] Y.-H. Park and H.-W. Nam, "Clinical features and treatment of ocular toxoplasmosis," *The Korean Journal of Parasitology*, vol. 51, no. 4, pp. 393–399, 2013.

[6] M.-H. Heinemann, J. M. W. Gold, and J. Maisel, "Bilateral toxoplasma retinochoroiditis in a patient with acquired immune deficiency syndrome," *Retina*, vol. 6, no. 4, pp. 224–227, 1986.

[7] K. F. Tabbara, "Ocular toxoplasmosis," *International Ophthalmology*, vol. 14, no. 5-6, pp. 349–351, 1990.

[8] F. J. San-Andres, R. Rubio, J. Castilla et al., "Incidence of acquired immunodeficiency syndrome-associated opportunistic diseases and the effect of treatment on a cohort of 1115 patients infected with human immunodeficiency virus, 1989–1997," *Clinical Infectious Diseases*, vol. 36, no. 9, pp. 1177–1185, 2003.

[9] C. Renold, A. Sugar, J. P. Chave et al., "Toxoplasma encephalitis in patients with the acquired immunodeficiency syndrome," *Medicine (Baltimore)*, vol. 71, no. 4, pp. 224–239, 1992.

[10] S. B. Porter and M. A. Sande, "Toxoplasmosis of the central nervous system in the acquired immunodeficiency syndrome," *The New England Journal of Medicine*, vol. 327, no. 23, pp. 1643–1648, 1992.

[11] B. J. Luft and J. S. Remington, "Toxoplasmic encephalitis in AIDS," *Clinical Infectious Diseases*, vol. 15, no. 2, pp. 211–222, 1992.

[12] E. S. Neves, L. N. Bicudo, A. L. Curi et al., "Acute acquired toxoplasmosis: clinical-laboratorial aspects and ophthalmologic evaluation in a cohort of immunocompetent patients," *Memórias do Instituto Oswaldo Cruz*, vol. 104, no. 2, pp. 393–396, 2009.

[13] L. E. H. Bosch-Driessen, T. T. J. M. Berendschot, J. V. Ongkosuwito, and A. Rothova, "Ocular toxoplasmosis: clinical features and prognosis of 154 patients," *Ophthalmology*, vol. 109, no. 5, pp. 869–878, 2002.

[14] S. Borna, M. Shariat, M. Fallahi, and L. Janani, "Prevalence of immunity to toxoplasmosis among Iranian childbearing age women: systematic review and meta-analysis," *Iranian Journal of Reproductive Medicine*, vol. 11, no. 11, pp. 861–868, 2013.

[15] Y. A. Al-Zahrani, H. A. Al-Dhibi, and A. A. Al-Abdullah, "Atypical presentation of ocular toxoplasmosis: a case report of exudative retinal detachment and choroidal ischemia," *Middle East African Journal of Ophthalmology*, vol. 23, no. 1, pp. 150–152, 2016.

[16] A. Faridi, S. Yeh, E. B. Suhler, J. R. Smith, and C. J. Flaxel, "Retinal detachment associated with ocular toxoplasmosis," *Retina*, vol. 35, no. 2, pp. 358–363, 2015.

[17] F. Kianersi, A. Naderi Beni, H. Ghanbari, and F. Fazel, "Ocular toxoplasmosis and retinal detachment: five case reports," *European Review for Medical and Pharmacological Sciences*, vol. 16, Suppl 4, pp. 84–89, 2012.

[18] V. K. Sashindran and R. Thakur, "Malnutrition in HIV/AIDS: aetiopathogenesis," in *Nutrition and HIV/AIDS*, N. Dumais, Ed., IntechOpen, Rijeka, 2020.

[19] T. J. Stokkermans and S. J. Havens, *Toxoplasma Retinochoroiditis*, StatPearls Publishing, 2021, http://www.ncbi.nlm.nih.gov/pubmed/29630234. Accessed April 15, 2021.

[20] S. B. Murugan, "Commentary: ocular toxoplasma: from bench-side to clinical practice!," *Indian Journal of Ophthalmology*, vol. 66, no. 10, pp. 1489-1490, 2018.

14

Multimodal Imaging of Subfoveal Pachydrusen Containing a Blood Flow Signal

Naoko Ishiguro,[1] Takaaki Hayashi,[1,2] Yoshiko Yamawaki,[1] Kei Mizobuchi,[1] Tsutomu Yasukawa,[3] Shigeru Honda,[4] and Tadashi Nakano[1]

[1]*Department of Ophthalmology, The Jikei University School of Medicine, Tokyo, Japan*
[2]*Department of Ophthalmology, Katsushika Medical Center, The Jikei University School of Medicine, Tokyo, Japan*
[3]*Department of Ophthalmology and Visual Science, Nagoya City University Graduate School of Medical Sciences, Aichi, Japan*
[4]*Department of Ophthalmology and Visual Sciences, Osaka City University Graduate School of Medicine, Osaka, Japan*

Correspondence should be addressed to Takaaki Hayashi; taka@jikei.ac.jp

Academic Editor: Stephen G. Schwartz

Individuals with pachydrusen, larger than 125 μm, have a significantly thicker choroid than do those with soft drusen or reticular pseudodrusen. Little is known about cases of abnormal blood flow within pachydrusen. The purpose of this report was to demonstrate a blood flow signal within pachydrusen using optical coherence tomography (OCT) angiography. A 76-year-old Japanese woman presented with innumerable drusen/pachydrusen in both posterior poles. Her visual acuity was good. OCT showed subfoveal pachydrusen in the left eye, but no exudative changes. The subfoveal choroidal thickness was increased to 274 μm in the left eye. OCT angiography revealed a blood flow signal within the pachydrusen. However, fluorescein and indocyanine green angiographies indicated no abnormal hyperfluorescent lesion in the macula of the left eye. During the 13-month follow-up, the blood flow signal in OCT angiography did not change in diameter, and no exudative change was observed. The blood flow signal may have properties of capillary blood vessels derived from the choriocapillaris, rather than angiogenic vessels from choroidal neovascularization or polypoidal choroidal vasculopathy/aneurysmal type 1 neovascularization.

1. Introduction

Drusen are the accumulation of yellow deposits between the retinal pigment epithelium (RPE) and Bruch's membrane due to abnormalities of the RPE. Soft drusen, which are an essential precursor of age-related macular degeneration, are defined as drusen with a diameter of ≥63 μm or more [1]. Cases of soft drusen are often accompanied by thinning of the choroid. In 2018, Spaide [2] reported relatively large (≥125 μm) pachydrusen with choroidal thickening, and Cheung et al. [3] demonstrated that patients with pachydrusen had a significantly thicker choroid than did those with soft drusen or reticular pseudodrusen. To the best of our knowledge, there are no reported cases of a blood flow signal within the pachydrusen in the absence of exudative changes as indicated by optical coherence tomography (OCT) angiography (OCTA). Here, we report a case of a patient in whom a blood flow signal was detected within subfoveal pachydrusen using OCTA.

2. Case Presentation

A 76-year-old Japanese female patient presented with blurred vision in her left eye. At presentation, her decimal best-corrected visual acuity was 1.0 (Snellen equivalent 20/20) in the right eye and 1.5 (Snellen equivalent 20/13) in the left eye with +3.00 diopter sphere, and her intraocular pressure was 15 mmHg in the right and 18 mmHg in the left eyes. There were no remarkable findings in the anterior segment and media, aside from mild cataracts in both eyes. On fundoscopy, innumerable drusen/pachydrusen were found in the posterior poles of both eyes (Figures 1(a) and 1(b)). Pachydrusen was found in the fovea of the left eye (Figure 1(c)). Fundus autofluorescence imaging using a

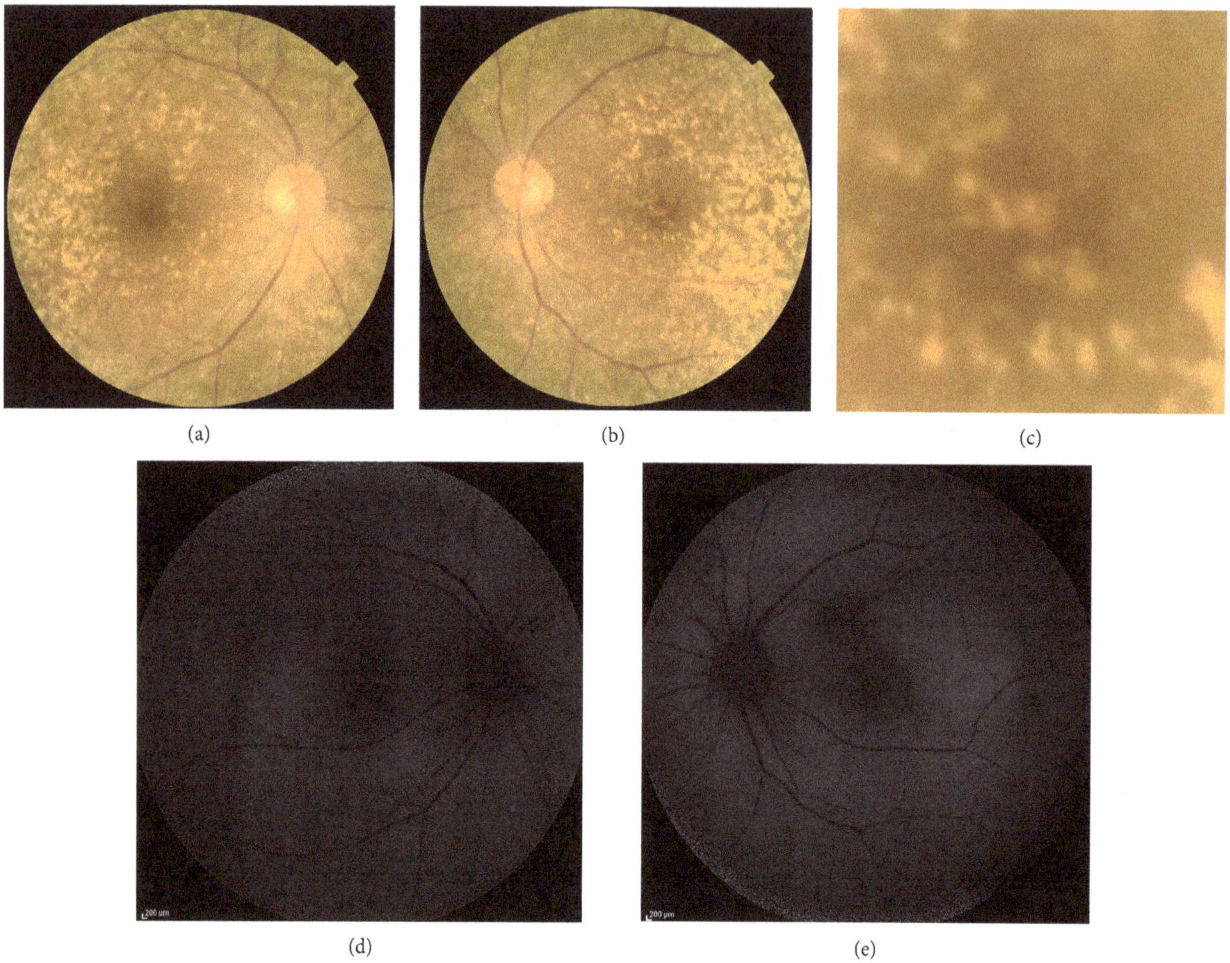

Figure 1: Color fundus photographs of the right (a) and left (b) eyes and the left macula (c). Fundus autofluorescence of the right (d) and left (e) eyes.

confocal scanning laser scanning ophthalmoscope (Spectralis HRA, Heidelberg Engineering, Heidelberg, Germany) showed autofluorescence of the drusen on the temporal side of the macula of both eyes (Figures 1(d) and 1(e)). OCT (Cirrus 5000 Carl Zeiss Meditec, Dublin, CA) showed that the pachydrusen located at the RPE level were subfoveal in the left eye (Figure 2(a)). OCTA identified a blood flow signal in the subfoveal pachydrusen (Figure 2(b)). The horizontal diameter of the flow signal was 208 μm. Fluorescein angiography (Figures 3(a) and 3(b)) and indocyanine green angiography (Figures 3(c) and 3(d)) revealed no hyperfluorescence/leakage, abnormal vasculature, vascular network, or polypoidal/aneurysmal lesions at the macula in the left eye in the early (Figures 3(a) and 3(c)) to late phase images (Figures 3(b) and 3(d)).

One month after presentation, her decimal best-corrected visual acuity was 1.5 in the left eye, and the size of the flow signal remained unchanged (Figures 4(a) and 4(b)). During the 13-month follow-up, the blood flow signal in OCTA did not change in horizontal diameter, and no exudative changes were observed (Figure 4(c)). At 13 months after presentation, her decimal best-corrected visual acuity was 1.0 in the left eye. On swept-source OCT (Triton, Topcon, Tokyo, Japan), subfoveal pachydrusen were clearly observed between the RPE and Bruch's membrane (Figure 5(a)), and the blood flow signal was detected within the pachydrusen (Figure 5(b)). The subfoveal choroidal thickness was 274 μm. Clinical timeline of the patient is described in Figure 6.

3. Discussion

In this report, we describe a female patient in whom a blood flow signal was detected within the subfoveal pachydrusen on OCTA.

A Korean population-based cohort study on choroidal thickness in Asia demonstrated that the mean subfoveal choroidal thickness of 255 older people aged 65-99 years (mean age, 76.6 years) was 182 μm [4]. In our patient, the subfoveal choroidal thickness was increased to 274 μm. Recently, Cheung et al. investigated the association between choroidal thickness and drusen subtypes in Asian and white populations [3]. The Asian population included 145 older patients (mean age, 71.6 years) with drusen; the mean subfoveal choroidal thickness was significantly thicker in the pachydrusen group ($n = 37$, 265.5 μm) than in the soft drusen group

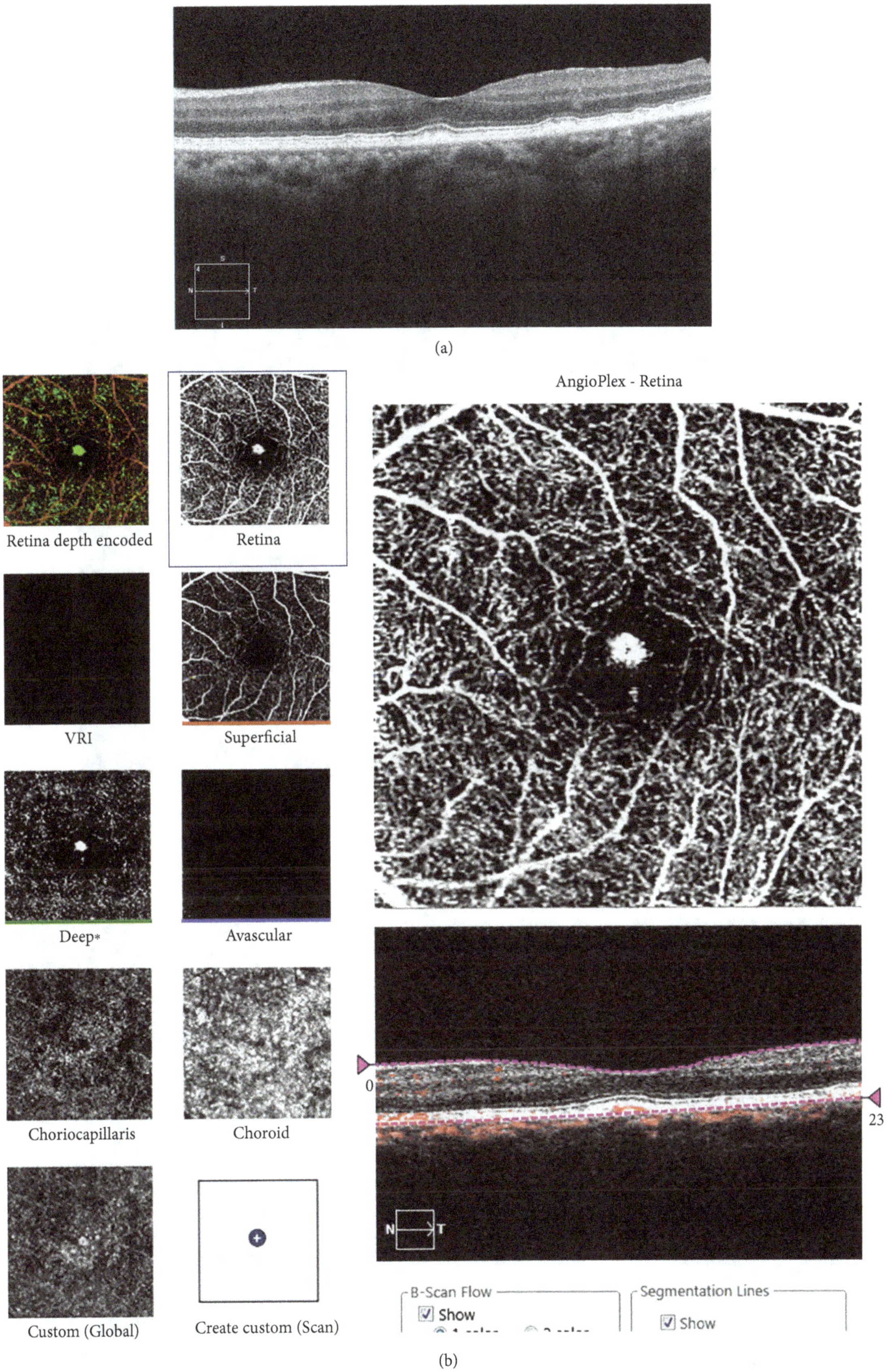

FIGURE 2: Horizontal optical coherence tomography (OCT) B-scan of the left eye (a) and OCT angiography of the left eye (b).

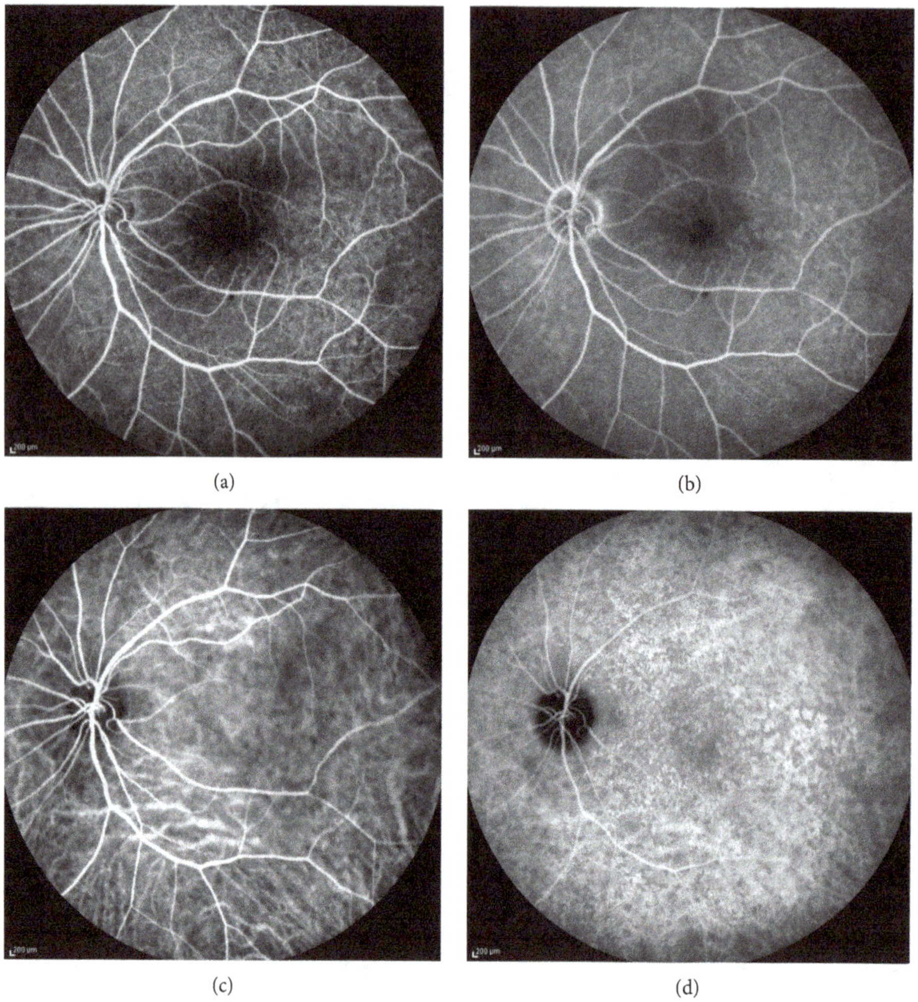

Figure 3: Fluorescein angiograms of the early (a) and late (b) phases in the left eye. Indocyanine green angiograms of the early (c) and late (d) phases in the left eye.

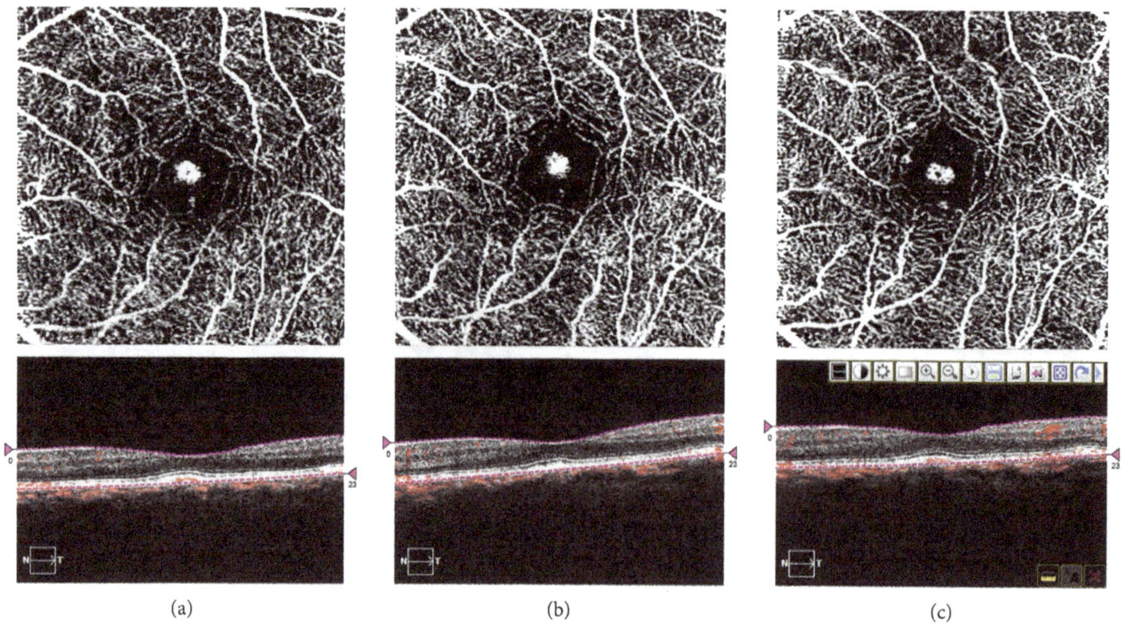

Figure 4: Optical coherence tomography angiography at baseline (a), 1 month later (b), and 13 months later (c) in the left eye.

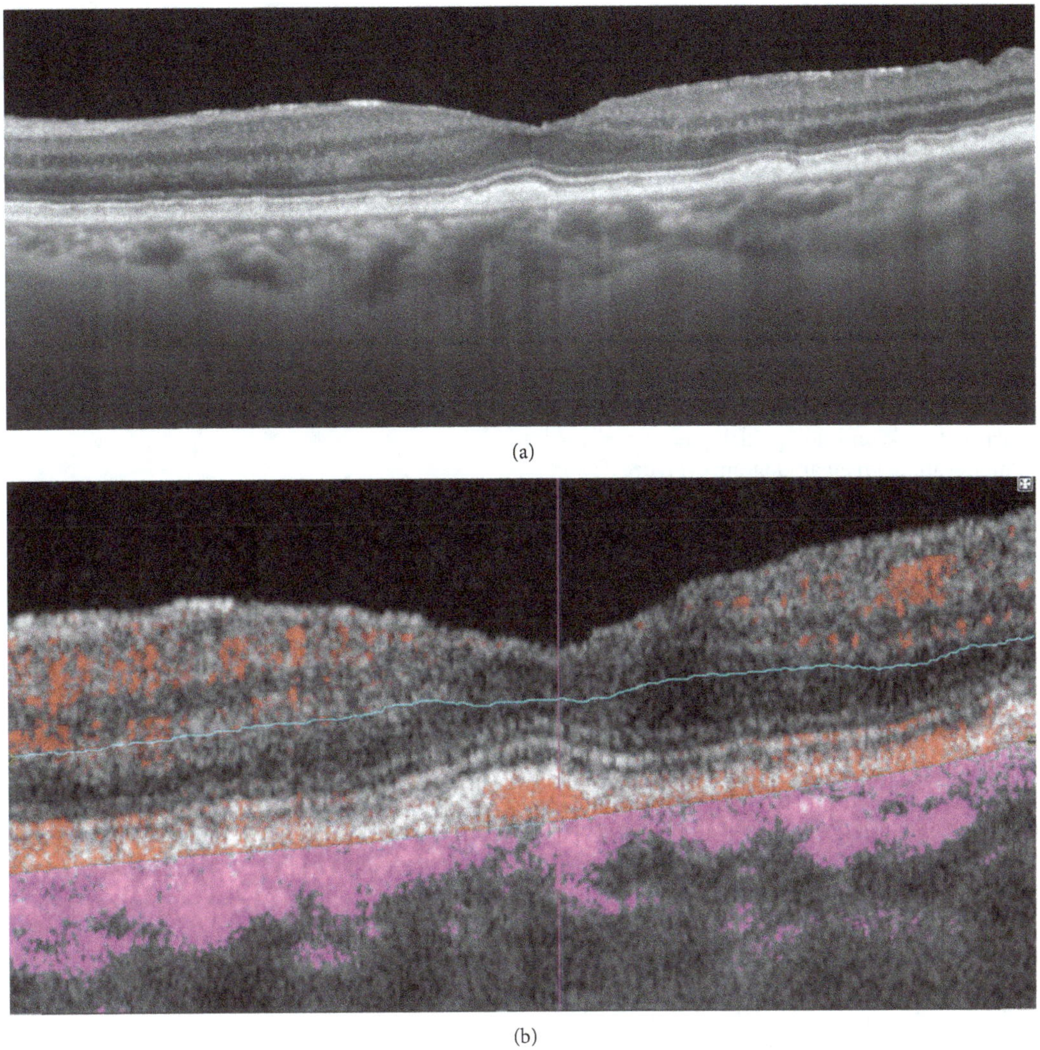

Figure 5: Horizontal swept-source optical coherence tomography (SS-OCT) B-scan (a) and horizontal B-scan SS-OCT angiography (b) at 13 months after presentation in the left macula.

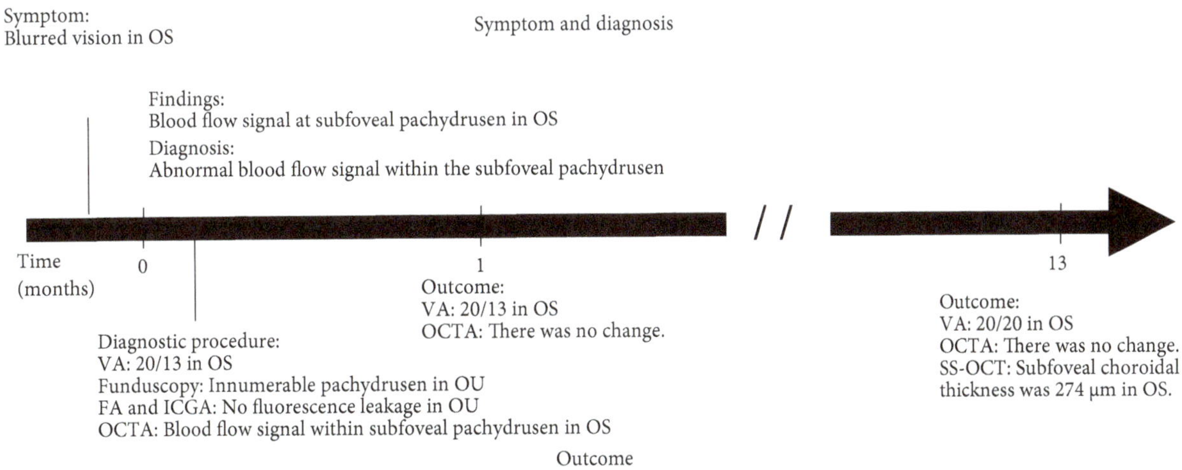

Figure 6: Clinical timeline of the female patient. OU: both eyes; FA: fluorescein angiography; ICGA: indocyanine green angiography; OCT: optical coherence tomography; OCTA: OCT angiography; SS-OCT: swept source OCT; VA: corrected visual acuity.

($n = 83$, 218.0 μm) and the pseudodrusen group ($n = 25$, 151.4 μm). Similar outcomes were reported in a study of older Japanese patients [5]. Interestingly, in the Asian cohort [3], patients with polypoidal choroidal vasculopathy (also known as aneurysmal type 1 neovascularization), a pachychoroid spectrum disease [6], were more likely to have a thicker choroid and pachydrusen.

We believe that the blood flow signal (Figures 2, 4, and 5) in our patient originated from the choriocapillaris (or less likely from choroidal vessels directly). However, the signal was distinct from that of typical angiogenic vessels from choroidal neovascularization or a polypoidal/aneurysmal lesion in polypoidal choroidal vasculopathy because of the absence of fluorescein leakage in the fluorescein angiograms (Figure 3), vascular network, and polypoidal/aneurysmal vasculature on the indocyanine green angiograms (Figure 3) and any exudative changes on OCT (Figures 2 and 5). Thus, our multimodal imaging data demonstrated that the blood flow signal may have properties of capillary blood vessels containing endothelial cells, such as retinal capillaries. Although no apparent break in Bruch's membrane was observed on OCT (Figures 2 and 5), the blood flow would penetrate Bruch's membrane from the choriocapillaris and may have been associated with vulnerability of Bruch's membrane due to aging and/or the formation of pachydrusen. However, it cannot be denied that the flow signal may have been an indication of very early stage choroidal neovascularization or polypoidal choroidal vasculopathy. A recent retrospective cross-sectional study using OCTA has demonstrated that called vascularized drusen (presence of flow within the drusen) were seen in 5.5 percent of 128 patients with intermediate nonexudative age-related macular degeneration [7]. In that study [7], the vascularized drusen exhibited a uniform sub-RPE hyperreflectivity in OCT and lacked neovascular nature in fluorescein angiography. On the other hand, it was not mentioned whether pachydrusen patients are included. The subsequent consecutive study has revealed that 2 eyes with the vascularized drusen developed CNV during 24-month follow up [8].

In this report, we observed a blood flow signal within the subfoveal pachydrusen, but the actual cause remains unclear. Continued follow-up will be required to assess both OCT and OCTA findings and to elucidate the mechanism of development of the flow signal.

References

[1] R. F. Spaide and C. A. Curcio, "Drusen characterization with multimodal imaging," *Retina*, vol. 30, no. 9, pp. 1441–1454, 2010.

[2] R. F. Spaide, "Disease expression in nonexudative age-related macular degeneration varies with choroidal thickness," *Retina*, vol. 38, no. 4, pp. 708–716, 2018.

[3] C. M. G. Cheung, A. Gan, Y. Yanagi, T. Y. Wong, and R. Spaide, "Association between choroidal thickness and drusen subtypes in age-related macular degeneration," *Ophthalmol Retina*, vol. 2, no. 12, pp. 1196–1205, 2018.

[4] N. K. Ryoo, S. J. Ahn, K. H. Park et al., "Thickness of retina and choroid in the elderly population and its association with complement factor H polymorphism: KLoSHA eye study," *PLoS One*, vol. 13, no. 12, article e0209276, 2018.

[5] Y. Fukuda, Y. Sakurada, S. Yoneyama et al., "Clinical and genetic characteristics of pachydrusen in patients with exudative age-related macular degeneration," *Scientific Reports*, vol. 9, no. 1, p. 11906, 2019.

[6] S. Borooah, P. Y. Sim, S. Phatak et al., "Pachychoroid Spectrum Disease," *Acta Ophthalmologica*, vol. 99, no. 6, pp. e806–e822, 2021.

[7] C. Or, J. S. Heier, D. Boyer et al., "Vascularized drusen: a cross-sectional study," *International Journal of Retina and Vitreous*, vol. 5, no. 1, p. 36, 2019.

[8] K. Ramezani, O. Abu-Qamar, J. S. Heier et al., "Longitudinal follow-up of vascularized drusen [ARVO Annual Meeting Abstract]," *Investigative Ophthalmology & Visual Science*, vol. 62, no. 8, p. 298, 2021.

15

Subepithelial Corneal Deposits Associated with Exemestane

Annahita Amireskandari, Elena Nguyen, David Hinkle, and Thomas Mauger

Department of Ophthalmology, West Virginia University, USA

Correspondence should be addressed to Annahita Amireskandari; annahita.rezai@gmail.com

Academic Editor: Nicola Rosa

This is a case report of corneal deposits noted in a 69-year-old female patient taking the aromatase inhibitor, exemestane, after undergoing a mastectomy and chemotherapy for breast cancer. The patient presented to our eye clinic for a new-onset floater in one eye, and bilateral subepithelial opacities were found incidentally on exam. The patient completed a 5-year course of the medication shortly after her initial visit with us and was noted to have a slight improvement in the density of the opacities on a follow-up visit 3 months later. We believe these corneal changes were most likely secondary to exemestane. The effect of aromatase inhibitors on the eye deserves further exploration as an increasing number of patients are prescribed these medications.

1. Introduction

Exemestane (trade name Aromasin (Pfizer)) is an irreversible aromatase inhibitor (AI) used as an adjuvant treatment for postmenopausal women with estrogen receptor-positive breast cancer [1–3]. Several studies have reported on the ocular side effects of aromatase inhibitors, with the most common being ocular surface disease [4–6]. A case report by Papathanassiou et al. [5] reported corneal epithelial deposits associated with exemestane. Here, we discuss a patient on exemestane with development of subepithelial corneal opacities.

2. Case Report

A 69-year-old female presented to the ophthalmology clinic with a new onset of a floater in her right eye. Her medical history was notable for stage 1 estrogen, progesterone, and HER2/neu-positive invasive ductal carcinoma of the left breast diagnosed 5 years prior. She had completed 12 weeks of adjuvant chemotherapy with Taxol (paclitaxel, Bristol-Myers Squibb) and Herceptin (trastuzumab, Roche) and was in her fifth and final year of Aromasin (exemestane) when she presented to us. The only other medication she was taking at the time of presentation to our clinic was bisoprolol-hydrochlorothiazide for hypertension, which was well controlled. She had no other significant systemic illnesses. Additionally, she denied a personal or family history of eye disease.

At her initial visit to the retina clinic, she was noted to have uncorrected Snellen distance visual acuities of 20/30-2 OD and 20/25-2 OS. Her lids, adnexa, and conjunctiva were all normal. She was noted to have bilateral diffuse subepithelial corneal opacities. The deposits ranged in size from pinpoint to 0.5 mm with poorly demarcated edges. They were hazy and whitish in color, varying in density, and best visualized with a narrow slit beam. The corneal stroma and endothelium appeared normal. There was no staining with fluorescein dye. Schirmer's testing with anesthetic was 8 mm on the right and 5 mm on the left. Corneal sensation was intact bilaterally. On dilated fundus exam, she was noted to have inferotemporal retinoschisis bilaterally. The decision was made to observe the retinoschisis, and she was referred to the cornea service for further evaluation. It was thought that the subepithelial corneal irregularities were most likely secondary to exemestane. She completed 5 years of exemestane the following month, was seen at a follow-up visit, and was noted to have a posterior vitreous detachment in the right eye. The corneal findings were stable. She was seen again 3 months later after stopping the exemestane, and the

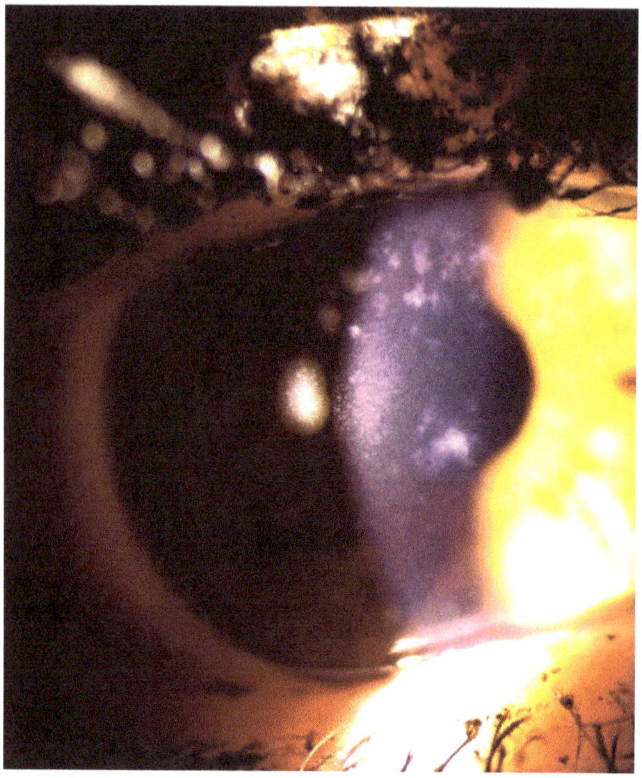

Figure 1: Slit lamp photograph of the right cornea.

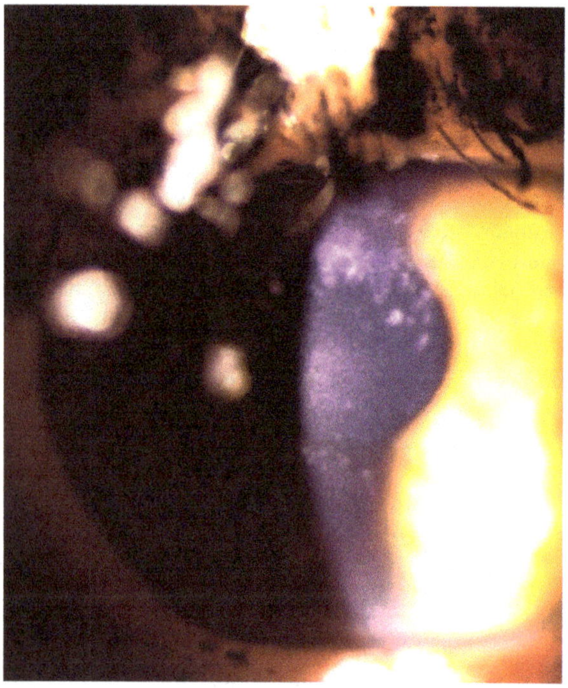

Figure 2: Slit lamp photograph of the left cornea.

subepithelial opacities were noted to have a more annular pattern and were less dense compared to prior visits. Slit lamp photographs of the right (Figure 1) and left eyes (Figure 2) were taken at this visit.

3. Discussion

The corneal abnormalities noted in this patient were found incidentally when she presented with a new-onset floater. We were unable to obtain any ophthalmologic records from the patient's previous eye care providers so the duration of her clinical findings remains unknown. Given the use of exemestane at the time of diagnosis and improvement after cessation of the medication, we believe this was the most likely cause of the subepithelial opacities noted on her exam.

Exemestane is an irreversible inhibitor of aromatase, the enzyme responsible for the conversion of androgens to estrogens. Although estrogen receptors are more readily associated with reproductive organs, they are also known to be present in the cornea, lens, retina, meibomian glands, and the lacrimal glands [7–11]. Several studies have reported on adverse ocular effects of AIs [12–14]. Inglis et al. [4] used the Ocular Surface Disease Index questionnaire and found a significantly higher rate of self-reported dry eye disease in patients taking AIs compared to controls. Gibson et al. noted no significant difference in ocular surface symptoms in AI users compared to controls but did note worse meibomian gland expressibility and pain perception in AI users [13]. Others have also reported increased rates of anterior segment pathology including meibomian gland dysfunction [14], blepharitis, superficial punctate keratitis, conjunctival injection [6, 14], and Sjögren's syndrome in AI users [15]. One isolated case report documented epithelial deposits associated with exemestane use [5]. These deposits were described as intraepithelial microcysts, while those of our patient appeared to be subepithelial opacities. Papathanassiou et al. [5] hypothesized that the corneal changes noted in their patient were a sign of impaired epithelium due to an inhibitory effect of exemestane on limbal stem cells, citing research that estrogens enhance stem cell survival and proliferation [16].

Eisner et al. [17] examined the effects of anastrazole, another commonly used AI, on the posterior segment. They observed an increased rate of retinal hemorrhages and vitreoretinal traction in patients taking anastrazole compared to patients taking tamoxifen and controls [17]. They hypothesized that the hemorrhages were a result of traction, and the higher rate of traction was likely due to accelerated aging from estrogen depletion, noting that posterior vitreous detachments and macular holes are more common in postmenopausal women than men [18]. Epstein also reported a case of a macular hole associated with the initiation of exemestane [19]. Interestingly, our patient initially presented with a new floater, was noted to have retinoschisis, and was subsequently found to have a posterior vitreous detachment. Though there are no published reports of retinoschisis and AI use, it is difficult to assess whether either of these posterior segment changes was the result of normal aging or if this process was accelerated by a reduction in circulating estrogen.

The exact role of estrogen on the eye is still being investigated. Though many studies attribute the adverse effects of AIs to low estrogen levels, the mechanism is likely more complex and related to the balance between estrogens, androgens, and other circulating hormones [10, 20–22].

It is also worth discussing Taxol (paclitaxel) and Herceptin (trastuzumab) as our patient had previously been treated with these agents. Given that these medications had been completed more than 4 years prior to her presentation, we believe that they were unlikely to be the cause of her corneal findings. And, while retinal and optic nerve toxicities are known adverse effects of paclitaxel, we are not aware of corneal toxicity as a reported side effect [23–27]. Herceptin and related drugs, however, have been associated with adverse effects on the anterior segment with dry eye, epiphora, blurred vision, and conjunctivitis being the most common [12, 28, 29]. It is not surprising that these drugs might have an effect on the ocular surface given the expression of HER receptors by the corneal, limbal, and conjunctival epithelia [30] and the role of HER family tyrosine kinase receptors on cell differentiation, proliferation, and migration [31, 32].

Tamoxifen, a selective estrogen receptor modulator which is commonly given prior to initiation of exemestane, has been associated with corneal deposits [33, 34], as well as corneal pigmentation changes [35]. However, our patient had not taken this medication.

As the rate of breast cancer diagnosis increases, the number of patients taking these medications continues to rise. With AIs in particular, there are often issues with adherence to therapy due to side effects [36], and at the same time, higher rates of adverse effects have been associated with lower risk of breast cancer recurrence [37]. It is important that we continue to investigate the effects of these agents and the resulting hormonal changes on various tissues in the body in order to better detect and manage any possible adverse effects.

Consent

Informed consent was obtained from the patient for publication of this case report and all accompanying images.

References

[1] R. C. Coombes, L. S. Kilburn, C. F. Snowdon et al., "Survival and safety of exemestane versus tamoxifen after 2–3 years' tamoxifen treatment (Intergroup Exemestane Study): a randomised controlled trial," *The Lancet*, vol. 369, no. 9561, pp. 559–570, 2007.

[2] E. D. Deeks and L. J. Scott, "Exemestane," *Drugs*, vol. 69, no. 7, pp. 889–918, 2009.

[3] A. Robinson, "A review of the use of exemestane in early breast cancer," *Therapeutics and Clinical Risk Management*, vol. 5, no. 1, pp. 91–98, 2008.

[4] H. Inglis, F. M. Boyle, M. L. Friedlander, and S. L. Watson, "Dry eyes and AIs: If you don't ask you won't find out," *The Breast*, vol. 24, no. 6, pp. 694–698, 2015.

[5] M. Papathanassiou, E. Nikita, P. Theodossiadis, G. P. Theodossiadis, and I. Vergados, "Exemestane-induced corneal epithelial changes," *Cutaneous and ocular toxicology*, vol. 29, no. 3, pp. 209–211, 2010.

[6] K. Turaka, J. M. Nottage, K. M. Hammersmith, P. K. Nagra, and C. J. Rapuano, "Dry eye syndrome in aromatase inhibitor users," *Clinical & Experimental Ophthalmology*, vol. 41, no. 3, 2012.

[7] B. Esmaeli, J. T. Harvey, and B. Hewlett, "Immunohistochemical evidence for estrogen receptors in meibomian glands," *Ophthalmology*, vol. 107, no. 1, pp. 180–184, 2000.

[8] C. Munaut, V. Lambert, A. Noël et al., "Presence of oestrogen receptor type beta in human retina," *The British Journal of Ophthalmology*, vol. 85, no. 7, pp. 877–882, 2001.

[9] H. Spelsberg, M. Klueppel, T. Reinhard et al., "Detection of Oestrogen receptors (ER) _α_ and _β_ in conjunctiva, lacrimal gland, and tarsal plates," *Eye*, vol. 18, no. 7, pp. 729–733, 2004.

[10] D. A. Sullivan, "Tearful Relationships? Sex, Hormones, the Lacrimal Gland, and Aqueous- Deficient Dry Eye," *The Ocular Surface*, vol. 2, no. 2, pp. 92–123, 2004.

[11] T. Suzuki, Y. Kinoshita, M. Tachibana et al., "Expression of sex steroid hormone receptors in human cornea," *Current Eye Research*, vol. 22, no. 1, pp. 28–33, 2009.

[12] J. C. B. Chiang, I. Zahari, M. Markoulli et al., "The impact of anticancer drugs on the ocular surface," *The Ocular Surface*, vol. 18, no. 3, pp. 403–417, 2020.

[13] E. Gibson, F. Stapleton, R. Dear, J. S. Wolffsohn, and B. Golebiowski, "Dry eye signs and symptoms in aromatase inhibitor treatment and the relationship with pain," *The Ocular Surface*, vol. 18, no. 1, pp. 108–113, 2020.

[14] I. Chatziralli, T. Sergentanis, F. Zagouri et al., "Ocular surface disease in breast cancer patients using aromatase inhibitors," *The Breast Journal*, vol. 22, no. 5, pp. 561–563, 2016.

[15] M. Laroche, S. Borg, S. Lassoued, B. De Lafontan, and H. Roché, "Joint pain with aromatase inhibitors: abnormal frequency of Sjögren's syndrome," *The Journal of Rheumatology*, vol. 34, no. 11, pp. 2259-2263, 2007.

[16] R. Ray, N. M. Novotny, P. R. Crisostomo, T. Lahm, A. Abarbanell, and D. R. Meldrum, "Sex steroids and stem cell function," *Molecular Medicine*, vol. 14, no. 7-8, pp. 493–501, 2008.

[17] A. Eisner, E. J. Thielman, J. Falardeau, and J. T. Vetto, "Vitreoretinal traction and anastrozole use," *Breast Cancer Research and Treatment*, vol. 117, no. 1, pp. 9–16, 2009.

[18] J. Y. Chuo, T. Y. Y. Lee, H. Hollands et al., "Risk factors for posterior vitreous detachment: a case-control study," *American Journal of Ophthalmology*, vol. 142, no. 6, pp. 931–937.e1, 2006.

[19] R. J. Epstein, "Visual impairment in myopic patients with breast cancer receiving adjuvant therapy with aromatase inhibitors," *Clinical Breast Cancer*, vol. 9, no. 3, pp. 184–186, 2009.

[20] D. A. Sullivan, R. V. Jensen, T. Suzuki, and S. M. Richards, "Do sex steroids exert sex-specific and/or opposite effects on gene expression in lacrimal and meibomian glands?," *Molecular Vision*, vol. 15, pp. 1553–1572, 2009.

[21] P. Versura and E. C. Campos, "Menopause and dry eye: a possible relationship," *Gynecological Endocrinology*, vol. 20, no. 5, pp. 289–298, 2009.

[22] S. B. Wang, K. M. Hu, K. J. Seamon, V. Mani, Y. Chen, and K. Gronert, "Estrogen negatively regulates epithelial wound healing and protective lipid mediator circuits in the cornea," *The FASEB Journal*, vol. 26, no. 4, pp. 1506–1516, 2011.

[23] M. H. L. Amigo, P. Falabella, Â. Bettarello, and W. Ghirelli, "Irreversible visual loss after use of paclitaxel," *Revista Brasileira de Oftalmologia*, vol. 74, no. 4, pp. 254–256, 2015.

[24] L. S. Hofstra, E. G. de Vries, and P. H. Willemse, "Letters to the editor: Ophthalmic toxicity following paclitaxel infusion," *Annals of Oncology*, vol. 8, no. 10, p. 1053, 1997.

[25] M. M. Joshi and B. R. Garretson, "Paclitaxel maculopathy," *Archives of Ophthalmology*, vol. 125, no. 5, pp. 709-710, 2007.

[26] Y. Li, Y. Li, J. Li, G. Pi, and W. Tan, "Paclitaxel- and/or cisplatin-induced ocular neurotoxicity: a case report and literature review," *OncoTargets and Therapy*, vol. 7, pp. 1361–1366, 2014.

[27] V. Scaioli, A. Caraceni, C. Martini, S. Curzi, G. Capri, and G. Luca, "Electrophysiological evaluation of visual pathways in paclitaxel-treated patients," *Journal of Neuro-Oncology*, vol. 77, no. 1, pp. 79–87, 2006.

[28] H. A. Burris III, H. S. Rugo, S. J. Vukelja et al., "Phase II study of the antibody drug conjugate trastuzumab-DM1 for the treatment of human epidermal growth factor receptor 2 (HER2)-positive breast cancer after prior HER2-directed therapy," *Journal of Clinical Oncology*, vol. 29, no. 4, pp. 398–405, 2011.

[29] M. Untch, M. Rezai, S. Loibl et al., "Neoadjuvant treatment with trastuzumab in HER2-positive breast cancer: results from the GeparQuattro study," *Journal of Clinical Oncology*, vol. 28, no. 12, pp. 2024–2031, 2010.

[30] Z. Liu, M. Carvajal, C. A. Carothers Carraway, K. Carraway, and S. C. Pflugfelder, "Expression of the receptor tyrosine kinases, epidermal growth factor receptor, ErbB2, and ErbB3, in human ocular surface epithelia," *Cornea*, vol. 20, no. 1, pp. 81–85, 2001.

[31] M. Olayioye, R. Neve, H. Lane, and N. Hynes, "New EMBO members' review: the ErbB signaling network: receptor heterodimerization in development and cancer," *The EMBO Journal*, vol. 19, no. 13, pp. 3159–3167, 2000.

[32] N. Prenzel, O. M. Fischer, S. Streit, S. Hart, and A. Ullrich, "The epidermal growth factor receptor family as a central element for cellular signal transduction and diversification," *Endocrine-Related Cancer*, vol. 8, no. 1, pp. 11–31, 2001.

[33] M. Orkun, U. Ö. Özlenen, and K. Ayfer, "Clinical and in vivo confocal microscopy findings in patients receiving tamoxifen citrate," *Eye Contact Lens*, vol. 32, no. 5, pp. 228–232, 2006.

[34] S. Tarafdar, L. T. Lim, C. E. Collins, and K. Ramaesh, "Tamoxifen keratopathy as seen with in-vivo confocal microscopy," *Seminars in Ophthalmology*, vol. 27, no. 1-2, pp. 27-28, 2012.

[35] M. I. Kaiser-Kupfer and M. E. Lippman, "Tamoxifen retinopathy," *Cancer Treatment Reports*, vol. 62, no. 3, pp. 315–1978.

[36] R. L. Sedjo and S. Devine, "Predictors of non-adherence to aromatase inhibitors among commercially insured women with breast cancer," *Breast Cancer Research and Treatment*, vol. 125, no. 1, pp. 191–200, 2011.

[37] J. Cuzick, I. Sestak, D. Cella, and L. Fallowfield, "Treatment-emergent endocrine symptoms and the risk of breast cancer recurrence: a retrospective analysis of the ATAC trial," *The Lancet Oncology*, vol. 9, no. 12, pp. 1143–1148, 2008.

16

Iris Vascular Malformation with 360-Degree Iridocorneal Angle Affectation

Cristina Calleja-García, Jorge Suárez-Baraza, and Enrique Mencía-Gutiérrez

Ophthalmology Department, 12 de Octubre Hospital, Complutense University, 28041 Madrid, Spain

Correspondence should be addressed to Enrique Mencía-Gutiérrez; emencia.hdoc@salud.madrid.org

Academic Editor: Cristiano Giusti

Vascular iris lesions are rare and can sometimes be associated to systemic vascular lesions. They usually cause spontaneous recurrent hyphema. The differential diagnosis should be considered primarily with iris rubeosis and with highly vascular tumors as iris melanoma. Generally, vascular lesions of hemangioma type are located in the iris without extension to iridocorneal angle. We present a case of a 77-year-old male with an iris vascular lesion suggestive of racemose hemangioma, who is asymptomatic, and with 360-degree iridocorneal angle affectation showing no lesions at any other location.

1. Introduction

There are a variety of tumors and iridian lesions that range from cystic tumors to even solid melanocytic and nonmelanocytic tumors. According to Shields et al., the nonmelanocytic lesions constitute 11% of iridian tumors, and of these, the vascular type constitutes 2% [1]. Different types of iridian hemangiomas can be distinguished: racemose, cavernous, capillary, and pupil rim microhemangioma, and they must be distinguished from other arteriovenous alterations such as iris rubeosis among others [2].

2. Case Report

A 77-year-old male was referred for a possible study of unilateral iris rubeosis in right eye (RE) found in a routine exploration previous to cataract surgery. The patient was asymptomatic and did not refer any previous ocular pathology except divergent strabismus since childhood with left eye amblyopia. The patient had a personal history of arterial hypertension with renal repercussion, metabolic syndrome, auricular fibrillation, prostatic syndrome, and moderate chronic obstructive pulmonary emphysema. In the exploration, he presented a visual acuity (VA) (decimal scale) of the RE of 0.5 and in the left eye (LE) of 0.15, as well as divergent strabismus. In a slit lamp, we observed radial iridian vascular engorgement at 5 to 7 o'clock location in RE. The vessels seem to originate from the iris stroma and then extended circumferentially (Figure 1(a)). Gonioscopic examination showed a graded IV open angle with a vascular racemose net of 360 degrees in the iridocorneal angle (Figures 1(b) and 1(c)). No sentinel vessels were found at the episcleral level, and the presence of masses at other sites of the iris was ruled out. Intraocular pressure in the RE was 10 mmHg and in the LE, 12 mmHg. LE examination was normal. Ocular fundus showed in the RE an oblique papilla, myopic coriorretinitis, without exudates, hemorrhages, or neovascularization (Figure 2). There were not any clinical signs of pathology that could cause retinal ischemia such as diabetic retinopathy, central or branch vein, or central artery obstruction.

Peripheral tumor masses, such as choroidal melanoma, retinoblastoma, metastasis, or ciliary body lesions, were ruled out by fundus examination with indentation and maximum midriasis.

Supra-aortic trunk exam with ecoDoppler showed no other causes of ocular ischemia. No carotid stenosis with hemodynamic significance was observed. In the differential diagnosis, entities such as sickle-cell anemia, Takayasu disease, giant cell arteritis, or carotid-cavernous fistula were also proposed, but additional tests were not requested since they have low probability in the patient's clinical context.

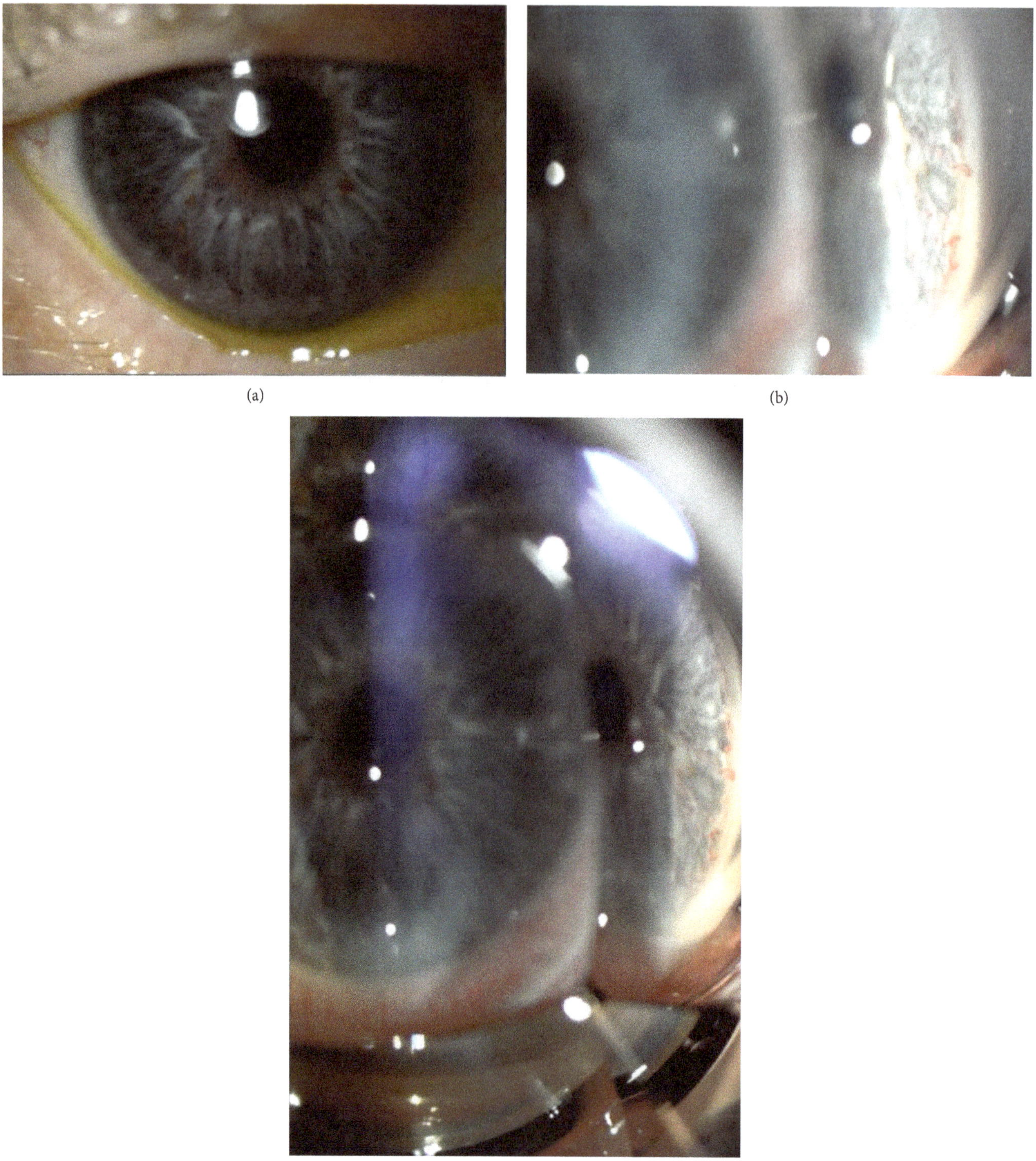

FIGURE 1: (a) Radial iridian vascular engorgement at 5 to 7 o'clock location in RE. (b, c) Gonioscopic examination shows a graded IV open angle with a vascular racemose net of 360 degrees in the iridocorneal angle.

An anterior segment optic coherence tomography was performed to refine the characterization of the lesion, and poorly defined intrastromal hyporeflective spaces were observed coinciding with the lumen of the vessels (Figure 3).

For the differential diagnosis between neovascularization and tumor/vascular malformation, a fluorescein angiography (FA) was performed and normal contrast uptake was demonstrated without extravasation of the latter at the level of the iridian, iridocorneal angle, and retinal vessels (Figures 4(a) and 4 (b)). An early filling of the iridian vessels was observed without contrast diffusion, thus ruling out retinal ischemia and neovessels.

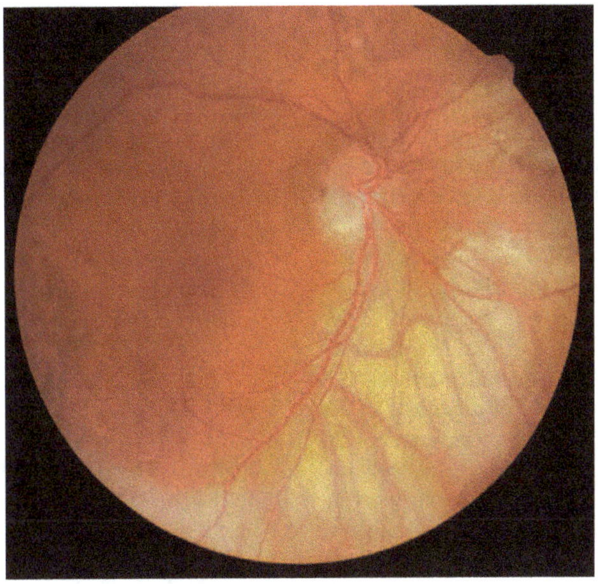

FIGURE 2: RE ocular fundus shows an oblique papilla and myopic coriorretinitis without other findings.

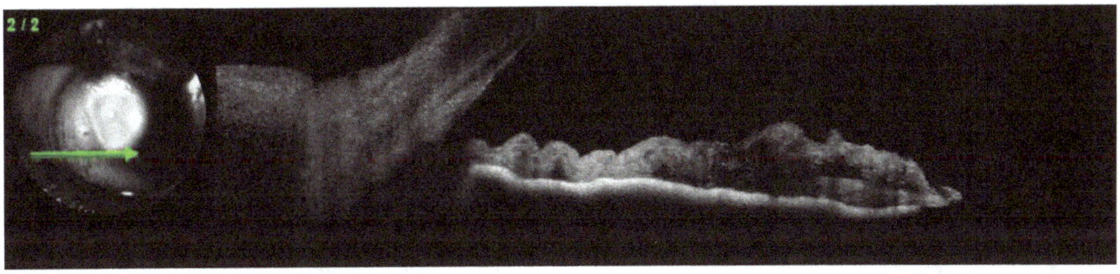

FIGURE 3: RE anterior segment optic coherence tomography shows intrastromal hyporeflective spaces corresponding to the iris vessels.

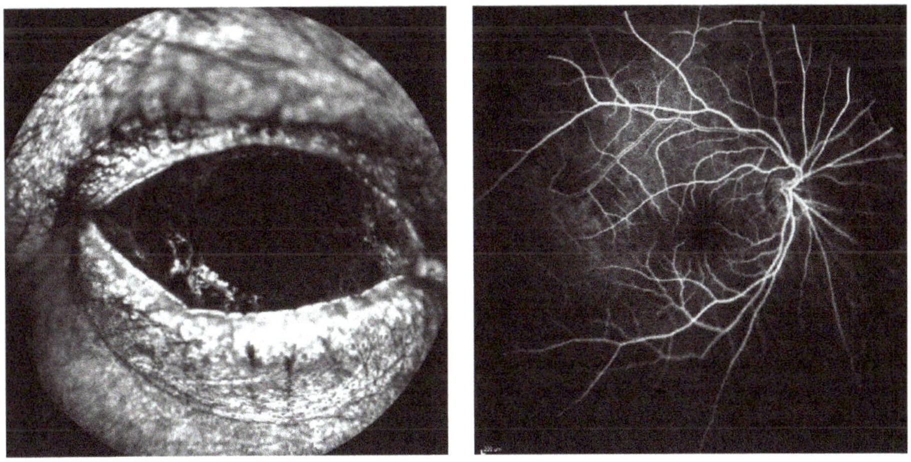

(a) (b)

FIGURE 4: (a, b) RE fluorescein angiography shows an early filling of the vessels without contrast diffusion in the iris, angle, and retina vessels.

3. Discussion

Vascular malformations of the iris are those in which there is a connection between an artery and a vein without an interposed capillary plexus, and they are very rare. They can cause spontaneous hyphemas associated with ocular hypertension. These lesions must be distinguished from other arteriovenous alterations such as iris rubeosis, juvenile xanthogranuloma, iris varix, and highly vascular melanoma [2]. Different types of iridian hemangiomas can be distinguished: racemose, cavernous, capillary, and pupil rim microhemangioma. The racemose hemangioma can be associated with the presence of dilated episcleral vessels that are related to the presence of a ciliary body melanoma [3]. As for the cavernous hemangioma, Shields et al. cast doubt on its existence since they consider that it can be part of a spectrum of lesions, including thrombosed iris varicose veins. However, these may be associated with lesions of the cavernous hemangioma at the brain level. Capillary hemangioma is extremely rare and is usually more frequent in childhood, associated with ipsilateral cutaneous lesions [3]. Iris microhemangiomas are the most frequent vascular lesions of the iris, and they are diagnosed when spontaneous hyphema is associated. This subtype of hemangioma is related by an unknown mechanism with myotonic dystrophy and with diabetes mellitus [3].

Shields et al. [2] reported a mean age of diagnosis of 55 years, all lesions being unilateral. They are more frequent in clear eyes, probably because they are easier to visualize, and are usually located in the temporal region, although there is no clear explanation for this. It is not clear if they are congenital or acquired lesions. Of the 14 cases of arteriovenous iris malformations studied by Shields et al., none of them were associated with systemic diseases/syndromes. In 50% of cases, a sentinel episcleral vessel was located, which could have been a sign of a melanoma of the underlying ciliary body, but in all cases, its presence was ruled out.

These vascular-type lesions must be distinguished from other arteriovenous alterations such as iris rubeosis. For this, it is essential to detect those risk factors for ocular ischemia: venous thrombosis, diabetic retinopathy, central retinal artery obstruction, ocular ischemia syndrome (carotid stenosis, Takayasu disease, giant cell arteritis, and carotid-cavernous fistula), vasculopathies such as sickle-cell anemia or Eales disease, and tumors (choroidal melanoma and highly vascular iris).

FA plays a fundamental role in detecting the presence of neovascularization and areas of retinal ischemia. In iridian vascular malformations, FA is characterized by an early hyperfluorescence that may also be visible later and, unlike rubeosis, it will not produce contrast extravasation. FA is a very useful but invasive test, so new diagnostic methods such as optical coherence tomography angiography allow us to perform a more precise exploration of the iridian vasculature in a noninvasive way [4].

In the literature, there have been no reported cases of iridian vascular lesions of the hemangioma type in which the vascular malformation extends 360 degrees through the iridocorneal angle. Shields et al. [3] did not report cases of hemangiomas with the extension of the iridocorneal angle. The study by de Corral et al. [5] describes a case of spontaneous hyphema due to an anomalous vessel in the iridocorneal angle that does not present hemangioma characteristics.

In general, the management of these lesions consists of observation without any specific treatment, since most of them are asymptomatic, as in this case. In cases where there has been spontaneous bleeding, improvement has been reported after treatment with argon laser photocoagulation applied directly over the vascular lesion [5]. In case of doubt or diagnoses of melanoma or when they cause recurrent hyphema, a sectoral iridectomy can be performed with excision of the lesion.

4. Conclusion

Vascular malformations of the iris are very rare and can sometimes be associated with vascular lesions at other locations; however, in our case, we describe the existence of a vascular malformation known as racemose hemangioma type iris, with 360-degree extension by the iridocorneal angle without any other lesions. These are asymptomatic lesions that require follow-up and a differential diagnosis, mainly with iris rubeosis and neovascular glaucoma. Tumors such as ciliary body melanoma, although rare, should be ruled out.

Consent

Consent for the publication of ophthalmic images was obtained from the patient.

References

[1] C. L. Shields, P. W. Shields, J. Manalac, C. Jumroendararasame, and J. A. Shields, "Review of cystic and solid tumors of the iris," *Oman Journal of Ophthalmology*, vol. 6, no. 3, pp. 159–164, 2013.

[2] J. A. Shields, T. F. Streicher, J. H. Spirkova, M. Stubna, and C. L. Shields, "Arteriovenous malformation of the iris in 14 cases," *Archives of Ophthalmology*, vol. 124, no. 3, pp. 370–375, 2006.

[3] J. A. Shields, C. Bianciotto, B. E. Kligman, and C. L. Shields, "Vascular tumors of the iris in 45 patients," *Archives of Ophthalmology*, vol. 128, no. 9, pp. 1107–1113, 2010.

[4] J. L. Chien, K. Sioufi, S. Ferenczy, E. A. T. Say, and C. L. Shields, "Optical coherence tomography angiography features of iris racemose hemangioma in 4 cases," *JAMA Ophthalmology*, vol. 135, no. 10, pp. 1106–1110, 2017.

[5] L. R. de Corral, M. Conway, G. A. Peyman, and A. Constanteras, "Argon laser treatment of an abnormal angle vessel producing recurrent hyphema," *International Ophthalmology*, vol. 8, no. 3, pp. 179–182, 1985.

17

Photodynamic Therapy of Presumed Choroidal Metastasis Secondary to Colorectal Carcinoma: Literature Review

Laurentino Biccas Neto,[1] José Z. Pulido,[2] Gustavo B. Melo,[3,4] Luiz H. Lima,[4] and Eduardo B. Rodrigues[4,5]

[1]*Ocular Oftalmologia, Vitória, Brazil*
[2]*Department of Oncology, Hospital Evangélico, Cachoeiro do Itapemirim, Brazil*
[3]*Hospital de Olhos de Sergipe, Aracaju, Brazil*
[4]*Department of Ophthalmology, Universidade Federal de São Paulo, São Paulo, Brazil*
[5]*Department of Ophthalmology, Saint Louis University School of Medicine, Saint Louis, MO, USA*

Correspondence should be addressed to Eduardo B. Rodrigues; rodriguesretina@gmail.com

Academic Editor: Stefano Baiocchi

Colorectal cancer may yield metastasis to the choroid. Its management may be challenging, since there is no consensus about treatment. We describe a case of a 70-year-old male with colon cancer who complained of worsening visual acuity of his better-seeing eye to 20/40 secondary to a nonpigmented choroidal mass of medium reflectivity under the inferior temporal arcade and neurosensory foveal detachment. Besides systemic chemotherapy, local treatment with verteporfin photodynamic therapy (vPDT) was performed. After one month, visual acuity improved to 20/25 and subretinal fluid faded. In conclusion, vPDT may be a useful adjuvant treatment modality for choroidal metastasis secondary to colorectal cancer.

1. Introduction

Colorectal cancer (CRC) consists of the development of cancer from the colon or rectum. Various histology types of CRC have been described, whereas adenocarcinoma comprises over 95% of the cases. About 20% of the patients with CRC present with metastases at diagnosis, and the most common sites include the liver, lung, peritoneum, and bones [1–3].

Ocular and periocular metastases in patients with CRC have been described in the medical literature, with the choroid being the main site [4–8]. Choroidal metastasis may be uni- or bilateral and may comprise around 4% of CRC sites of metastasis [8, 9]. Management of such choroidal lesions may be challenging, since there is no consensus about treatment. It might include observation, radiotherapy, or other modalities of local therapy, like vascular endothelial growth factor inhibitors.

The primary purpose of this paper was to report on a case of presumed choroidal metastasis in a patient with colon carcinoma treated by photodynamic therapy with verteporfin (vPDT). The secondary goal of the paper was to present a review of medical literature about epidemiology, clinical features, and multimodal imaging findings, with special emphasis on the management options of choroidal and retinal metastasis secondary to CRC.

2. Case Report

A 70-year-old male was referred with a complaint of complete and sudden visual loss in the left eye (LE) immediately following a cardiac surgery (mitral valve exchange). The patient informed previous diagnosis of a spinal lesion following a spinal cord abscess on T9 which led to paraplegy. On ophthalmic examination, best-corrected visual acuity (BCVA) was 20/20 in the right eye (RE) and no light perception in the LE, which showed a relative afferent pupillary defect (RAPD). Intraocular pressure (IOP) was 15 mmHg in both eyes (BE). Multimodal imaging demonstrated acute

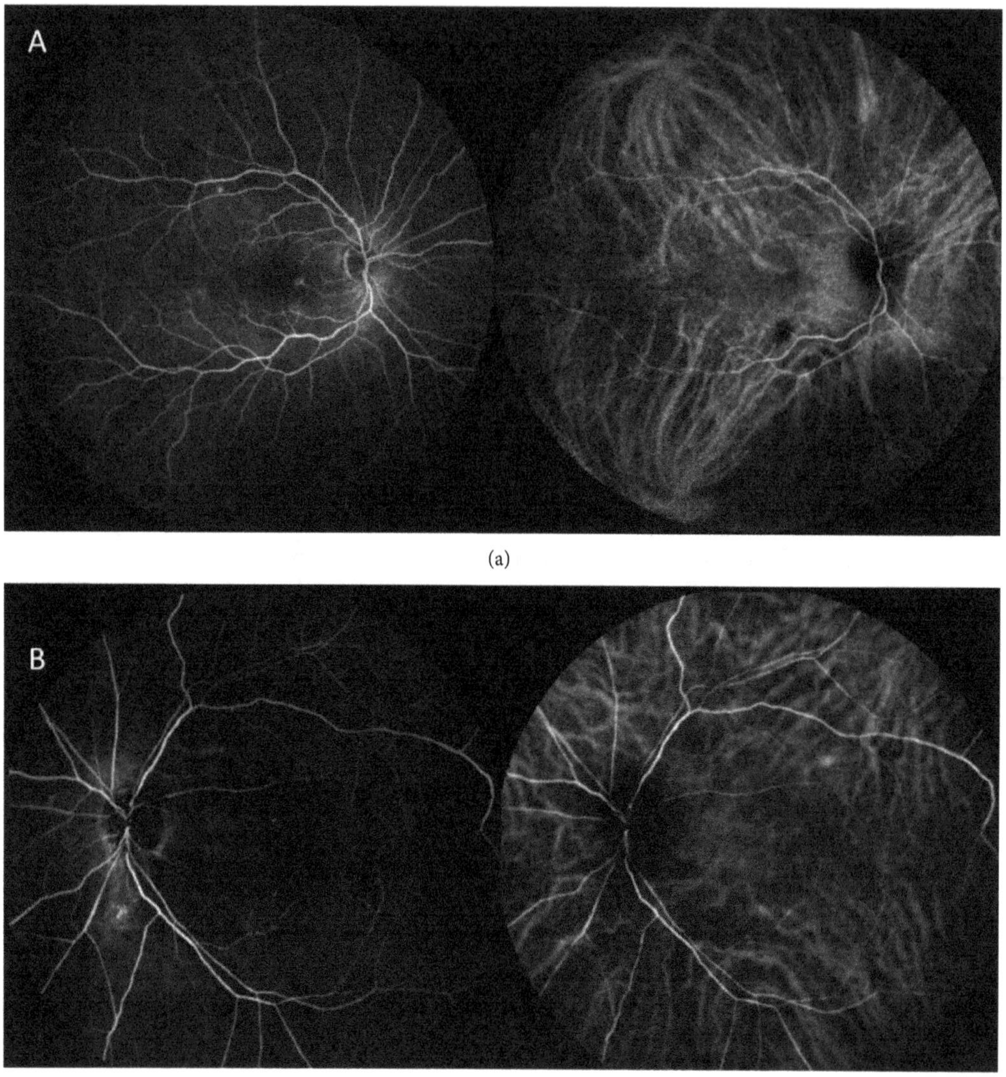

(a)

(b)

Figure 1: Images 5 months before the diagnosis of the metastatic lesion in the right eye (RE). (a) Midphase wide field FA and ICG of the RE showing discrete hyperfluorescent spots (transmission defects) in the arcades. Hypofluorescent plaque on ICG in the inferior temporal vascular arcade, with no relevant findings on multimodal OCT. (b) Late arterial phase FA and ICG of the left eye showing narrow arterial vessels and horizontal hyperfluorescent tracks due to RPE atrophy in the central macula.

central retinal artery occlusion in the LE; in the RE, there were discrete soft drusen throughout the macula. A small area of hypofluorescence was seen on ICG angiography near the inferior temporal vascular arcade in the RE but was deemed to be irrelevant (Figure 1). No intraocular masses were seen in the macular area on Spectral Domain OCT (SDOCT). Blue autofluorescence imaging was unremarkable in the RE.

Five months later, the patient returned to the ophthalmology office complaining of worsening of vision in the RE (better-seeing eye). In the meantime, he was diagnosed with colon adenocarcinoma at a metastatic stage (multiple lesions in the liver and lungs recently discovered) and treated with endovenous chemotherapy. The assistant oncologist informed that the chemotherapeutic regimen (bevacizumab+FOLFIRINOX) had led to a partial reduction of the systemic metastasis (estimated around 30%). FOLFIRINOX is a chemotherapy regimen for the treatment of advanced pancreatic cancer made up of the following four drugs: folinic acid (leucovorin), fluorouracil (5-FU), irinotecan, and oxaliplatin. At the second ophthalmic examination, BCVA was 20/40 in the RE and no light perception in the LE; anterior segment was normal in BE; there was a shallow neurosensory foveal detachment seen on SDOCT, along with a choroidal mass of medium reflectivity superior to the inferior temporal arcade in the RE (Figure 2). The choroidal lesion was nonpigmented, measuring $6 \times 7 \times 1.5$ mm by ultrasound, without hemorrhages, hard exudates, or calcification. There was moderate pigment clumping and atrophy overlying the lesion, showing mottled areas of hypo- and hyperautofluorescence in the blue spectrum. Fundus examination of the LE revealed diffuse vascular attenuation and two parallel

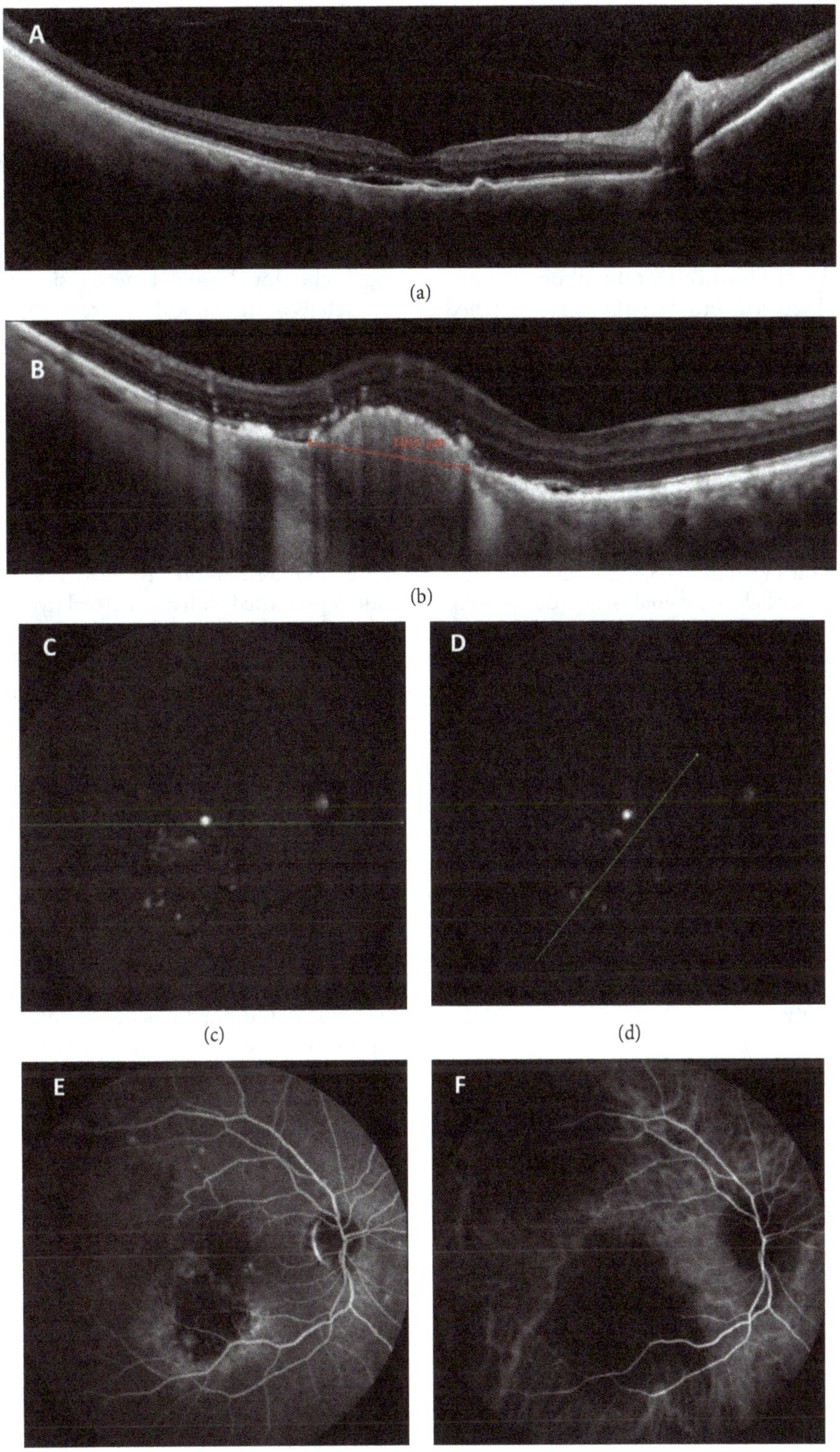

(a) (b) (c) (d) (e) (f)

Figure 2: A metastatic lesion appears in the right eye five months later. (a) Horizontal OCT showing a small neurosensory macular detachment, with discrete thickening of the RPE and of the outer foveal lines over the detachment. Scattered hyperreflective foci within the retina. Note the loss of typical choroidal texture under the serous detachment. (b) OCT showing a choroidal mass with moderate internal reflectivity on OCT superior to the inferior temporal arcade, measuring 1,912 μm in diameter, with no overlying choriocapillaris. Overlying hyperreflective foci and contiguous neurosensory foveal detachment are seen. (c, d) IR image depicts numerous whitish subretinal clumps suggesting fibrin along both vascular arcades. The green lines represent the axial orientation of the B-scans of images (a) and (b), respectively. (e) FA shows a hypofluorescent plaque surrounded by mottled hyperfluorescence in the inferior temporal arcade. (f) Hypofluorescent plaques on ICG along the superior and inferior vascular arcades.

hyperfluorescent horizontal streaks in the macula as a result of the central arterial occlusion (unchanged from the previous examination 5 months before). On ICG, there were two new areas (compared to the previous exam) of hypofluorescence in the RE, one corresponding to the choroidal mass and a second one under the superior temporal arcade (Figure 2). SDOCT, matched to the superior hypofluorescent area, showed no evident tumor, but there was loss of the choroidal texture, as if no vessels could be seen in this layer.

Potential risks and benefits of verteporfin photodynamic therapy (vPDT) were discussed with the patient, and a signed informed consent was obtained. As the RE was the only seeing eye of the patient, it was decided that only the inferior lesion should be treated, fearing collateral damage by extensive vPDT in a single session. Laser settings and treatment guidelines of vPDT were performed according to the guidelines of the Treatment of Age-related Macular Degeneration with Photodynamic Therapy study protocol: standard full-fluence PDT was performed using a 6 mg/m^2 dose of verteporfin and a 689 nm laser (Visulas 690S; Carl Zeiss Meditec, Inc.) with 50 J/cm^2 of laser light delivered over a duration of 83 seconds on the area of the tumor. The spot size was adjusted to as wide as possible, in order to cover the largest diameter of the tumor with a 0.5 mm free margin. Three overlapping spots were necessary to cover the entire lesion.

One month after vPDT, we observed a significant reduction in choroidal tumor thickness and in subretinal fluid. BCVA improved to 20/25 in the RE after successful vPDT. Fluorescein angiography disclosed a hypofluorescent plaque under the tumor region with mottled hyperfluorescent spots (Figure 3). ICG angiography revealed reduction in hyperfluorescent spots and enhancement in the hypofluorescent area. OCT over the tumor area showed an intraretinal dense hyperreflective band with underlying RPE irregularities and choroidal hyperreflectivity.

3. Main Text

Adenocarcinomas make up about 95% of CRC. Other less common tumors are lymphomas and sarcomas. The 5-year survival rate for patients with stage I colon cancer is about 90%, while those with a more advanced disease, such as in stage IV CRC, have an estimated survival rate of 10%. CRC may lead to a variety of distance metastases including the lung, liver, peritoneum, brain, and bones [1, 3, 10, 11]. Less common sites of metastasis secondary to CRC include the bladder, brain, adrenals, spleen, and the eye and its adnexa, whereas some isolated reports found metastatic disease in the orbit, periocular skin, retina, and choroid [4–7, 12–28]. Carcinoma can metastasize to the uvea from any portion of the colon, although the sigmoid colon and rectum appear to be most highly represented [19, 29].

Gastrointestinal metastases are relatively uncommon in the uvea [9, 29, 30]. This implies either a molecular property that makes the uvea particularly attractive to breast and lung cancers or a molecular difference between lung, breast, and gastrointestinal primary tumors that allows breast and lung cancers to metastasize more readily to the uvea.

The incidence of metastasis of CRC to the choroid and retina is not yet clear, even though a survey by Shields determined that 4% of all uveal metastases (43 eyes of 40 patients) are caused by tumors of the gastrointestinal tract in a survey of 2214 tumors in 1111 patients [8]. In 2014, Tei et al. [31] published one case of choroidal metastasis secondary to rectum carcinoma plus a review of thirteen case reports of the literature with a discussion about ophthalmic and systemic features. However, a deeper analysis on the therapeutic approaches for choroidal metastasis was not provided [31].

Details of the clinical features such as laterality and types of masses of choroidal metastasis can be obtained from case reports. Papers such as those published by Ma et al., Ha et al., Khawaja et al., and Lin et al. showed unilateral single choroidal mass in reports of colorectal adenocarcinoma [5, 13, 19, 32]. Moreover, Maudgil et al. described two eyes with a single choroidal mass in patients with diagnosis of adenocarcinoma of the cecum, while Ward et al. reported single bilateral choroidal masses in a patient with presumed colon cancer [33, 34]. Similar to most previous publications, our patient presented with a unilateral hyperreflective and hyperechogenic choroidal mass in the inferior temporal arcade. Shields et al. demonstrated that 93% of patients with choroidal metastasis due to tumors of the gastrointestinal tract have unilateral masses [8]. Based on this evidence, one may assume that a choroidal metastasis due to CRC will most likely induce a unilateral focal lesion compared to other types of tumors like breast carcinoma that present an average of 1.9 tumors per eye.

Only four cases of retinal metastases occurring in patients with CRC have been published in the medical literature so far to our knowledge [12, 35–37]. The lesions also were unilateral and solitary. Kennedy et al. described one case in 1956 in a male patient who showed a small-sized well-demarcated and grayish-white lesion in the macula extending into the vitreous. It was associated with annular carcinoma of the rectosigmoid junction. A second case was reported in a woman with Muir-Torre syndrome that had multiple tumors including sebaceous adenomas of the face and neck and adenocarcinoma of the colon and retinal tumor. She underwent enucleation of the eye for a retinal tumor and histopathology revealed adenocarcinoma. The case by Spraul et al. was of an adenocarcinoma of the cecum which led to an exudative retinal detachment. The retinal mass was resected by pars plana vitrectomy [36]. Nookala et al. proposed that when a patient experiences metastasis to the retina, there is a high chance of cancer spreading to the central nervous system, which may mean less favorable prognosis [12].

Treatment of symptomatic choroidal metastasis depends on the systemic status and staging of the metastatic disease. Options include observation (in preterminal patients or when metastasis regresses with chemotherapy), chemotherapy, immunotherapy, hormone therapy, radiotherapy, and even enucleation for blind and painful eyes harboring metastatic tumors [38]. Local palliative treatment of choroidal metastasis may be efficient and yield good control of visual symptoms in patients with a metastatic neoplasm with little collateral damage, as with vPDT.

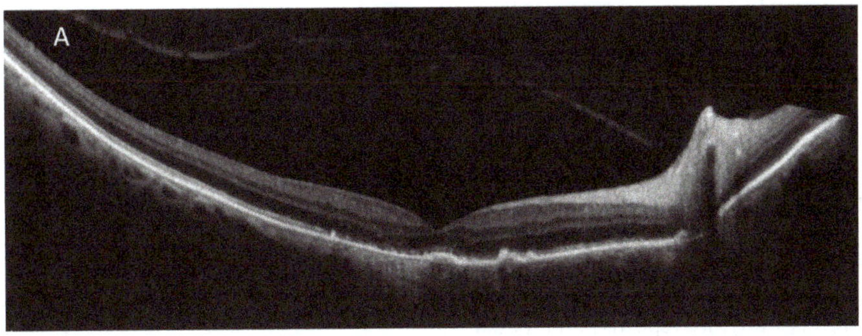

(a)

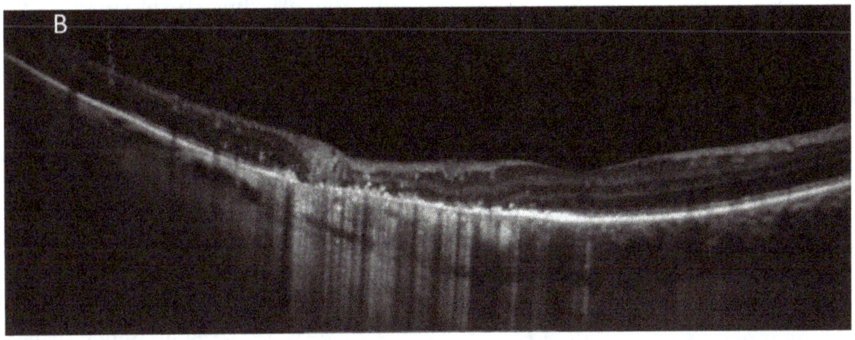

(b)

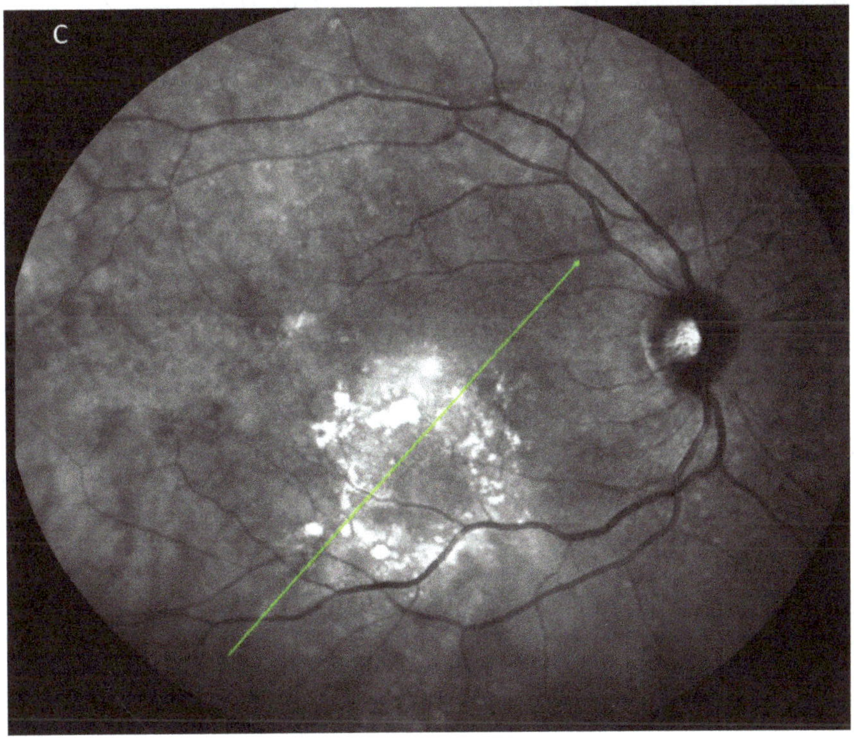

(c)

FIGURE 3: One month after photodynamic therapy. (a) Repeated OCT over the central macula (as seen in Figure 2(a)) showing complete resolution of the serous macular detachment. Some incomplete RPE and outer retinal atrophy (iRORA) are seen temporally along with irregularity and thickening of the RPE in the foveal region. (b, c) Coupled IR and OCT showing complete resolution of the choroidal mass under the inferior vascular arcade, with a broad complete RPE and retinal atrophy (cRORA) and subsidence of the inner retinal layers. No choroidal layer could be seen on this site. Green line (c) represents the axial orientation of the OCT scan in (b).

Photodynamic therapy is a nonthermal laser modality primarily employed in the treatment of vascular diseases, through light activation of the photosensitizing agent verteporfin. This therapy may also be employed in the treatment of ocular tumors through induction of necrosis and apoptosis, damage to the intratumoral vasculature, and local inflammatory reaction [38]. vPDT seems to be more effective in treating retroequatorial tumors with low to moderate exudative symptoms and with a thickness less than 3 mm and diameter less than 10 mm. Lesions that are too thick might not be eligible for vPDT, since the wavelength (689 nm) of the laser used will not penetrate the entire tumor. Moreover, visual acuity seems to improve after vPDT probably due to the decrease of subretinal fluid [39].

There have been sporadic reports of vPDT for choroidal metastasis secondary to other sites, such as the breast, with good results [40–43]. In this study, we reported on a patient with presumed choroidal metastasis secondary to colorectal cancer who showed an excellent response after one session of vPDT. Due to the severity of the primary metastatic disease and the lack of effective therapies to eliminate the presumed metastatic lesions in the macula without considerable collateral damage, after a comprehensive discussion with the patient, we decided to employ vPDT as a palliative measure to assure useful vision to this patient's only seeing eye.

In addition to vPDT, other reports discussed intravitreal bevacizumab for local therapy of a choroidal mass. Intravitreal treatment might be a good therapeutic option for patients with a metastatic disease as it preserves the quality of life without reducing clinical effectiveness. Mathis et al. suggested beginning with a single dose followed by a monthly as-needed regimen [39]. It could be proposed for multimetastatic patients under systemic chemotherapy with short life expectancy, as it improves or preserves the vision in most cases without time-consuming treatment. Furthermore, unlike vPDT, this treatment can be given in cases of exudative or large tumors. In summary, local therapy of choroidal metastasis due to CRC may provide ancillary support and a vision-saving treatment option.

Prognosis of patients with choroidal metastasis is usually not favorable. In many patients, metastatic disease may be found elsewhere, associated with a low survival rate. A high index of suspicion must be considered in choroidal masses of unknown systemic malignancies. Systemic control of colon carcinoma may aid in the ocular tumor regression.

In summary, we presented a case of a patient with presumed choroidal metastasis secondary to colon adenocarcinoma. Local vPDT therapy was performed with marked reduction of the subretinal mass and vision improvement. Choroidal metastasis secondary to CRC may be usually unilateral, with a single mass, and associated with advanced systemic spread of the disease.

Disclosure

None of the funders/sponsors had any role in the design and conduct of the study; collection, management, analysis, and interpretation of the data; preparation, review, or approval of the manuscript; and decision to submit the manuscript for publication.

Acknowledgments

This publication was supported by FAPESP (São Paulo, Brazil), CNPq (Brasília, Brazil), the Pan-American Association of Ophthalmology/Pan-American Ophthalmological Foundation, and the Paul Kayser/Retina Research Foundation Global Award (Pan-American Association of Ophthalmology/Pan-American Ophthalmological Foundation, Arlington, TX).

References

[1] L. G. van der Geest, J. Lam-Boer, M. Koopman, C. Verhoef, M. A. Elferink, and J. H. de Wilt, "Nationwide trends in incidence, treatment and survival of colorectal cancer patients with synchronous metastases," *Clinical & Experimental Metastasis*, vol. 32, no. 5, pp. 457–465, 2015.

[2] M. Riihimäki, A. Hemminki, J. Sundquist, and K. Hemminki, "Patterns of metastasis in colon and rectal cancer," *Scientific Reports*, vol. 6, no. 1, article 29765, 2016.

[3] M. Qiu, J. Hu, D. Yang, D. P. Cosgrove, and R. Xu, "Pattern of distant metastases in colorectal cancer: a SEER based study," *Oncotarget*, vol. 6, no. 36, pp. 38658–38666, 2015.

[4] P. J. Ostriker, "Metastasis of adenocarcinoma of colon to conjunctival surface of lid," *Archives of Ophthalmology*, vol. 57, no. 2, pp. 279–281, 1957.

[5] J. Y. Ha, E. H. Oh, M. K. Jung, S. E. Park, J. T. Kim, and I. G. Hwang, "Choroidal and skin metastases from colorectal cancer," *World Journal of Gastroenterology*, vol. 22, no. 43, pp. 9650–9653, 2016.

[6] M. D. Cole and N. B. Farah, "The choroid–an unusual site for metastasis in patients with adenocarcinoma of the rectum–a case report," *European Journal of Surgical Oncology*, vol. 11, no. 3, pp. 275–278, 1985.

[7] P. Linares, C. Castanon, S. Vivas et al., "Bilateral choroidal metastasis as the initial manifestation of a rectal cancer," *Journal of Gastroenterology and Hepatology*, vol. 19, no. 6, pp. 726-727, 2004.

[8] C. L. Shields, R. J. Welch, K. Malik et al., "Uveal metastasis: clinical features and survival outcome of 2214 tumors in 1111 patients based on primary tumor origin," *Middle East African Journal of Ophthalmology*, vol. 25, no. 2, pp. 81–90, 2018.

[9] C. L. Shields, J. A. Shields, N. E. Gross, G. P. Schwartz, and S. E. Lally, "Survey of 520 eyes with uveal metastases," *Ophthalmology*, vol. 104, no. 8, pp. 1265–1276, 1997.

[10] E. Van Cutsem, B. Nordlinger, R. Adam et al., "Towards a pan-European consensus on the treatment of patients with colorectal liver metastases," *European Journal of Cancer*, vol. 42, no. 14, pp. 2212–2221, 2006.

[11] D. A. August, R. T. Ottow, and P. H. Sugarbaker, "Clinical perspective of human colorectal cancer metastasis," *Cancer Metastasis Reviews*, vol. 3, no. 4, pp. 303–324, 1984.

[12] R. Nookala, V. V. Batchu, H. M. Lee, A. Loghmani, and G. S. Chhabra, "Difficult Diagnosis of Colon Adenocarcinoma Metastasis to Retina: A case report and literature review," *International journal of hematology-oncology and stem cell research*, vol. 10, no. 3, pp. 186–190, 2016.

[13] L. Ma, N. Wolkow, and F. A. Jakobiec, "Choroidal mucinous metastatic adenocarcinoma from the colon: a diagnostic challenge," *Ocular Oncology and Pathology*, vol. 5, no. 1, pp. 66–74, 2019.

[14] M. García-Fernández, J. Castro-Navarro, A. Saiz-Ayala, and C. Álvarez-Fernández, "Orbital metastases in colorectal

cancer: a case report," *Archivos de la Sociedad Española de Oftalmología*, vol. 87, no. 7, pp. 216–219, 2012.

[15] E. B. Ludmir, S. J. McCall, B. G. Czito, and M. Palta, "Radiosensitive orbital metastasis as presentation of occult colonic adenocarcinoma," *Case Reports*, vol. 2014, article bcr2014206407, 2014.

[16] E. M. Hobdy, T. E. Ciesielski, and S. Kummar, "Unusual sites of colorectal cancer metastasis," *Clinical Colorectal Cancer*, vol. 3, no. 1, pp. 54–57, 2003.

[17] G. L. Wang, M. Y. Wang, and W. B. Wei, "Clinical features and treatment of choroidal metastasis," *Zhonghua Yan Ke Za Zhi*, vol. 45, no. 3, pp. 229–233, 2009.

[18] P. A. Schneider and C. Bosshard, "Metastasis from the colon to the choroid (author's transl)," *Klinische Monatsblätter für Augenheilkunde*, vol. 172, no. 4, pp. 513–516, 1978.

[19] M. R. Khawaja, J. T. Minturn, A. J. Spittler, and E. G. Chiorean, "Ocular metastasis of colorectal cancer: an uncommon presentation of a common malignancy," *Hematology/Oncology and Stem Cell Therapy*, vol. 8, no. 4, pp. 176–180, 2015.

[20] C. L. Shields, J. F. McMahon, H. T. Atalay, M. Hasanreisoglu, and J. A. Shields, "Retinal metastasis from systemic cancer in 8 cases," *JAMA Ophthalmology*, vol. 132, no. 11, pp. 1303–1308, 2014.

[21] S. Tano, H. Hayashi, and S. Momoeda, "Metastasis of rectal carcinoma to the choroid: a case report," *Nihon Ganka Kiyo*, vol. 40, pp. 1284–1288, 1989.

[22] M. Shinjo, "Iridochoroidal carcinoma metastatic from the cecum," *Rinsho Ganka*, vol. 44, pp. 23–26, 1990.

[23] H. Endo, T. Tajika, H. Takebayashi, H. Shiota, M. Yoshida, and E. Kudo, "A case report of choroidal metastasis from rectal cancer," *Ganka Rinsho Iho*, vol. 91, p. 1141, 1997.

[24] H. Nakamura, A. Harada, T. Sakakibara, T. Ishikawa, T. Yaguchi, and Y. Murakami, "Metastatic choroidal tumor from cancer of the ascending colon-A case report," *Nihon Rinsho Geka Gakkai Zasshi (Journal of Japan Surgical Association)*, vol. 63, no. 4, pp. 1031–1035, 2002.

[25] T. Fujiwara, S. Machida, K. Murai, Y. Tazawa, Y. Baba, and O. Shimooki, "A case of choroidal tumor metastasized from rectal cancer," *Ganka*, vol. 46, pp. 1099–1103, 2004.

[26] R. B. Hisham, H. Thuaibah, and Y. A. Gul, "Mucinous adenocarcinoma of the rectum with breast and ocular metastases," *Asian Journal of Surgery*, vol. 29, no. 2, pp. 95–97, 2006.

[27] H. Sashiyama, Y. Abe, S. Sasagawa et al., "A case of choroidal metastasis from rectal cancer manifesting visual loss as the initial recurrence symptom," *The Japanese Journal of Gastroenterological Surgery*, vol. 43, no. 7, pp. 746–751, 2010.

[28] E. Miyake, M. Moriwaki, T. Sunada, and J. Takemura, "Regression of choroidal metastasis from rectal cancer following chemotherapy," *Atarashii Ganka (J Eye)*, vol. 29, pp. 701–704, 2012.

[29] A. P. Ferry and R. L. Font, "Carcinoma metastatic to the eye and Orbit," *Archives of Ophthalmology*, vol. 92, no. 4, pp. 276–286, 1974.

[30] N. C. Charles, D. D. Ng, and C. I. Zoumalan, "Signet cell adenocarcinoma of the rectum metastatic to the orbit," *Ophthalmic Plastic and Reconstructive Surgery*, vol. 28, no. 1, pp. e1–e2, 2012.

[31] M. Tei, M. Wakasugi, and H. Akamatsu, "Choroidal metastasis from early rectal cancer: case report and literature review," *International Journal of Surgery Case Reports*, vol. 5, no. 12, pp. 1278–1281, 2014.

[32] C. J. Lin, K. H. Li, J. F. Hwang, and S. N. Chen, "The effect of intravitreal bevacizumab treatment on choroidal metastasis of colon adenocarcinoma–case report," *Eye*, vol. 24, no. 6, pp. 1102-1103, 2010.

[33] A. Maudgil, K. S. Sears, P. A. Rundle, I. G. Rennie, and S. M. Salvi, "Failure of intravitreal bevacizumab in the treatment of choroidal metastasis," *Eye*, vol. 29, no. 5, pp. 707–711, 2015.

[34] S. D. Ward, B. J. Byrne, M. C. Kincaid, and E. S. Mann, "Ultrasonographic evidence of a mushroom-shaped choroidal metastasis," *American Journal of Ophthalmology*, vol. 130, no. 5, pp. 681-682, 2000.

[35] R. J. Kennedy, W. D. Rummel, J. L. McCarthy, and J. B. Hazard, "Metastatic carcinoma of the retina; report of a case and the pathologic findings," *Archives of Ophthalmology*, vol. 60, no. 1, pp. 12–18, 1958.

[36] C. W. Spraul, G. E. Lang, H. E. Grossniklaus, and G. K. Lang, "Metastatic adenocarcinoma to the retina in a patient with Muir-Torre syndrome," *American Journal of Ophthalmology*, vol. 120, no. 2, pp. 248–250, 1995.

[37] R. S. Apte, C. Dibernardo, J. R. Pearlman et al., "Retinal metastasis presenting as a retinal hemorrhage in a patient with adenocarcinoma of the cecum," *Archives of Ophthalmology*, vol. 123, no. 6, pp. 850–853, 2005.

[38] E. Cerman and O. Çekiç, "Clinical use of photodynamic therapy in ocular tumors," *Survey of Ophthalmology*, vol. 60, no. 6, pp. 557–574, 2015.

[39] T. Mathis, P. Jardel, O. Loria et al., "New concepts in the diagnosis and management of choroidal metastases," *Progress in Retinal and Eye Research*, vol. 68, pp. 144–176, 2018.

[40] S. Kaliki, C. L. Shields, S. A. Al-Dahmash, A. Mashayekhi, and J. A. Shields, "Photodynamic therapy for choroidal metastasis in 8 cases," *Ophthalmology*, vol. 119, no. 6, pp. 1218–1222, 2012.

[41] D. H. Ghodasra and H. Demirci, "Photodynamic therapy for choroidal metastasis," *American Journal of Ophthalmology*, vol. 161, pp. 104–109.e2, 2016.

[42] P. Soucek and I. Cihelkova, "Photodynamic therapy with verteporfin in subfoveal choroidal metastasis of breast carcinoma (a controlled case)," *Neuro Endocrinology Letters*, vol. 27, no. 6, pp. 725–728, 2006.

[43] V. Isola, A. Pece, and L. Pierro, "Photodynamic therapy with verteporfin of choroidal malignancy from breast cancer," *American Journal of Ophthalmology*, vol. 142, no. 5, pp. 885–887, 2006.

18

Conjunctival Tarsal Actinic Keratosis Treated with Interferon Alfa-2b: A Rare Case Report and Literature Review

Mónica Gimeno-Carrero,[1] María-Jesús Suárez-Fernández,[1] Beatriz Alonso-Martín,[1] Almudena de-Pablo-Cabrera,[1] María-Concepción Garrido-Ruíz,[2] and Enrique Mencía-Gutiérrez[1]

[1]*Ophthalmology Department, 12 de Octubre Hospital, Complutense University, 28041 Madrid, Spain*
[2]*Pathology Department, 12 de Octubre Hospital, Complutense University, 28041 Madrid, Spain*

Correspondence should be addressed to Enrique Mencía-Gutiérrez; emencia.hdoc@salud.madrid.org

Academic Editor: Cristiano Giusti

Conjunctival neoplasia is one of the most frequent tumors in the eye. Actinic keratosis (AK) or solar keratosis is a precancerous lesion that is included with other epithelial tumors. This alteration does not break the basal membrane. There is enough evidence of successful outcomes to consider interferon alfa-2b (IFN alfa-2b) as the first choice of treatment for this type of tumors. In addition, side effects are mild and uncommon. We report a case in an 83-year-old woman who was referred to evaluate a leukoplakia in the tarsal conjunctiva of the lower left eyelid that measured 1 cm in diameter. Pathological study revealed AK. After the INF alfa-2b treatment, we observed conjunctival hyperemia, noninfiltrated upper nasal de-epithelization, and inferior nasal bulla. AK with presentation in conjunctiva is rarely described and in tarsal conjunctiva is exceptional. It is the first case published with only tarsal conjunctiva affectation.

1. Introduction

Actinic keratosis (AK) or solar keratosis is a hyperkeratotic plaque-like lesion (leukoplakia) with defined borders and squamous surface (it is a premalignant lesion because it includes dysplasia keratinocytes). It is frequent in the elderly population and in the light skin since its main risk factor is sun exposure [1]. Due to that fact the presentation in the tarsal conjunctiva is very unusual [2], the tarsal conjunctiva is not directly exposed to ultra violet (UV) radiation, the usual etiological cause of its development. Yearly AK to squamous cell carcinoma progression rates of 0-6% have been reported [3].

Individuals with Fitzpatrick type I or II (I-VI) skin characteristics, such as fair skin, freckles, light-colored eyes (blue or green), and blonde or red hair, are more likely to develop AKs, as they are more sensitive to damage from chronic sun exposure [4].

Interferons are a set of glycoproteins identified in 1957 and produced naturally by the body for their antiviral, antiproliferative, and immunomodulatory properties [5]. To achieve tumor remission, surgical treatment with wide free margins has been performed classically, followed by cryotherapy at the base of the lesion [6]. However, the recurrence rate is high because of the difficulty of achieving noninfiltrated margins.

In addition, the surgical procedure involves a higher cost and causes greater stress and trauma to the patient [5]. Topical treatment with IFN alfa-2b has been shown to have excellent results, so the use of topical treatments like INF alfa-2b is becoming widespread.

The use of topical INF alfa-2b is considered safe, effective, and generally well tolerated. However, side effects due to its systemic absorption have been found. These include flu-like symptoms, migraine or fatigue, and others due to its topical use such as follicular conjunctivitis, conjunctival injection, or superficial punctate keratitis [6–8]. All of them usually remit spontaneously within one month after treatment completion. None of the aforementioned adverse effects constitutes a sufficient reason to discontinue treatment. Few cases affecting the conjunctiva have been published [9], one only with conjunctival eyelid margin involvement [2] and none localized on the tarsal conjunctiva.

2. Case Presentation

An 83-year-old female referred from the outpatient clinic for a leukoplakia measuring 1 cm in its wide diameter on the tarsal conjunctiva of the lower eyelid of the left eye (Figure 1). The patient had not had prolonged exposure to the sun during her life. She had no history of skin cancer. She was not immunosuppressed. An incisional biopsy of the lesion was sent to the pathology department. The results showed acanthosis with epidermal hyperplasia and slight papillomatosis and hypergranulosis in superficial layers (Figure 2). Focal keratinocyte atypia was observed (Figures 3(a) and 3(b)). A diagnosis of presumed conjunctival AK was made. Treatment with INF alfa-2b one million IU/ml eye drops every 6 hours was started. After one month, the lesion had practically disappeared entirely, so IFN alfa-2b treatment was changed to 1 drop every 12 hours for 15 days and 1 drop every 24 hours for another 15 days (Figure 4). However, the patient came to the emergency room 15 days later presenting conjunctival hyperemia, noninfiltrated upper nasal circular de-epithelization, and inferior nasal bulla (Figures 5(a) and 5(b)); thus, discontinuation of interferon was decided. After 5 days without the INF alfa-2b treatment, the clinical picture was almost resolved, with complete disappearance of the conjunctival hyperemia, near-complete superior nasal reepithelization, and marked reduction of the inferior nasal bulla, with complete disappearance of the symptoms after one month (Figure 6). Follow-up after 18 months showed no recurrence of the lesion or the adverse event that had occurred.

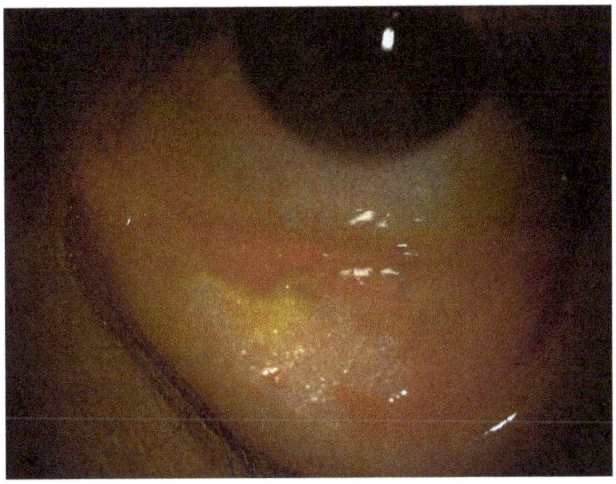

FIGURE 1: Image with the presence of a leukoplakia measuring 1 cm in length on the lower left eyelid tarsal conjunctiva.

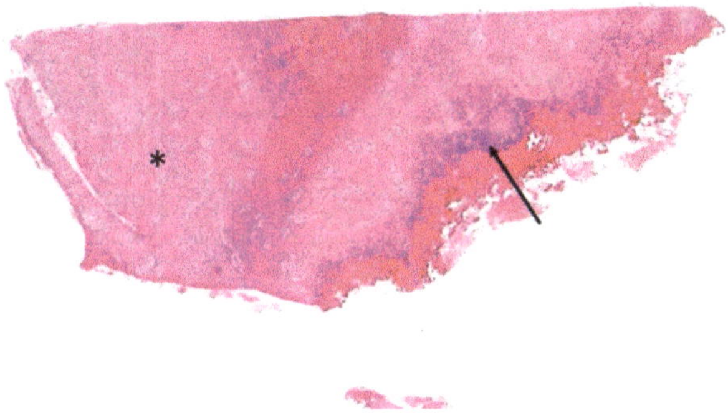

FIGURE 2: Conjunctival tarsal biopsy fragment showing acanthosis with epidermal hyperplasia (asterisk) and slight papillomatosis and hypergranulosis in superficial layers (arrow). Hematoxylin and Eosin, 4x magnification.

3. Discussion

AK (premalignant lesion) is described as neoplastic transformation and proliferation of keratinocytes within the epidermis that does no breach the basal membrane [1]. The histopathology of the keratotic plaque shows acanthosis of the epithelium and keratinization of the conjunctival epithelium and parakeratosis. The AK shows a similar histopathologic aspect with prominent keratosis and usually appears as a chronic inflammation. It must be treated due to the risk of developing SCC. Since they represent the initial stage in the evolution of SCC, recognition and treatment are important. Clinically conjunctival AK and intraepithelial neoplasia (IEN) are indistinguishable. Histopatologically conjunctival AK occurs as a localized, minimally aggressive lesion confined to the surface epithelium. Conjunctival IEN is characterized by a partial-thickness replacement of the surface epithelium by anaplastic epithelial cells that lack normal maturation [1]. They account for less than 1% of conjunctival lesions [1]. Although the most important cause is direct UV radiation exposure, other risk factors have been described: fair skin, advanced age, exposure to carcinogens, immunosuppression, and genetic conditions [10].

To achieve tumor remission, surgical treatment with wide free margins has been performed classically, followed by cryotherapy at the base of the lesion [6]. However, because of the difficulty of achieving noninfiltrated margins, the recurrence rate was high. In addition, the surgical procedure involves a higher cost and causes greater stress and trauma to the patient [5]. In this case, due to the location and size of the lesion, surgical treatment would have required a long and complex procedure with high risk of complications and several follow-up visits, and the result would probably have been nonesthetic, with a worse quality of life. Chemotherapy with

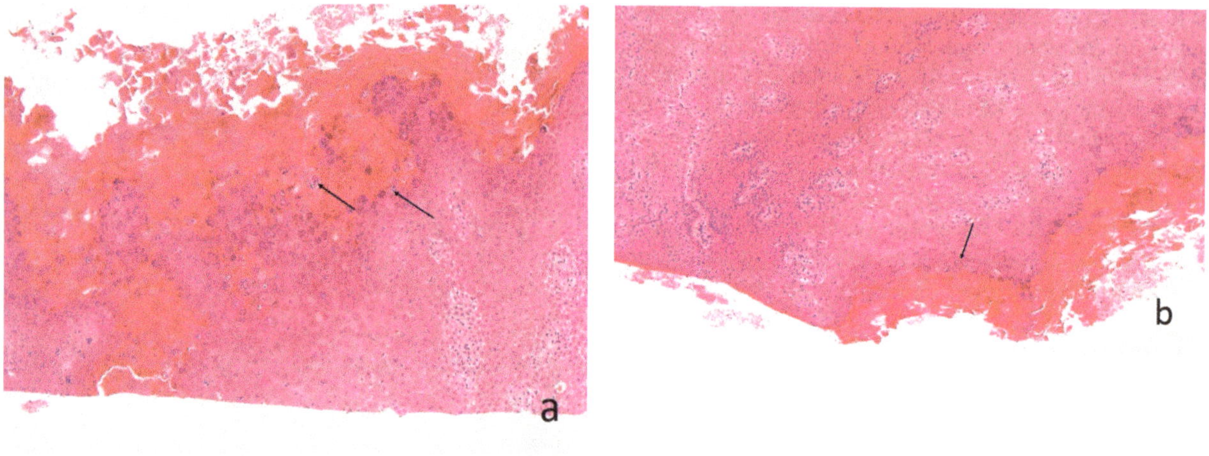

(a) (b)

FIGURE 3: (a, b) Keratinocyte atypia is observed focally (arrows). Hematoxylin and Eosin, 10x magnification.

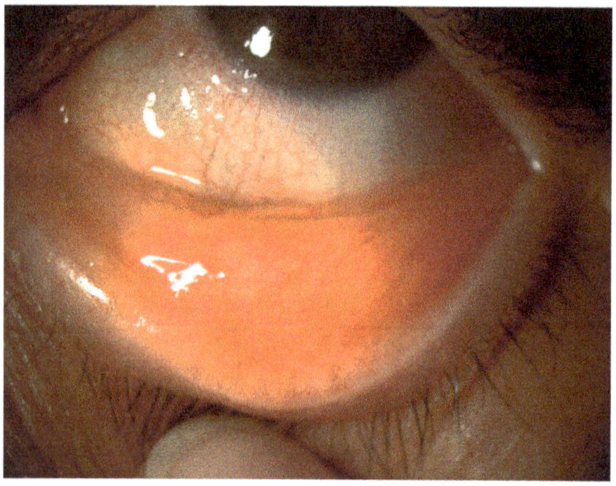

FIGURE 4: One month after the start of the treatment, the lesion has disappeared in the left eye.

INF alfa-2b eye drop treatment was chosen due to its proven effectiveness and despite being an expensive treatment [9]. Topical treatment with IFN alfa-2b has been shown to have excellent results, equal to or greater than those found with surgical excision. Because of these factors, the use of topical treatments like INF alfa-2b is becoming widespread.

The use of topical INF alfa-2b is considered safe, effective and generally well-tolerated. However, side effects due to its systemic absorption have been found; these include flu-like symptoms, migraine and fatigue; other side effects are due to its topical use, and include follicular conjunctivitis, conjunctival injection or superficial punctate keratitis [6–8]. All of them usually remit spontaneously within one month after treatment completion. None of the aforementioned adverse effects constitutes a sufficient reason to discontinue treatment [2]. The commonly used dose is 1 million IU/ml four times per day, as the dose of 3 million IU/ml four times per day has not demonstrated superiority in tumor eradication [7].

The use of topical interferon achieves a higher resolution rate than the use of surgery plus cryotherapy of the base of the lesions, due to the difficulty of completely resecting the lesion without leaving infiltrated borders. In addition, the convenience of topical versus surgical treatment has led to its becoming a widely used treatment nowadays [5]. Not rebiopsy was performed due to the total clinical disappearance of the lesion after topical treatment with INF alfa-2b. After more than 18 months of follow-up, there has been no recurrence. So, it is highly unlikely that remains of the AK exist, since they usually recur with great frequency when that is the case.

Adverse effects due to systemic absorption in the case of the topical administration of the drug are rare, although flu-like and fever conditions are described [7].

Alternatively, topical chemotherapeutic agents, 5-fluoracil, mitomycin C, imiquimod, photodynamic therapy, igenol mebutate, and diclofenac, have been effective [11].

It should be noted that there are no reported cases in the literature of the side effects such as those found in our patient, upper infiltrated upper nasal circular epithelialization and lower nasal congestion, and that these signs decreased drastically within 5 days of cessation of interferon exposure, and the patient was fully recovered from the previously described lesions within one month.

Few cases affecting the conjunctiva have been published [12], only one with conjunctival eyelid margin involvement [2] and none localized on the tarsal conjunctiva.

4. Conclusions

Conjunctival AK lesions are scarcely reported in the literature. They are premalignant lesions with the presence of dysplastic keratinocytes. The etiology is due to UV

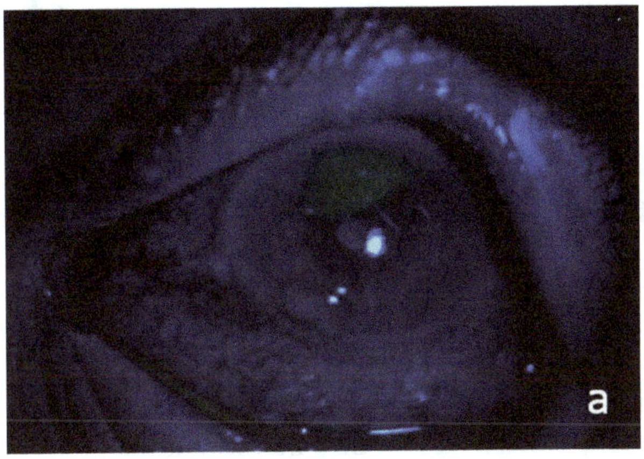

(a)

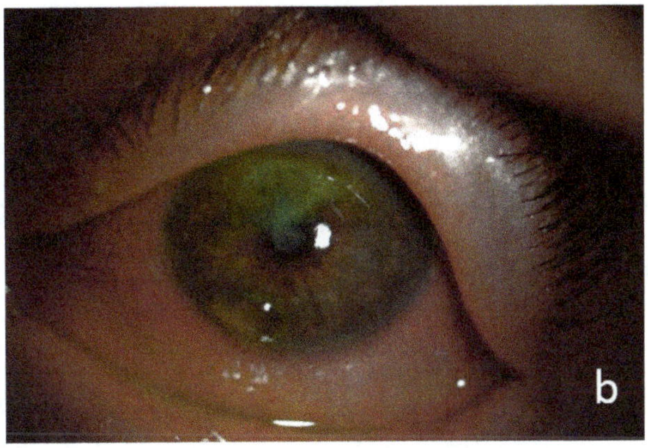

(b)

FIGURE 5: Slit-lamp image of the left eye with conjunctival hyperemia, noninfiltrated upper nasal de-epithelization, and inferior nasal bulla. (a) Image with fluorescein staining and blue filter and (b) image with white light.

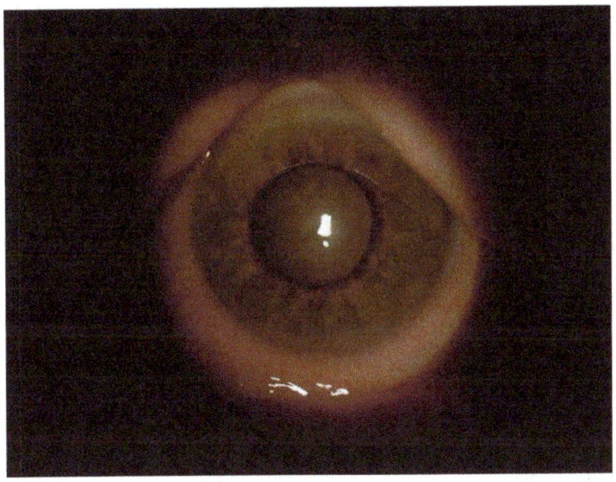

FIGURE 6: Slit-lamp image of the left eye five days after the cessation of alfa-2b interferon therapy with almost complete disappearance of the signs.

radiation in elderly patients. The treatment of choice is excision with clearance of margins to avoid possible transformation in SCC. Other treatments have been described in the conjunctiva, such as INF alfa-2b, as in this case report. The form of presentation in the tarsal conjunctiva is not described to this day.

Consent

Consent for the publication of ophthalmic images was obtained from the patient.

References

[1] J. A. Shields and C. L. Shields, *Eyelid conjunctival and orbital tumors. An Atlas and Textbook*, Philadelphia: Lippincott Williams & Wilkins, 2nd edition, 2008.

[2] S. Khan and M. Chak, "A rare presentation of actinic keratosis affecting the tarsal conjunctiva and review of literature," *Case Reports in Ophthalmological Medicine*, vol. 2018, Article ID 4375354, 2018.

[3] T. L. Diepgen and V. Mahler, "The epidemiology of skin cancer," *British Journal of Ohthalmology*, vol. 146, Supplement 61, pp. 1–6, 2002.

[4] R. Rossi, M. Mori, and T. Lotti, "Actinic keratosis," *International Journal of Dermatology*, vol. 46, no. 9, pp. 895–904, 2007.

[5] B. A. Schechter, A. Schrier, R. S. Nagler, E. F. Smith, and G. E. Velasquez, "Regression of presumed primary conjunctival and corneal intraepithelial neoplasia with topical interferon alpha-2b," *Cornea*, vol. 21, no. 1, pp. 6–11, 2002.

[6] A. A. Nanji, C. S. Moon, A. Galor, J. Sein, P. Oellers, and C. L. Karp, "Surgical versus medical treatment of ocular surface squamous neoplasia: a comparison of recurrences and complications," *Ophthalmology*, vol. 121, no. 5, pp. 994–1000, 2014.

[7] B. A. Schechter, A. F. Koreishi, C. L. Karp, and W. Feuer, "Long-term follow-up of conjunctival and corneal intraepithelial neoplasia treated with topical interferon alfa-2b," *Ophthalmology*, vol. 115, no. 8, pp. 1291–1296.e1, 2008.

[8] C. L. Shields, S. Kaliki, H. J. Kim et al., "Interferon for ocular surface squamous neoplasia in 81 Cases," *Cornea*, vol. 32, no. 3, pp. 248–256, 2013.

[9] H. Endo, S. Kase, Y. Suzuki, and M. Kase, "Coincidence of inflamed conjunctival carcinoma in situ and primary pterygium," *Case Reports in Ophthalmology*, vol. 7, no. 3, pp. 208–212, 2017.

[10] J. Anwar, D. A. Wrone, A. Kimyai-Asadi, and M. Alam, "The development of actinic keratosis into invasive squamous cell carcinoma: evidence and evolving classification schemes," *Clinics in Dermatology*, vol. 22, no. 3, pp. 189–196, 2004.

[11] P. W. Hashim, T. Chen, D. Rigel, N. Bhatia, and H. Kircik, "Actinic keratosis: current therapies and insights into new treatments," *Journal of Drugs in Dermatology*, vol. 18, no. 5, pp. s161–166., 2019.

[12] M. A. Rowlands, J. N. Giacometti, J. Servat, M. A. Materin, and F. Levin, "Topical imiquimod in the treatment of conjunctival actinic keratosis," *Ophthalmic Plastic and Reconstructive Surgery*, vol. 33, no. 1, pp. e21–e23, 2017.

19

Clinical Presentation and Management Strategies in Intraorbital Foreign Bodies

Samreen Khanam, Ayushi Agarwal, Ruchi Goel, Neha Rathie, Akash Raut, Shweta Raghav, Sumit Kumar, Mohit Chhabra, Sonam Singh, and Sushil Kumar

Guru Nanak Eye Centre, Maulana Azad Medical College, New Delhi, India

Correspondence should be addressed to Ayushi Agarwal; ayushiagarwal.2110@gmail.com

Academic Editor: Nicola Rosa

The authors present a retrospective, observational case study of seven patients, who presented with retained Intra-Orbital Foreign Bodies (IOrbFBs) following penetrating orbital injury at a tertiary eye hospital over a period of one year. Cases were reviewed for epidemiological features, mechanism of injury, nature of foreign body, clinical features, imaging modality, associated complications, management outcomes, and the final prognosis. The mean age of presentation was 27.43 years. Amongst the seven patients, two were children (aged <10 years). The male : female ratio was 4 : 3. Of the seven retained IOrbFBs, two were plastic, two wooden, and three metallic in nature (one gunshot injury, one ball projectile (commonly referred to as BB) injury, and one with knife). Two out of seven had no light perception at presentation. The periocular location of the foreign bodies was inferior in 4 cases and medial in 3 cases. Computed Tomography scan confirmed the diagnosis in five cases and Magnetic Resonance Imaging (MRI) was diagnostic in one. Surgical intervention was done in five cases, and two cases were managed conservatively. The authors conclude that favourable outcome can be achieved even without surgical removal in cases of inert metallic/inorganic IOrbFBs. The properties of plastic FBs can frequently render them invisible on imaging, or they may mimic chronic inflammatory conditions like tuberculosis. Long-standing wooden IOrbFBs evade identification radiologically due to prolonged hydration. The ultimate choice of intervention must be individualised, weighing the risks of retention against the risk of iatrogenic damage.

1. Introduction

Ocular trauma is a significant cause of blindness all over the world. Approximately 16% cases of orbital trauma are associated with a foreign body [1]. Intra-Orbital Foreign Bodies (IOrbFBs), though commonly encountered in routine ophthalmology practice, may have unusual presentations. They may occasionally accompany trivial trauma, such as in children while playing. The diagnosis and management of IOrbFBs are often a conundrum for most ophthalmologists. For a better understanding, the authors present their experience of seven cases of retained IOrbFBs and discuss their presentations as well as diagnostic and management dilemmas.

2. Methods

This is a retrospective analysis of seven patients, diagnosed with retained IOrbFBs following penetrating injury, who presented to a tertiary eye hospital in New Delhi, India, between December 2018-19. The epidemiological characteristics, clinical features, mechanism of injury, nature of foreign body, diagnostic imaging, associated complications, management outcome, and the long-term prognosis were evaluated.

3. Results

Seven patients diagnosed with IOrbFB were studied (Table 1). The mean age of presentation was 27.43 years.

Table 1: Summary of clinical profile and management outcomes of cases with IOrbFBs.

No.	Age/sex	Nature of FB (location)	Mode of injury	Time between injury and presentation	Presenting features	Investigation	BCVA	Treatment/ surgical findings	Status at last follow-up (duration)
1	4 y/M	Plastic FB (medial extending up to the apex)	Trauma while playing with pen	5 months	Right: Chronic discharging sinus at the medial canthal region with orbital cellulitis	CT: linear nonmetallic foreign body extending up to the posterior orbit. MRI: not done. Culture: *Staphylococcus aureus*	OD: not following light. Fundus suggestive of optic atrophy OS: following light. Refraction suggestive of hyperopia (+5D)	Intravenous antibiotics given Surgical removal of the 30 mm × 3 mm plastic FB done	OD: not following light EOM OU: full and free Discharging sinuses with orbital cellulitis resolved (5 months)
2	10 y/M	Plastic FB (inferior orbit, extending up to the apex)	Trauma while playing with pen	10 days	OD: traumatic superior orbital fissure syndrome with traumatic optic atrophy Entry wound seen 6 mm below the right lower lid margin	Initial CT inconclusive Repeat CT: nonmetallic linear IOrbFB (24 × 5 mm) between the floor and IR extending from the mid orbit to SOF, abutting the ipsilateral optic nerve MRI: FB extending up to the orbital apex abutting the optic nerve associated with right orbital floor fracture and fat herniation	OD: NLP OS: 20/20	Intravenous steroids given for TON Patient refused surgery in view of guarded visual prognosis	BCVA: OD NLP OS: 20/20 EOM OU: full and free Ptosis resolved Fundus OD: optic atrophy (10 months)
3	27 y/F	Metallic FB (inferior)	Gunshot	3 hours	OD: vitreous hemorrhage and limitation of movement in upgaze OS: circumferential limbal perforation with uveal tissue prolapse with NLP	CT: metallic FB in relation to the right orbital floor in close proximity to the IR along with a fracture of the right orbital floor, lateral wall, and medial wall. Comminuted fracture of frontal bone along with roof, medial wall, and floor of the left orbit. MRI: not done	OD: 20/200 OS-NLP	OD: surgery deferred Conservative management done OS: evisceration	BCVA: OD 20/40 OS: prosthetic eye EOM OD: full and free No significant enophthalmos noted (1 year)
4	30 y/M	Metallic FB (medial)	BB injury	6 hours	Referred for ophthalmic evaluation in view of BB injuries at multiple sites. Asymptomatic with entry wound at left glabellar area	CT: metallic FB in the anterior orbit adjacent to the medial rectus	OU: 20/20	Surgical exploration done. Intraoperative canalicular injury noted. Repair with silicon intubation done. FB could not be retrieved intraoperatively. Postoperative CT suggestive of posterior migration. No further surgical intervention done	Asymptomatic OU: 20/20 EOM OU: full and free Syringing: patent (6 months)

Table 1: Continued.

No.	Age/sex	Nature of FB (location)	Mode of injury	Time between injury and presentation	Presenting features	Investigation	BCVA	Treatment/ surgical findings	Status at last follow-up (duration)
5	35 y/F	Wooden FB (anterior orbit extending up to the posterior orbit)	Undetermined	3 years	OS: diminution of vision associated with inferolateral swelling with limitation of extraocular movements in all gazes Left hypotropia with chemosis and congestion noted	CT: posterior orbital mass in the lateral half of posterior orbital fat. MRI: focal well-defined lesion in the posteroinferior aspect of the left orbit between LR and IR muscle with peripheral enhancement postcontrast suggestive of FB granuloma	OD: 20/20 OS: 5/200 PR accurate	Surgical exploration with histopathological examination A, 3.8 cm × 0.5 cm , wooden foreign body removed surgically	BCVA OU: 20/20 EOM OD: full and free OS: improvement in extraocular movements. Left hypotropia present. No diplopia seen Complete resolution of inflammatory signs (2 months)
6	36 y/F	Wooden FB (medial orbit)	Trauma while cutting wooden log	8 months	Left lower lid recurrent abscess Syringing patent	USG: inferior orbital abscess. CT/MRI: not done Culture: sterile	OU: 20/20	Surgical exploration: abscess drainage done. FB found and removed. Postoperative MRI showed no evidence of IOrbFB	BCVA OU: 20/20 EOM OU: full and free Complete resolution of signs and symptoms (1 year)
7	50 y/M	Metallic FB (inferior orbit)	Physical assault with a knife	1 day	OD: pain with entry wound 7-8 mm below the right lower lid margin OS: mature cataract	X-ray and NCCT orbit: suggestive of a linear metallic FB running along the right orbital floor	OD: 20/20 OS: PL positive PR accurate	Successful surgical removal of the linear foreign body (knife) OS: cataract surgery done a few days later	BCVA OD: 20/20 OS: 20/20 (8 months)

FB: foreign body; BCVA: best-corrected visual acuity; EOM: extraocular muscles; NLP: no light perception; CT: computed tomography; MRI: magnetic resonance imaging; PR: projection of rays; IR: inferior rectus; LR: lateral rectus.

Amongst the seven patients, two were children (aged <10 years). The male : female ratio was 4 : 3. Of the seven retained IOrbFBs, two were plastic foreign bodies, two wooden, and three metallic in nature (one gunshot injury, one ball projectile (commonly referred to as BB) injury, and one injury with knife). The time of presentation varied from as early as three hours to a delayed presentation of three years. Only one of these patients was asymptomatic with a Best-Corrected Visual Acuity (BCVA) of 20/20 whereas one of them was diagnosed as Traumatic Orbital Apex Syndrome (TOAS) with a retained posterior foreign body (FB) and no light perception (NLP). Surgical intervention was recommended in six patients. The periocular location of the foreign body was inferior in 4 cases and medial in 3 cases. Three patients presented with features of inflammation including discharging sinuses. Traumatic optic neuropathy was seen in two patients (cases 1 and 2). Initial Computed Tomography (CT) scan could confirm the diagnosis in five cases whereas in one case, a repeat scan was helpful. MRI was diagnostic in one case (Figure 1).

3.1. Illustrative Case 1. A 4-year-old male patient presented with features of orbital inflammation, impaired motility, and relative afferent pupillary defect (RAPD) in the right eye. Fundoscopy was suggestive of right optic atrophy. The left eye was unremarkable. A history of trauma to the right eye, while playing with a pen 5 months prior to presentation, was present. A provisional diagnosis of orbital cellulitis was made, and the patient was started on broad-spectrum antibiotics (linezolid 10 mg/kg IV q8 hr, metronidazole 10 mg/kg IV q8 hr and ceftriaxone 50 mg/kg IVq12 hr). Purulent discharge, sent for culture and sensitivity examination, from the superomedial aspect of the orbit was positive for *Staphylococcus aureus* and negative for AFB (Acid Fast Bacilli) staining. CT scan of the orbit was suggestive of soft tissue thickening with inflammatory changes more prominent in the extraconal, medial compartment of the right orbit. No abscess or foreign body could be identified. Empirical treatment resulted in clinical improvement. However, there was persistence of discharging sinus on the superomedial aspect of the right orbit. A review of the scan was requested, and a linear non-metallic FB running posteriorly along the medial orbital wall was identified. Surgical exploration was done, and a cylindrical plastic FB, measuring 30 mm × 3 mm, was successfully removed (Figure 2). The patient was continued on post-operative antibiotics. At 5-month follow-up, complete resolution of discharging sinuses and infection was achieved with no change in BCVA and fundoscopy.

3.2. Illustrative Case 2. A 10-year-old male presented with sudden diminution of vision in the right eye for the past six days, following trauma from a ballpoint pen while playing at home. On examination, the right eye had NLP. An entry wound, 6 mm below the right lower lid, was noted. Right EOMs were limited in all gazes with ptosis, accompanied by hypoesthesia along the right forehead and upper lid region. A grade II RAPD with disc pallor was noted in the right eye. The rest of the examination was unremarkable. Initial Non-Contrast Computed Tomography (NCCT) scan was inconclusive. A repeat scan revealed a nonmetallic linear FB, 24 mm × 5 mm, lying in the posterior orbit. It was extraconal, posteriorly reaching up to the superior orbital fissure (SOF), inferiorly lifting the inferior rectus belly, and abutting the ipsilateral optic nerve. Fracture of the right orbital floor with fat herniation was also visualised. Magnetic Resonance Imaging (MRI) orbit further confirmed the CT findings. A Flash-Visual Evoked Potential (VEP) showed prolonged latency and low P-wave amplitude in the right eye. A confirmatory diagnosis of right TOAS was made. The patient was advised surgical removal of the IOrbFB due to its compressive effects and the FB being a potential source of infection. However, the patient's family refused surgery in view of increased perioperative morbidity and possibility of no significant gain in vision. Complete resolution of ptosis with full and free EOMs in the right eye was seen at a follow-up of 10 months with no change in BCVA (Figure 3).

3.3. Illustrative Case 3. A 27-year-old female presented with painful swelling in both eyes. At presentation, she was disoriented to time, place, and person. Her husband gave a history of gunshot injury few hours back. On examination, circumferential limbal perforation with uveal tissue prolapse was noted in the left eye with no light perception (NLP). The right eye had lower lid swelling and a vision of 20/200 with vitreous hemorrhage and limited extraocular movements in upgaze. The patient was referred to the neurosurgery emergency department for adequate systemic management. NCCT scan of the head, orbit, and paranasal sinuses revealed a metallic density foreign body (suggestive of bullet) in relation to right orbital floor and in close proximity to the inferior rectus muscle with fat entrapment. It also showed fracture of the anterior and posterior wall of the frontal sinus, bilateral nasal bone and septum, and bilateral ethmoid along with fracture of the medial wall, lateral wall, and floor of the right orbit. Comminuted fracture of frontal bone on the left side involving the roof, medial wall, and floor of the left orbit was seen with no obvious entrapment of fat or muscle (Figure 4). The patient's left eye was eviscerated one day following presentation.

Her right eye was initailly planned for orbital floor reconstruction with foreign body removal.

A final visual acuity of 20/40 was, however, achieved with conservative management at one-year follow-up. Right extraocular movements were restored with no diplopia or significant enophthalmos.

3.4. Other Cases (Figure 1, Table 1)

3.4.1. Case 4. A 30-year-old male with BB injuries at multiple sites and an entry wound at the glabella presented for ophthalmic evaluation within six hours of injury. An NCCT scan was suggestive of a metallic FB in the anterior orbit, adjacent to the left medial rectus. On surgical exploration, the FB could not be retrieved, and a coexisting lower canalicular injury was repaired with silicon tube intubation. The postoperative CT scan was suggestive of posterior migration of the foreign body. No further intervention was attempted. The

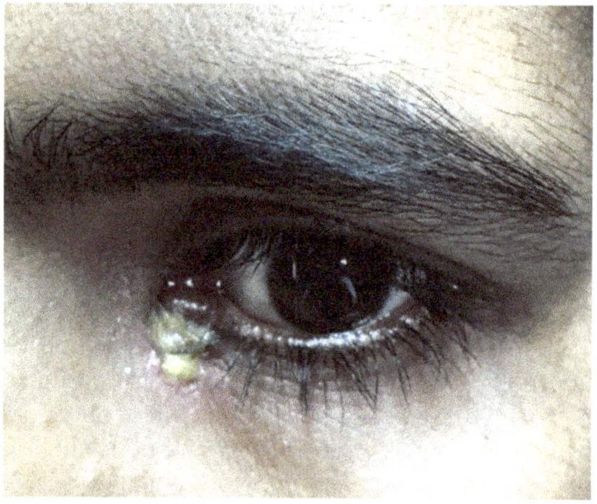

(a)

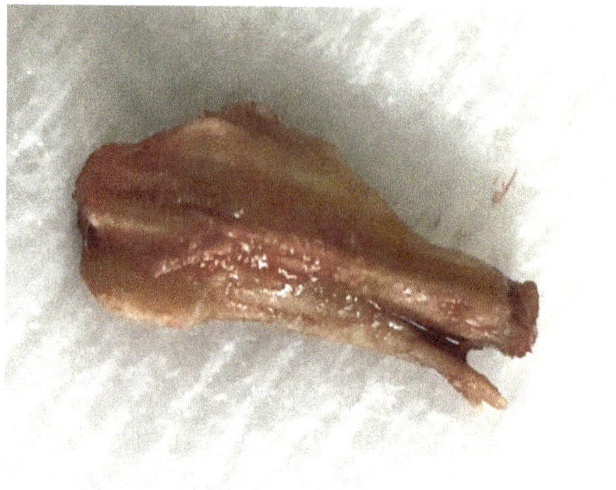

(b)

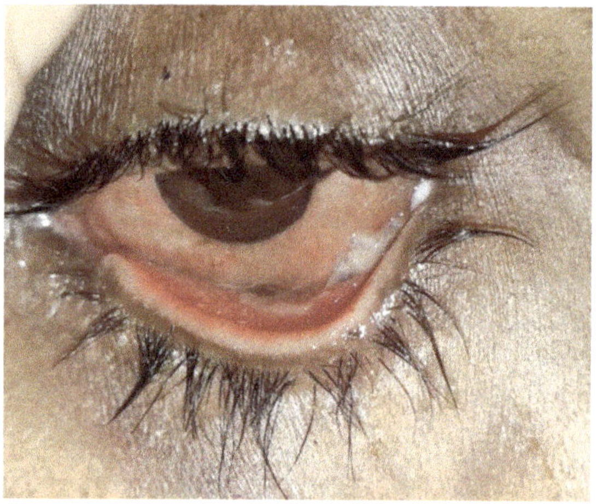

(c)

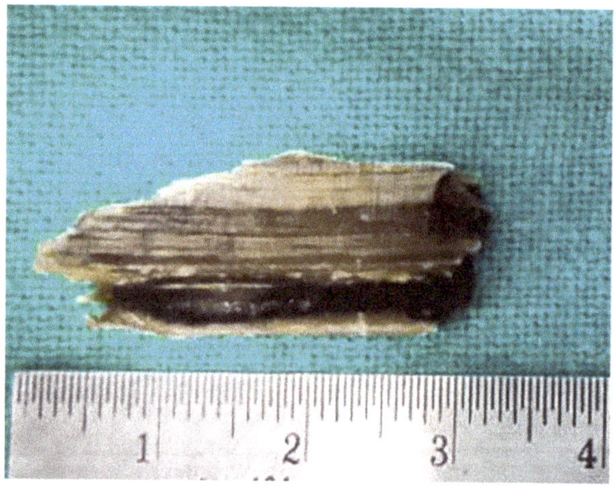

(d)

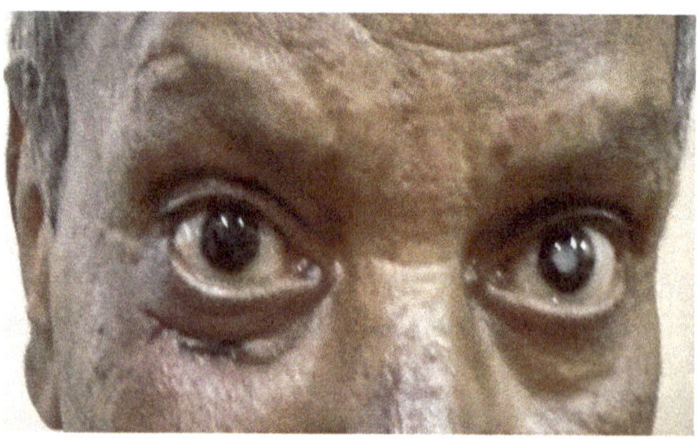

(e)

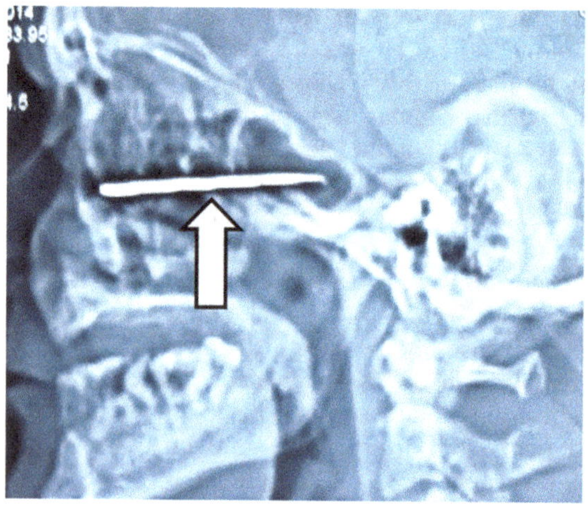

(f)

FIGURE 1: Continued.

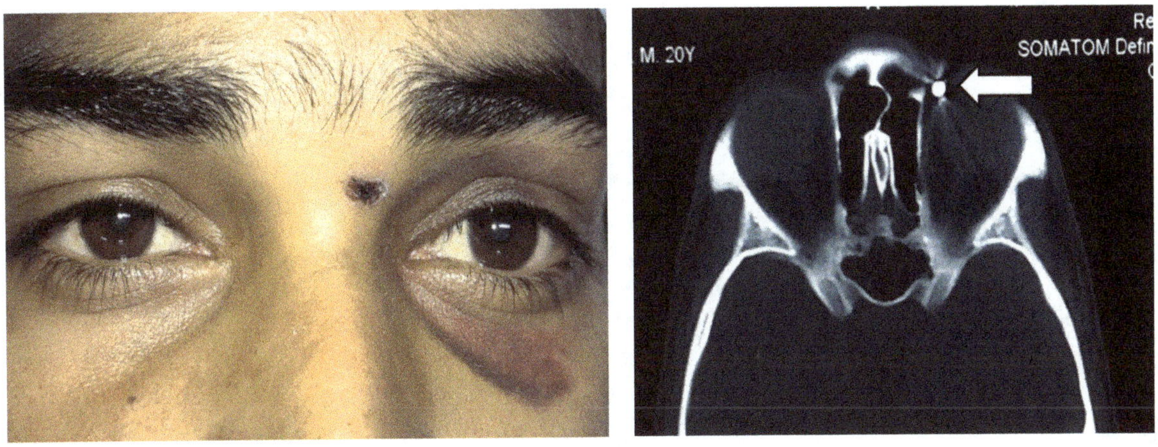

(g) (h)

Figure 1: (a) Clinical photograph showing purulent discharge in the left medial canthal area and (b) retrieved wooden IOrbFB in case 6. (c) Clinical image showing orbital inflammation and (d) retrieved wooden IOrbFB in case 5. (e) Clinical picture depicting an entry wound below the right lower lid and (f) radiological image showing a linear metallic foreign body along the orbital floor in case 7. (g) An entry wound in the glabellar region and (h) noncontrast CT orbit (axial view) suggestive of a metallic foreign body post-BB injury in case 4.

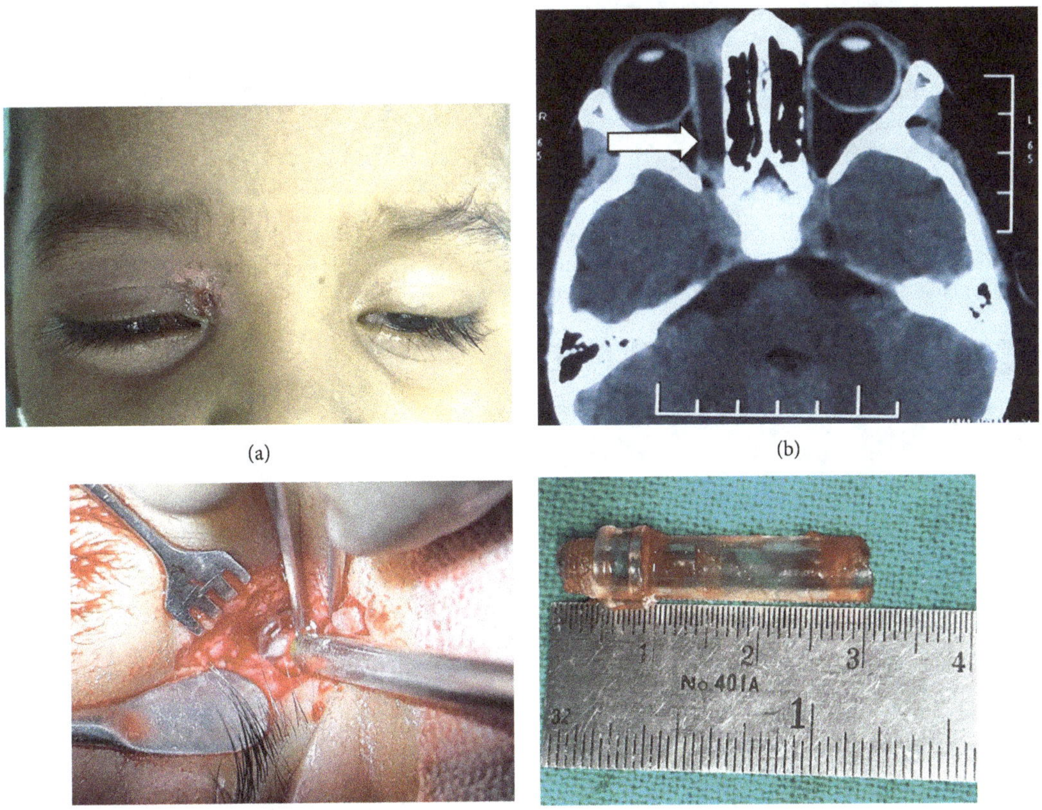

(a) (b) (c) (d)

Figure 2: Illustrative case 1: (a) preoperative photograph revealing chronic discharging sinus in the right superomedial region; (b) NCCT orbit suggestive of a linear nonmetallic foreign body along the right medial wall of the orbit (arrow); (c) surgical exploration was performed; (d) retrieved plastic foreign body.

BCVA was 20/20 OU, pre- as well as post-operatively. No extraocular motility limitations were seen.

3.4.2. Case 5. A 35-year-old female presented with intermittent pain, discharge, and swelling in the left eye for three years with acute exacerbation of symptoms for 15 days. On examination, the left eye was hypotropic with associated chemosis, congestion, and limited extraocular movements in all gazes. The BCVA was 20/20 OD and 5/200 OS. The patient was started on empirical antibiotic therapy. Imaging was

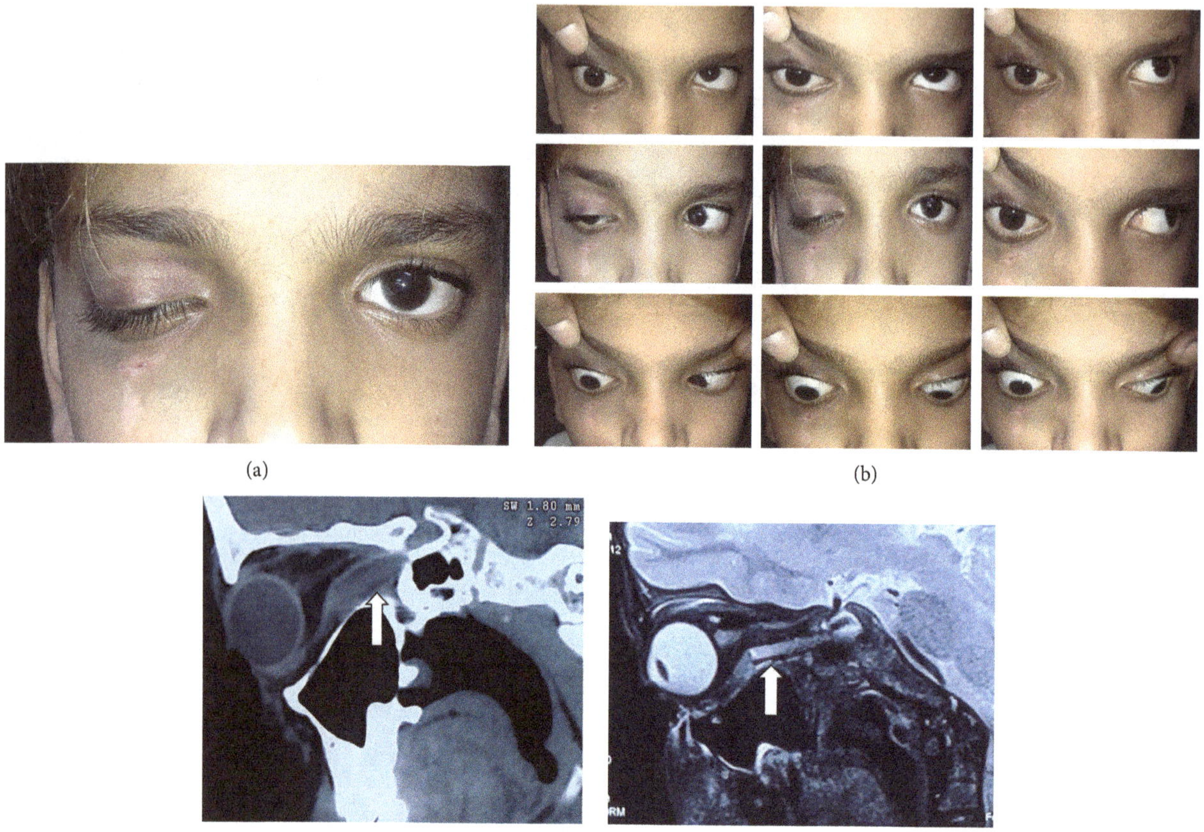

(a) (b) (c) (d)

Figure 3: Illustrative case 2: (a, b) clinical examination showing ptosis, limitation of right extraocular movements, and an entry wound below the right lower lid; (c) NCCT orbit and (d) MRI orbit, sagittal view, reveal a nonmetallic object extending up to the apex (white arrow).

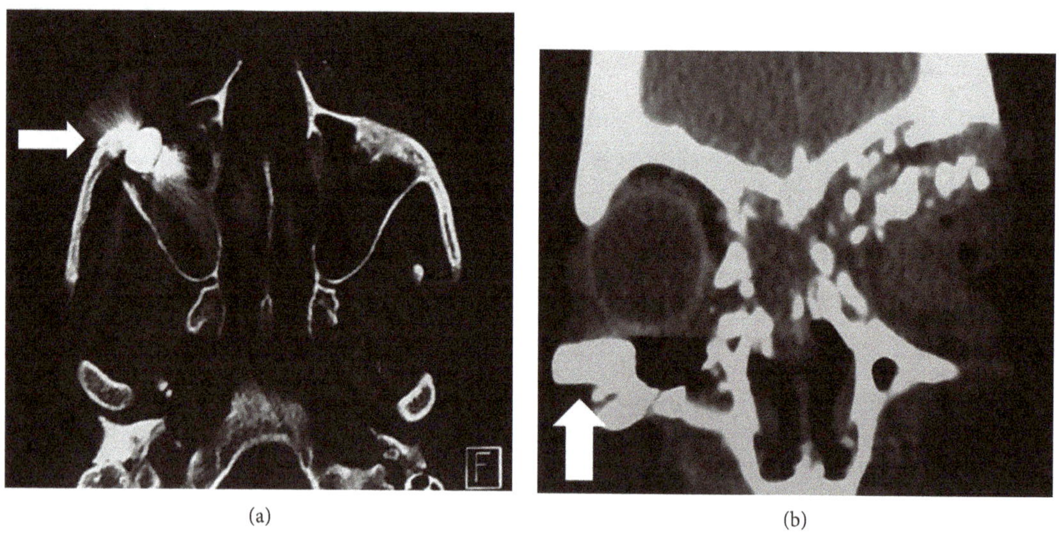

(a) (b)

Figure 4: NCCT orbit: (a) axial view showing metallic density foreign body (white arrow); (b) coronal view showing metallic density foreign body in relation to the right orbital floor and in close proximity to the inferior rectus muscle (white arrow).

suggestive of a well-defined lesion in the posterior aspect of the left orbit between lateral and inferior recti with post-contrast enhancement. On surgical exploration, a flat wooden IOrbFB (3.8 cm × 0.5 cm) was obtained. On further questioning, the patient vaguely recalled an episode of trauma to the left eye while cutting firewood 3 years back. After completion of antibiotic therapy, there was complete resolution of inflammation and improvement in extraocular motility in the left eye along with restoration of BCVA to 20/20 OU.

3.4.3. Case 6. A 36-year-old female presented with recurrent swelling in the left lower lid. There was an associated history of trauma to the left eye while cutting a wooden log 8 months back. The lacrimal apparatus was patent on syringing. Ultrasonography features were suggestive of left inferomedial orbital abscess. The abscess was drained surgically, and a wooden foreign body, measuring 2 cm × 1 cm × 0.3 cm, was retrieved.

3.4.4. Case 7. A 50-year-old male presented with a history of physical assault with a knife to the right eye 1 day back. There was an entry wound 7 to 8 mm below the right lower lid, and the BCVA was 20/20 OD. No impairment of ocular motility was seen. NCCT orbit was suggestive of a linear metallic IOrbFB running along the right orbital floor which was successfully removed with surgical intervention.

4. Discussion

Cases of trauma involving the orbit and periorbital region are commonly encountered in clinical settings. Both trivial and severe cases may be accompanied by a FB retained in the orbit. However, the diagnosis and management of a retained IOrbFB are frequently a challenging exercise for the treating ophthalmologist. In patients who present early, clinical suspicion and appropriate imaging may be conclusive in most cases. However, a late presentation with a vague history of trivial trauma can prove to be particularly difficult. Studies have documented a time lapse of up to 50 years [2]. In our study, the time of presentation of one patient was as late as 3 years.

The presenting features of IOrbFBs include clinical signs of orbital cellulitis, orbital hematoma, proptosis, impaired motility, diplopia, visual field loss, orbital abscess, optic neuropathy/atrophy, SOF syndrome, or TOAS. It is imperative to enquire about history of trauma in such patients. The most common presenting features in our series were the signs of orbital inflammation (swelling, pain, abscess, sinuses), impaired motility, and disc pallor. IOrbFBs can settle in the orbit via transocular route and can have concurrent intraocular foreign body along with vitreous hemorrhage, retinal/-choroidal detachment, uveitis, endophthalmitis, and panophthalmitis. The most interesting presentation in one of our cases was a plastic FB associated with chronic suppurative discharging sinus masquerading as a tuberculous osteomyelitis.

The nature of FB plays a decisive role in diagnosis and management. On the basis of composition, foreign bodies in the orbit can be metallic (iron, aluminium, lead), inorganic non-metallic (plastic, glass, rock, concrete), or organic (wood, thorns, bones) [3]. A plain X-ray film is helpful in detecting a metallic FB, except aluminium due to its relative radiolucency [4]. Ultrasonography (USG), being noninvasive and inexpensive, is considered the preferred imaging modality for initial evaluation, especially for anterior IOrbFBs. A meticulously performed standardized USG (combined A-scan and B-scan) can ascertain the nature and location of the foreign body and the presence of associated ocular damage [5, 6]. However, it requires expertise and detection can be difficult due to masking by surrounding inflammatory and fibroadipose tissue [7]. In fact, USG has not been shown to yield significant results in most reports [2] and there is a high possibility of missing IOrbFB, as can be seen in case 6, where the FB was discovered only during the incision and drainage of the abscess.

CT scan, a more readily available imaging modality with a shorter acquisition time, is the investigation of choice [8]. Thin axial and coronal views allow accurate localization of high-density FB like metal or glass. Identification of low-density objects such as wood can be challenging. The minimum size of FB that can be detected by CT scan is 0.3 mm for metal and 0.5 mm for glass. Imaging of intraorbital wooden FB (IOrbWFB) is quite complex and depends upon several factors like size, type, and hydration. Dry wood appears hypodense and can frequently be confused with entrapped air as both have similar densities. On the other hand, fresh wood appears isodense with fat, posing a diagnostic dilemma. Prolonged retention of wood may render it iso- or even hyperdense as imbibition of fluid and granulation both increase over a period of time, resulting in higher attenuation [9–13]. In one of our patients, (case 5), the presentation was delayed for three years and difficulty was encountered in identifying the wood on the basis of MRI scan. This may be ascribed to hydration over a period of time. It has been observed that specific parameters like 4000 HU (Hounsfield unit) width/400 HU level are more effective for detection of IOrbWFB, and radiologists should be requested for these settings where retained wood is suspected [14]. If an object that is less dense than water is suspected, the parameters should be set to a level of -500 HU and a window width of 1500 HU to distinguish it from air [14].

MRI is considered the investigation of choice for organic FBs. In cases with a definitive history of injury with organic matter, it may be considered as the initial investigation of choice. For all other situations, initial CT to rule out metallic FB is advisable. An MRI scan allows for better assessment of soft tissue damage. Unlike CT, wood is usually hypointense relative to intraorbital fat on both T1- and T2-weighted sequences and does not show gadolinium enhancement. In T1-weighted images (T1-WI), a wooden FB gives a more uniform signal and is more discernible as compared to T2-weighted imaging (T2-WI). The possibility of getting motion artefacts is also higher in T2-WI [15, 16].

In our study, CT scan helped to clinch the diagnosis in 5 patients while MRI was the diagnostic requirement in only one case of wooden FB. Two of our patients had plastic IOrbFBs, in whom diagnostic difficulties were encountered during imaging. Initially missed on CT, the FB was identified on subsequent scans. This may be attributed to the highly variable radiolucency of plastic. In some cases, plastic has been seen to resemble bone, while in others, it has mimicked air [14, 17].

All patients with retained IOrbFBs should be given anti-tetanus prophylaxis and broad-spectrum antibiotics. For wooden IOrbFBs, initiation of empirical antifungal therapy has been advocated, owing to the frequent polymicrobial nature of the associated infection [18]. The decision to

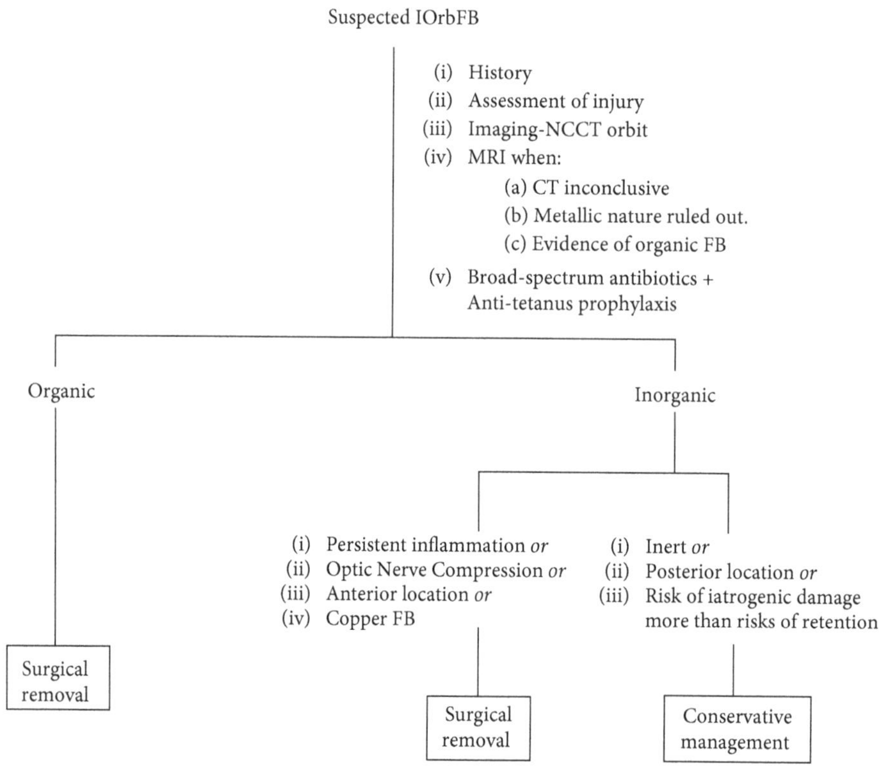

Note:

1. In case of organic FB, especially wood, post-operative check MRI to be considered to rule out residual fragments.
2. Follow-up necessary with patients of Iron IOrbFB till definitive surgery done.

Figure 5: Approach to an intraorbital foreign body (IOrbFB).

remove FB should be weighed against the risk of iatrogenic damage to the orbital structures. Retention of organic IOrbFB has a much higher rate of infection and inflammation than nonorganic IOrbFB and should be removed in all cases. Wooden IOrbFBs are notorious for fragmenting intraoperatively. One must be careful not to leave behind splinters/fragments in such cases. A postoperative MRI must be advised to look for residual fragments, thereby ensuring complete removal. Nonorganic IOrbFBs have a lower rate of infection, and the decision to remove must be based on their location and the associated complications. Anteriorly placed FBs are generally more easily removed. Metallic compounds containing copper can incite intense inflammatory reaction, and removal is, therefore, necessary. Iron-containing IOrbFBs may cause siderosis, and in cases where conservative management is chosen, the patient should be routinely assessed with electroretinography [19]. Removal of a metallic FB also eliminates the contraindication of MRI, if the latter is required in the future.

One patient in our study had injury with a BB pellet (case 4). It should be noted that orbital injury with a projectile metal such as a pellet or bullet can extend up to the cranial cavity. Shock waves from the projectile may cause chorioretinitis sclopetaria, even in the absence of direct trauma to the eyeball [20]. Air gun pellets are made of 0.5% antimony, while BB pellets are made of steel coated with zinc or copper. These are generally well-tolerated, as seen in our case. Bullets are heavier with faster velocities and are more likely to be associated with severe damage. Shots in shotguns are usually made of lead, and their retention in the orbit, theoretically, may cause lead poisoning, although any such case has not been reported [21].

Foreign objects at the orbital apex and those extending beyond the superior orbital fissure are frequently associated with optic neuropathy and permanent damage to the neurovascular structures. Owing to their proximity to the apex, they are likely to contribute to significant ocular morbidity. FBs at the apex may present as Superior Orbital Fissure syndrome (SOF), OAS, Cavernous Sinus Syndrome, or may be completely inert [22]. Surgical removal can be done via transcranial approach or a transnasal transethmoidal endoscopic approach that provides a safer and less invasive access to FBs lying in the extraconal medial compartment of the orbit [23]. There are no clear-cut guidelines for the management of posterior IOrbFBs. The authors believe that in cases where inorganic posterior IOrbFBs are inert, surgical retrieval can be deferred due to an increased risk of causing damage to the surrounding structures, including the vascular supply.

Thus, in all cases of suspected IOrbFB, detailed examination of the eye and appropriate imaging should be performed to evaluate the site, size and nature of the FB, and the resultant damage incurred. Patients with IOrbFBs must be well-informed regarding the choices and the prognosis. Ultimately, inputs from both the ophthalmologist as well as the patient are important for the final decision. In the present study, both conservative and surgical management strategies have been adopted in different situations and based on these experiences, the authors conclude that every case behaves uniquely, and a tailored approach should be adopted by the surgeon (Figure 5).

Consent

A well-written informed consent was obtained from all patients, along with approval of the institutional ethics committee. An explicit written consent regarding publishing the photographs was taken from all patients.

References

[1] A. M. Nasr, B. G. Haik, J. C. Fleming, H. M. Al-Hussain, and Z. A. Karcioglu, "Penetrating orbital injury with organic foreign bodies," *Ophthalmology*, vol. 106, no. 3, pp. 523–532, 1999.

[2] O. O. Adesanya and D. M. Dawkins, "Intraorbital wooden foreign body (IOFB): mimicking air on CT," *Emergency Radiology*, vol. 14, no. 1, pp. 45–49, 2007.

[3] T. P. Fulcher, A. A. McNab, and T. J. Sullivan, "Clinical features and management of intraorbital foreign bodies," *Ophthalmology*, vol. 109, no. 3, pp. 494–500, 2002.

[4] A. Al-Mujaini, R. Al-Senawi, A. Ganesh, S. Al-Zuhaibi, and H. Al-Dhuhli, "Intraorbital foreign body: clinical presentation, radiological appearance and management," *Sultan Qaboos University Medical Journal*, vol. 8, no. 1, pp. 69–74, 2008.

[5] A. B. Callahan and M. K. Yoon, "Intraorbital foreign bodies: retrospective chart review and review of literature," *International Ophthalmology Clinics*, vol. 53, no. 4, pp. 157–165, 2013.

[6] K. C. Ossoinig, F. Bigar, S. L. Kaefring, and L. McNutt, "Echographic detection and localization of BB shots in the eye and orbit," *Bibliotheca Ophthalmologica*, vol. 83, pp. 109–118, 1975.

[7] K. C. Ossoinig, "Detection of wood foreign bodies," *Ophthalmology*, vol. 98, no. 3, pp. 274-275, 1991.

[8] S. Taş and H. Top, "Intraorbital wooden foreign body: clinical analysis of 32 cases, a 10-year experience," *Turkish Journal of Trauma and Emergency Surgery*, vol. 20, no. 1, pp. 51–55, 2014.

[9] A. Pinto, L. Brunese, S. Daniele et al., "Role of computed tomography in the assessment of intraorbital foreign bodies," *Seminars in Ultrasound, CT, and MR*, vol. 33, no. 5, pp. 392–395, 2012.

[10] A. Uchino, A. Kato, Y. Takase, and S. Kudo, "Intraorbital wooden and bamboo foreign bodies: CT," *Neuroradiology*, vol. 39, no. 3, pp. 213–215, 1997.

[11] M. Czarnowska, D. Studniarek, D. Socha-Korybalska, and K. Raczyńska, "Ciało obce w oczodole–trudności diagnostyczne–opis przypadku," *Polish Journal of Radiology*, vol. 70, no. 3, pp. 86–89, 2005.

[12] A. R. Bhavsar, D. S. Fong, B. Kerman, and M. O. Yoshizumi, "Intraorbital air simulating an intraocular foreign body," *American Journal of Ophthalmology*, vol. 123, no. 6, pp. 835–837, 1997.

[13] K. S. Nadella and O. Bansal, "Retained intraorbital foreign body imaging!," *BMJ Case Reports*, vol. 13, no. 9, article e237302, 2020.

[14] F. Mirzaei, F. Salehpour, G. Shokuhi, T. Asvadi Kermani, S. Salehi, and S. Parsay, "An unusual case of intra orbital foreign body; diagnosis, management, and outcome: a case report," *BMC Surgery*, vol. 19, no. 1, p. 76, 2019.

[15] Y. H. Kim, H. Kim, and E. S. Yoon, "Unrecognized intraorbital wooden foreign body," *Archives of Craniofacial Surgery*, vol. 19, no. 4, pp. 300–303, 2018.

[16] L. M. Nagae, W. R. Katowitz, L. T. Bilaniuk, W. V. Anninger, and A. N. Pollock, "Radiological detection of intraorbital wooden foreign bodies," *Pediatric Emergency Care*, vol. 27, no. 9, pp. 895-896, 2011.

[17] Z. P. Joos, L. G. Longenecker, and B. C. Patel, "Orbital foreign body masquerading as orbital air," *Clinical & Experimental Ophthalmology*, vol. 44, no. 7, pp. 637–639, 2016.

[18] J. N. Jabang, L. Dampha, B. Sanyang, C. A. Roberts, and B. Ceesay, "Management of a large intraorbital wooden foreign body: case report," *Surgical Neurology International*, vol. 11, p. 158, 2020.

[19] A. N. Siedlecki, E. Tsui, J. Deng, and D. M. Miller, "Long-term retention of an Intraorbital metallic foreign body adjacent to the optic nerve," *Case Reports in Ophthalmological Medicine*, vol. 2016, Article ID 3918592, 3 pages, 2016.

[20] M. Al-Amry, H. Al-Taweel, N. Al-Enazi, M. Alrobaian, and S. Al-Othaimeen, "Retained periorbital and intracranial air-gun pellets causing sclopetaria and visual loss," *Saudi Journal of Ophthalmology*, vol. 28, no. 3, pp. 228–233, 2014.

[21] M. Finkelstein, A. Legmann, and P. A. Rubin, "Projectile metallic foreign bodies in the orbit: a retrospective study of epidemiologic factors, management, and outcomes," *Ophthalmology*, vol. 104, no. 1, pp. 96–103, 1997.

[22] S. Yeh and R. Foroozan, "Orbital apex syndrome," *Current Opinion in Ophthalmology*, vol. 15, no. 6, pp. 490–498, 2004.

[23] D. E. Montatixe, J. M. V. Aubá, Á. S. Barrueco, B. S. Guijarro, and C. C. Español, "Transnasal, transethmoidal endoscopic removal of a foreign body in the medial extraconal orbital space," *Case Reports in Otolaryngology*, vol. 2016, Article ID 1981456, 4 pages, 2016.

20

Chlamydia trachomatis Mimicking COVID-19 Chronic Follicular Conjunctivitis

Sukhmandeep Kaur[1], **Zachary Raphael Teibel**[2], **Nada Farhat**[3], **Adam Atoot**[4] **and Brett Bielory**[5]

[1]*Touro College of Osteopathic Medicine, Harlem, USA*
[2]*Department of Medicine, Hackensack Meridian Health Palisades Medical Center, USA*
[3]*Department of Pathology, Mount Sinai Health System, USA*
[4]*Department of Medicine, Hackensack Meridian Health Palisades Medical Center, Riverside Medical Group, USA*
[5]*Department of Ophthalmology, New York Eye and Ear infirmary of Mount Sinai School of Medicine, Hackensack University Medical Center, Riverside Medical Group, USA*

Correspondence should be addressed to Sukhmandeep Kaur; skaur10@student.touro.edu

Academic Editor: Maurizio Battaglia Parodi

Purpose. To characterize the clinical presentation and report lab findings of *Chlamydia trachomatis* follicular conjunctivitis in two patients with a positive history of active COVID-19 infection. *Participants.* Two patients with follicular conjunctivitis with a recent history of COVID-19 infection. *Design.* Retrospective, noncomparative, case report. *Methods.* Demographic data including age, gender, and place of residence were recorded. A full exam with an emphasis on inflammatory characteristics and systematic workup. Sample follicles were surgically excised in selected cases, and molecular and histopathological analyses were performed. *Results.* Both patients were initially treated for viral conjunctivitis. After symptoms failed to resolve, biopsy results indicated that both patients were positive for chlamydia conjunctivitis and treated accordingly. *Conclusions.* These cases illustrate the role of biopsy as an investigative tool in chronic conjunctivitis and the importance of having a broad differential when treating patients with acute conjunctivitis.

1. Background

The primary causes of conjunctivitis in the United States are viral and bacterial etiologies. The primary cause of viral conjunctivitis is adenovirus. Other viral culprits include *Picornaviruses*, *Herpesvirus*, *HIV*, and even *Coronavirus* [1]. Bacterial etiologies most commonly involve Gram-positive bacteria including *Staphylococcus aureus* or *Streptococcus pneumoniae*. Gram-negative bacterial conjunctivitis is generally more severe, less common, and generally attributable to *Haemophilus influenzae* and *Moraxella Catarrhalis*.

Conjunctivitis symptom onset can be hyperacute, acute, or chronic, with 4 weeks being the cutoff for an acute classification. Patients generally present with a combination of eye redness, irritation, photophobia, blurred vision, and tearing with or without purulence. Ophthalmologists further categorize conjunctivitis as follicular or papillary depending on physical exam findings.

In Western countries, *C. trachomatis* infection affects 5-20% of sexually active adults. Transmission is via autoinoculation from genital secretions or eye-to-eye spread. Acute symptoms consist of unilateral or bilateral discharge and redness [2]. Patients present with preauricular lymphadenopathy, prominent follicles in the inferior fornix, or upper tarsal conjunctiva [3]. If left untreated, acute chlamydial conjunctivitis can become chronic, with scarring of the conjunctiva, xerosis, and entropion trichiasis [4]. Chlamydial conjunctivitis can be distinguished from other causes with

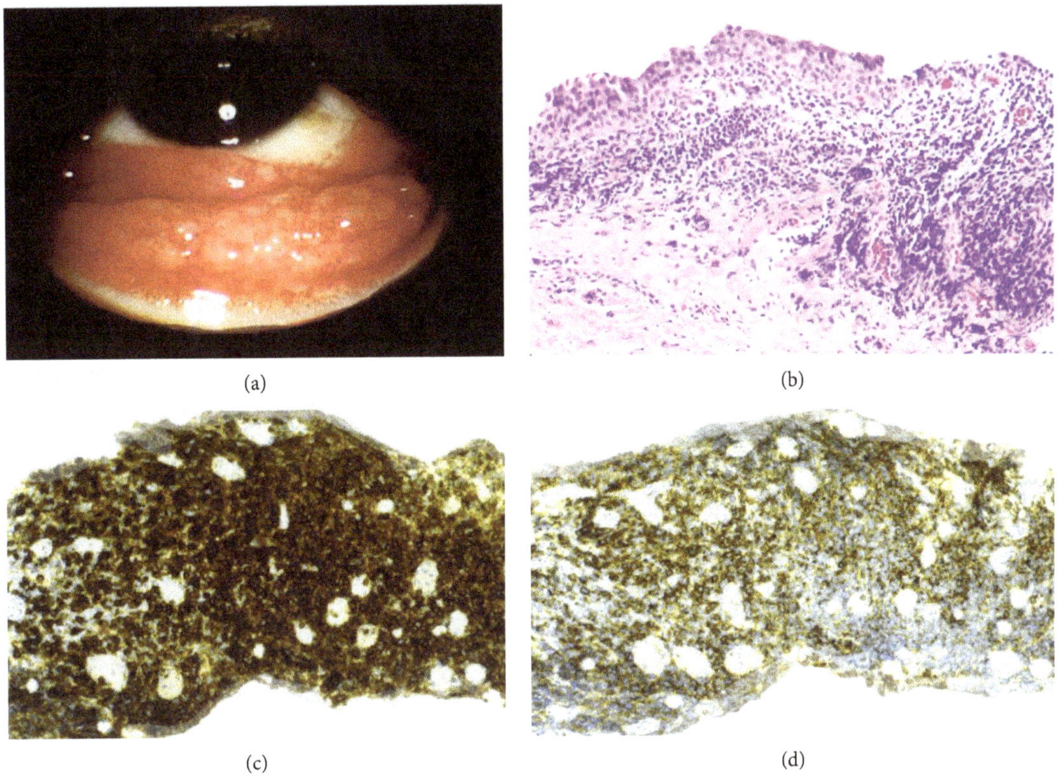

FIGURE 1: Clinical findings show prominent follicular reaction with conjunctival mucosa (a). Microscopically, a mixed chronic inflammatory infiltrate is seen within the subepithelium (b: H&E, 20x). Immunohistochemical studies highlight a mixture of B cells (c: CD20, 20x) and T cells (d: CD3; 20x).

nucleic acid amplification tests such as PCR or Giemsa staining of tarsal conjunctival scrapings [5].

Coronavirus conjunctivitis can be unilateral or bilateral and generally causes chemosis, watery discharge with or without systemic symptoms [6]. While *Adenovirus* is more common, the classification of COVID-19 as a pandemic by the World Health Organization (WHO) means it must be ruled out via RT-PCR and antibody testing before exploring other pathogens [7–9]. COVID-19-infected patients were found to contain Coronavirus RNA in their tears and conjunctival secretions [10, 11].

A study in China previously reported conjunctivitis in 0.8% COVID-19 patients (9 of 1099) [10]. COVID-19 penetrates into the conjunctiva the same way it does the lungs, using angiotensin-converting enzyme subtype 2 receptor on corneal epithelial cells via the assistance of heparan sulfate proteoglycan receptors [12]. If the condition persists without treatment, major complications such as punctate keratitis with subepithelial infiltrates, bacterial superinfection, conjunctival scarring, and symblepharon, severe dry eye, irregular astigmatism, corneal ulceration with persistent keratoconjunctivitis, corneal scarring, and chronic infection can occur [13]. Treatment includes supportive therapy such as cold compress, artificial tears, and antihistamines until the viral infection subsides.

2. Case Presentation

2.1. Case #1. A 25-year-old male presented with a 2-month history of bilateral eye redness, irritation, and tearing. One month prior to presentation, he was treated with a course of moxifloxacin eye drops but symptoms recurred 2 days thereafter. He had been diagnosed with COVID-19 using a nasopharyngeal specimen collected and analyzed via RT-PCR (LabCorp Inc., Raritan, NJ) in March 2020.

On exam, the patient had normal vision and intraocular pressure in both eyes and one 1.0 mm follicle on the right inferior tarsal of the right eye (OD) without discharge or injection. The left eye (OS) had one 1.5 mm follicle on the left inferior tarsal and ptosis of the left upper eyelid. There was bilateral bulbar and palpebral conjunctival injection.

Past medical history included a history of LASIK and genital herpes controlled with oral valacyclovir.

2.2. Case #2. A 19-year-old male presented with 1-month history of irritation and tearing in the left eye (OS) and redness in bilateral eyes (OU). The patient was initially treated with ciprofloxacin eye drops and erythromycin ointment, but his condition continued to worsen. He had been diagnosed with COVID-19 using a nasopharyngeal specimen collected and analyzed via RT-PCR. He had been diagnosed with COVID-19 via RT-PCR (Abbott Laboratories Inc., Lake Forest, IL) July 2020.

On exam, visual acuity was 20/60 bilaterally with normal intraocular pressure and bilateral redness of the bulbar conjunctiva. A prominent follicular reaction of the lower conjunctiva was seen, and superficial episcleral injection in both eyes without pain was noted (Figure 1).

Table 1: Patient-specific data that depicts coinfection of COVID-19 and chlamydia.

Pathogen tested	COVID-19	Chlamydia	HSV PCR	Adenovirus	Gonorrhea PCR
Case #1	Positive 3/2020	Positive 6/2020	Negative	Negative	Negative
Case #2	Positive 7/2020	Positive 8/2020	Positive 8/2020	Negative	Negative

Both patients had conjunctival biopsy and were tested for coinfections of chlamydia, HSV, adenovirus, and gonorrhea (Table 1). Biopsy of the left eye revealed benign epithelium with subepithelial tissue showing reactive lymphoid hyperplasia highlighted with B and T cell immunostains CD20 and CD3, respectively.

3. Diagnostics

3.1. Treatment. Both patients' symptoms resolved with a course of oral doxycycline and erythromycin.

3.2. Outcome and Follow-Up. Both patients recovered without recurrence or lasting visual complications. Of note, case 2 also had a biopsy-positive diagnosis of HSV and was started on a course of acyclovir.

4. Discussion

Viral and bacterial conjunctivitis often presents with many overlapping symptoms. Patients have redness, chemosis, and tearing. Physicians may be likely to attribute acute conjunctivitis to COVID-19 in patients with this as a preexisting diagnosis. However, like COVID-19, chlamydial conjunctivitis can also be spread via eye secretion and can also progress to a chronic form. Although supportive treatment is the current standard for COVID-19 conjunctivitis, chlamydia necessitates the use of oral antibiotics and, without proper treatment, it can cause conjunctival scarring, xerosis, and entropion trichiasis. As such, physicians must be cognizant of maintaining a broad differential for acute conjunctivitis in the post-COVID world [14].

5. Learning Points

(1) Consider tissue diagnosis via conjunctival biopsy when empiric therapy fails to resolve cases of acute or chronic conjunctivitis

(2) Secondary causes of conjunctivitis must be treated systemically along with assessing it from an ocular standpoint

Consent

This is a retrospective report that has no patient identifiable data included in this case report.

References

[1] J. Yannof and J. S. Duker, "Disorders of the conjunctiva and limbus," in *Ophthalmology*, pp. 397–412, Mosby, Spain, 2nd ed edition, 2004.

[2] A. A. Azari and N. P. Barney, "Conjunctivitis: a systematic review of diagnosis and treatment," *JAMA*, vol. 310, no. 16, pp. 1721–1729, 2013.

[3] J. J. Kanski and J. Menon, *Clinical Ophthalmology*, Butterworth-Heinemann, 2003.

[4] A. F. MacCallan, "Inclusion conjunctivitis," *The British Journal of Ophthalmology*, vol. 26, no. 6, pp. 271–275, 1942.

[5] J. Javaloy, C. Ferrer, M. T. Vidal, and J. L. Alió, "Follicular conjunctivitis caused by *Chlamydia trachomatis* in an infant Saharan population: molecular and clinical diagnosis," *The British Journal of Ophthalmology*, vol. 87, no. 2, pp. 142–146, 2003.

[6] S. Z. Scalinci and E. Trovato Battagliola, "Conjunctivitis can be the only presenting sign and symptom of COVID-19," *IDCases*, vol. 20, no. 774, article e00774, 2020.

[7] WHO, "Pandemic influenza preparedness and response: a WHO guidance document," in *The WHO pandemic phases*, vol. 4, World Health Organization, Geneva, 2009.

[8] WHO, "Director-General's opening remarks at the media briefing on COVID-19," 2020, https://www.who.int/dg/speeches/detail/who-direc tor-general-s-opening-remarks-at-the-media-briefing-on-covid-19%2D%2D-11-march-2020.

[9] WHO, "Update 27—one month into the global SARS outbreak: status of the outbreak and lessons for the immediate future," 2020, https://www.who.int/csr/sars/archive/2003_04_11/en/.

[10] L. Chen, M. Liu, Z. Zhang et al., "Ocular manifestations of a hospitalised patient with confirmed 2019 novel coronavirus disease," *British Journal of Ophthalmology*, vol. 104, no. 6, pp. 748–751, 2020.

[11] J. Xia, J. Tong, M. Liu, Y. Shen, and D. Guo, "Evaluation of coronavirus in tears and conjunctival secretions of patients with SARS-CoV-2 infection," *Journal of Medical Virology*, vol. 92, no. 6, pp. 589–594, 2020.

[12] S. K. Rao, H. N. Madhavan, P. Padmanabhan, G. S. Lakshmi, K. Natarajan, and D. Garg, "Ocular chlamydial infections. Clinicomicrobiological correlation," *Cornea*, vol. 15, no. 1, pp. 62–65, 1996.

[13] A. A. Panoutsopoulos, "Conjunctivitis as a sentinel of SARS-CoV-2 infection: a need of revision for mild symptoms," *SN Comprehensive Clinical Medicine*, vol. 2, no. 7, pp. 859–864, 2020.

[14] M. Thomas, "Upper respiratory tract infection. StatPearls. U.S. National Library of Medicine," 2020, https://www.ncbi.nlm.nih.gov/books/NBK532961/.

Commercial Cannabinoid Oil-Induced Stevens-Johnson Syndrome

Han Y. Yin,[1,2] **Nicholas Hadjokas**,[1] **Kanish Mirchia**,[3] **Robert Swan**,[1] **and Samuel Alpert**[1]

[1]*Department of Ophthalmology and Visual Sciences, SUNY Upstate Medical University, Syracuse, NY, USA*
[2]*Herbert Wertheim College of Medicine, Florida International University, Miami, FL, USA*
[3]*Department of Pathology, SUNY Upstate Medical University, Syracuse, NY, USA*

Correspondence should be addressed to Han Y. Yin; hhyin003@gmail.com

Academic Editor: Takaaki Hayashi

Purpose. To report an unusual presentation of commercial cannabidiol (CBD) oil-induced Stevens-Johnson Syndrome/toxic epidermal necrolysis (SJS-TEN). *Methods.* A 56-year-old woman presented with acute onset of a diffuse, blistering, maculopapular rash with over 30% total body surface area (BSA) involvement two days after taking CBD oil sublingually for chronic pain. Biopsy confirmed SJS-TEN. Ophthalmology was consulted and mild eye involvement was found. She was started on topical cyclosporine, prednisone, moxifloxacin, and erythromycin ointment to prevent progression, which was successful. She was otherwise treated with supportive therapy in the intensive care burn unit and ultimately passed away from septic shock. *Conclusion.* In this case, we described an unusual drug-induced SJS from a commercial, non-FDA-regulated cannabis product. The use of a commercial CBD product should be cautioned due to potential for series of drug reactions to the cannabis product and the risk for reaction to other unregulated other pharmacological components.

1. Background

Stevens-Johnson syndrome (SJS) and toxic epidermal necrolysis (TEN) are devastating mucocutaneous hypersensitivity reactions characterized by progressive severe exfoliative rash affecting mainly the skin and mucous membranes. Often, these are preceded by diffuse mucocutaneous tenderness and erythematous macules and blisters [1]. These two syndromes exist on a spectrum, with SJS involving less than 10% body surface area (BSA) and TEN involving greater than 30% BSA.

SJS-TEN have been reported in various age groups but occurs more frequently in females, HIV-infected patients, and the elderly. Common causes include medications including antibiotics and antiepileptics and infections such as mycoplasma; however, 50% of cases remain idiopathic [2]. The increased incidence in the elderly population is likely due to increased medication usage with age [3]. Drug hypersensitivity has been associated with genetic factors. In certain ethnic groups, medications like carbamazepine and allopurinol have a strong correlation with human leukocyte antigen- (HLA-) B*1502 and HLA-B*5801, respectively [4]. Unfortunately, the RegiSCAR study demonstrated that HLA-B*1502 is not a confirmatory marker for any of the high-risk drugs known to cause SJS-TEN in Europeans; so, these HLA markers cannot be used to confirm the diagnosis [2, 4].

Mortality rates for SJS-TEN range from 10 to 50%. Thus, prompt identification and discontinuation of the causative agent is vital. There have been reported cases of SJS from complementary and alternative products [5], but few from cannabis products. Cannabidiol (CBD) is one of the active ingredients of cannabis that stimulates cannabinoid receptors without causing psychotropic effects. It is currently being investigated for use in childhood epilepsy syndromes, anxiety, and chronic pain. Herein, we present an unusual case of drug-induced SJS from commercial CBD oil.

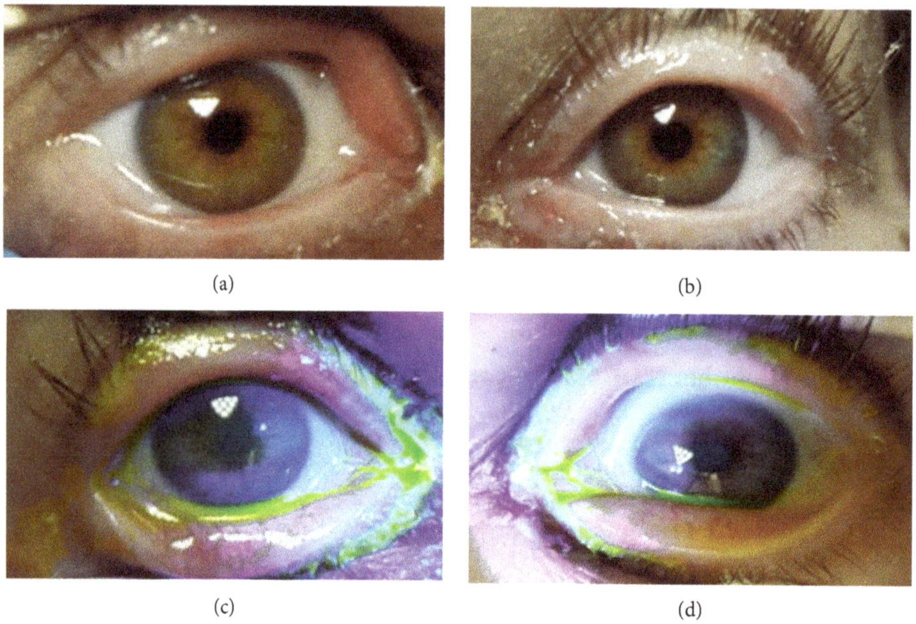

Figure 1: (a, b) External photo and (c, d) with fluorescein, without conjunctival injection, signs of pseudomembrane, or gross epithelial defect OU.

2. Case Report

A 56-year-old female with a past medical history of herniated disc with chronic pain, hypertension, and coronary artery disease presented to her local emergency room for diffuse vesicular rash and skin ulceration management. She denies prior history of dermatological rashes, or recent sick contacts, fever, or malaise prior to the onset of her symptoms. One week prior, she had tried a new liposomal CBD extract spray (Natural Native, Norman, Oklahoma, 73072) sublingually. Two days following the use of the new CBD product, she noticed a mild rash on her extremities, which was treated by her primary care physician with diphenhydramine and oral prednisone without improvement. Her symptoms progressed and she developed diffuse erythematous and vesicular rashes involving her entire body over the next 48 hours. She was transferred to a university hospital for a higher level of care. Her chronic outpatient medications for the past 5 years included famotidine, lisinopril-hydrochlorothiazide, and meloxicam. She had previously used other CBD products without any adverse effect.

On exam, she had diffuse erythematous macules and central necrosis with vesicles on her face. She had been experiencing crusting of the eyelashes and itching of the medial canthi, but she denied changes in vision and foreign body sensation. Her best corrected visual acuity was 20/20 with pinhole in both eyes, intraocular pressures were 16 in the right eye, 17 in the left eye, pupils were equal and briskly reactive without APD, and extraocular muscles were full. Her ophthalmic exam showed a maculopapular rash on the upper and lower eyelids without conjunctival injection, fibrin formation, or corneal epithelial defect in either eye (Figures 1(a)–1(d)). She had extensive oral mucosal ulceration (Figure 2(a)) and generalized erythematous macules and blisters with multiple ruptured bullae on her trunk and back (Figures 2(a) and 2(b)). In addition, she had extensive erythematous macules and central necrosis on all four extremities (Figures 3(a)–3(d)) along with urethral and labial involvement, totaling 30 percent BSA.

The patient was admitted to the burn intensive care service for presumed SJS-TEN and started on a wound care regimen and intravenous fluid. Her outpatient oral prednisone was discontinued in addition to all CBD products. She was started on topic cyclosporine drops OU.

BID, prednisolone OU QID for 1 week, and moxifloxacin OU QID for 1 week to prevent progression of ophthalmic involvement. Punch biopsy was obtained and was consistent with SJS (Figure 4). The patient expired about 1 month after initial presentation from septic shock.

3. Discussion

This case addresses some interesting considerations in the management and etiologies of SJS-TEN. Management usually consists of hospital admission, ideally with isolation in a burn unit to minimize potential hospital-acquired infections and provide supportive therapy including IV hydration for adequate nutrition. For drug-induced SJS-TENS, the offending agent is stopped immediately.

Medications for management of SJS-TEN at the acute stage are controversial. Some believe that T-cell-mediated immunologic responses are the cause of SJS-TEN and have consequentially administered high-dose glucocorticoids, cyclophosphamide, or cyclosporine as a means of arresting the progression of skin lesions [6]. These drugs, however, are of unproven benefit in the acute stage and may have systemic adverse effect when used at the chronic stage [7].

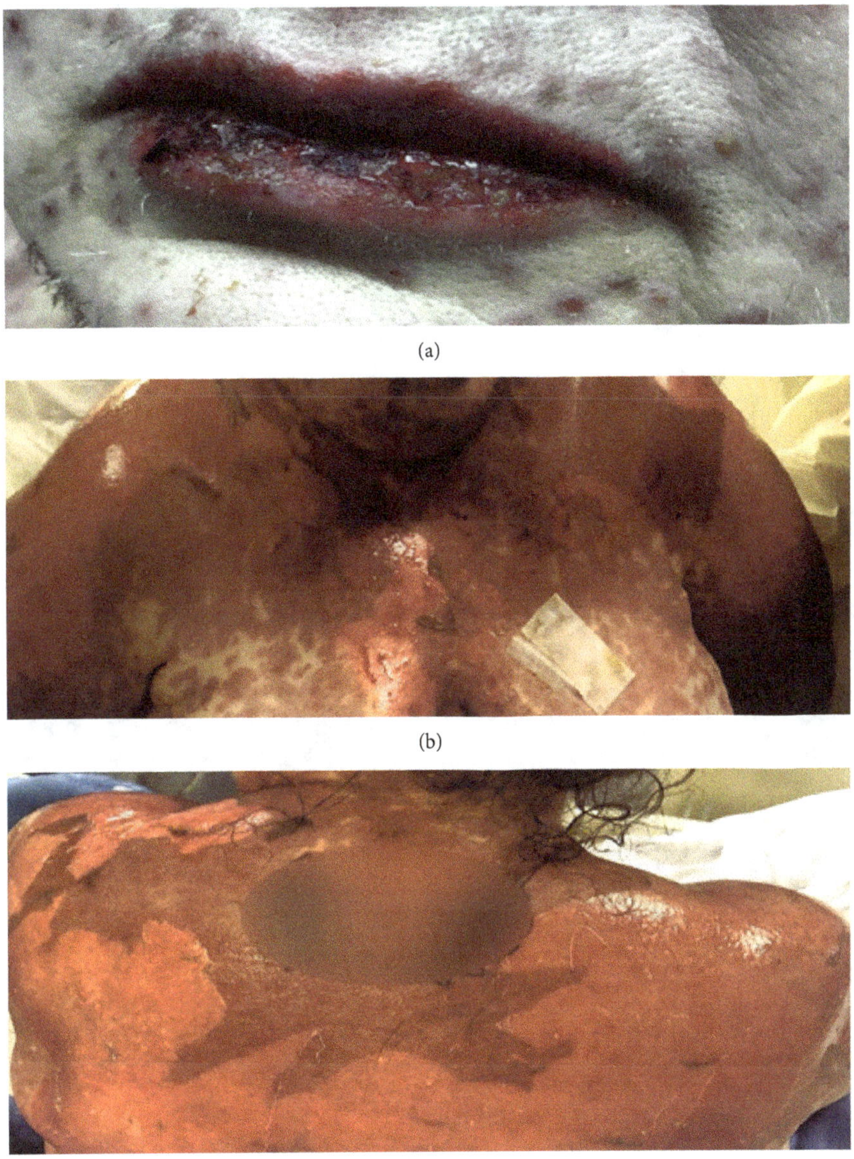

(a)

(b)

(c)

Figure 2: (a) External photo of diffuse oral ulceration and erythematous macules with vesicles on the trunk (b) and bullae and denudation on the back (c).

The use of systemic glucocorticoids is controversial. Many physicians no longer prescribe glucocorticoids, due to limited evidence to support their use. Others treat empirically under the assumption that such a short-term high dose of steroids can curb disease progression [6]. There is concern that systemic high-dose glucocorticoids may heighten the existing risk of inciting infections. Despite the associated risk with systemic steroids, some suggested that high dose of steroids (methylprednisolone 500 or 1000 mg/day for 3 to 4 days) within four days of disease onset has beneficial therapeutic effect in preventing ocular complications [8]. In addition, topical steroid also shows great promise for preventing corneal epithelial stem cell loss in the limbal region and cicatricial changes. Systemic therapeutic measures such as TNF-alpha inhibitor, thalidomide, and cyclophosphamide have been associated with increased mortality [9]. In our case, systemic steroids were not continued in the inpatient setting, due to passing the therapeutic window of 3 to 4 days since onset of her symptoms. However, topical steroids were prescribed to prevent further eye involvement.

The exact etiology of our patient's rash is unclear, but the temporal association of initiation of a new CBD oil and the onset of the rash is suggestive of association. There is an association between SJS and meloxicam which our patient had been taking. However, her chronic use of this medication (over 5 years) suggests that it is an unlikely trigger. Reports of systemic cannabis/cannabidiol hypersensitivity reaction are extremely rare. However, reports of marijuana associated with skin reactions such as allergic reactions, acute urticaria, and cannabis arteritis—a necrotic process presenting with ulceration of the lower extremities in the setting of chronic use [10]. There has been one case report of acute generalized

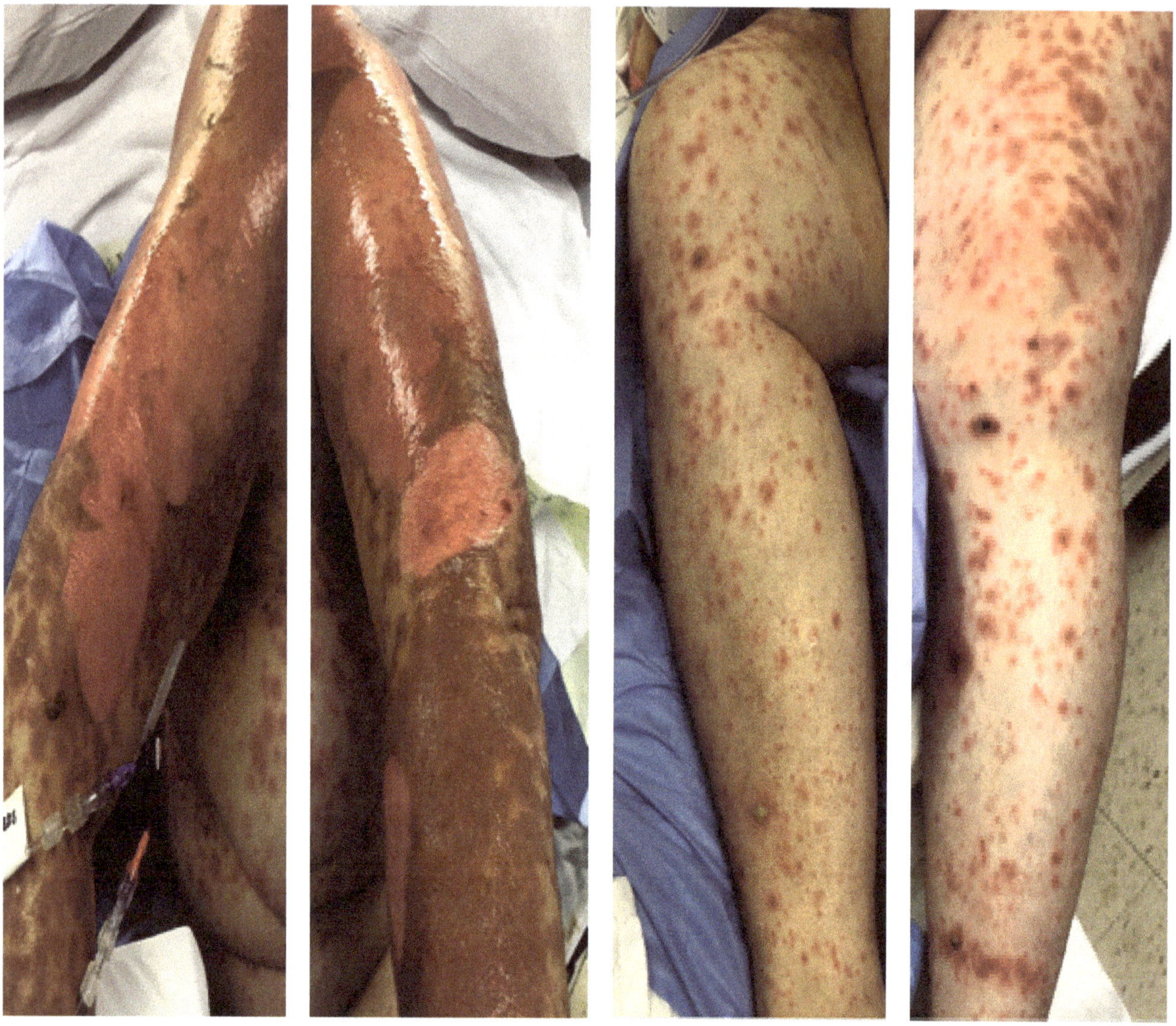

(a) (b) (c) (d)

Figure 3: External photo of diffuse ruptured vesicle and ulceration right and left upper extremities (a, b) and erythematous macules with central necrosis on the right and left lower extremities (c, d).

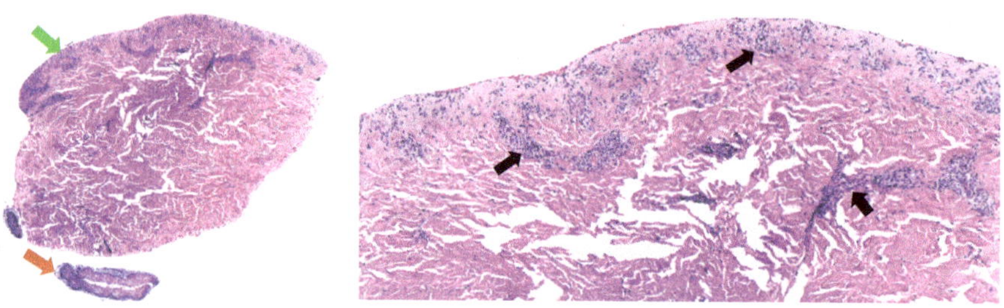

(a) (b)

Figure 4: Biopsy of the skin from the patient. Biopsy examination under 20x magnification (a): green—subepidermal blister, red—detached and necrotic epidermis and under 100x magnification (b): black arrows detailing chronic inflammation.

exanthematous pustulosis (AGEP) in the setting of CBD use which is a type IV hypersensitivity similar to SJS-TEN [11]. In our case, the patient has previously utilized other commercial CBD products without side effects or associated allergic reactions. This suggests involvement of other ingredients in this non-FDA-regulated product as the causative agent.

The complete chemical analysis from the patient's commercial CBD oil was not performed. In addition, our case also had minimal ocular involvement compared to other mucocutaneous surfaces.

We presented a case of a patient with CBD oil-induced SJS-TEN. Progression of ophthalmic involvement was prevented with cessation of the CBD oil product and initiation of an aggressive lubrication and topical anti-inflammatory regimen. It is unclear if marijuana-derived/CBD products can induce SJS-TEN. However, our case suggests an association. Further research and community surveillance is required to determine the risks of SJS-TEN from CBD products, especially given the severity and even potential fatality of this disease. Given the increased availability and use of commercial CBD products, clinicians should be aware of the possible association of CBD and SJS-TEN.

References

[1] M. Mockenhaupt, "The current understanding of Stevens-Johnson syndrome and toxic epidermal necrolysis," *Expert Review of Clinical Immunology*, vol. 7, pp. 803–813, 2011.

[2] A. O. J. Fakoya, P. Omenyi, P. Anthony et al., "Stevens - Johnson syndrome and toxic epidermal necrolysis; extensive review of reports of drug-induced etiologies, and possible therapeutic modalities," *Open Access Macedonian Journal of Medical Sciences*, vol. 6, no. 4, pp. 730–738, 2018.

[3] R. Schwartz, P. McDonough, and B. Lee, "Toxic epidermal necrolysis," *Journal of the American Academy of Dermatology*, vol. 69, no. 2, pp. 187.e1–187.e16, 2013.

[4] W. H. Chung, S. I. Hung, H. S. Hong et al., "A marker for Stevens-Johnson syndrome," *Nature*, vol. 428, no. 6982, p. 486, 2004.

[5] M. T. Ventura, M. Viola, G. F. Calogiuri, F. Gaeta, O. Pesole, and A. Romano, "Hypersensitivity reactions to complementary and alternative medicine products," *Current Pharmaceutical Design*, vol. 12, no. 26, pp. 3393–3399, 2006.

[6] S. C. G. Tseng, "Acute management of Stevens-Johnson syndrome and toxic epidermal necrolysis to minimize ocular sequelae," *American Journal of Ophthalmology*, vol. 147, no. 6, pp. 949–951, 2009.

[7] P. O. Fritsch and R. Ruiz-Moldanoda, "Stevens-Johnson syndrome - toxic epidermal necrolysis," in *Fitzpatrick's Dermatology in General Medicine*, I. M. Freedberg, A. Z. Eisen, K. Wolff, K. Frank Austen, L. A. Goldsmith, S. I. Katz, and T. B. Fitzpatrick, Eds., vol. 5, pp. 644–654, McGraw-Hill, 1999.

[8] Y. Araki, C. Sotozono, T. Inatomi et al., "Successful treatment of Stevens-Johnson Syndrome with steroid pulse therapy at disease onset," *American Journal of Ophthalmology*, vol. 147, no. 6, pp. 1004–1011.e1, 2009.

[9] S. Kohanim, S. Palioura, H. N. Saeed et al., "Stevens-Johnson Syndrome/Toxic Epidermal Necrolysis - a comprehensive review and guide to therapy. I. Systemic disease," *The Ocular Surface*, vol. 14, no. 1, pp. 2–19, 2016.

[10] G. Dhadwal and M. G. Kirchhof, "The risks and benefits of cannabis in the dermatology clinic," *Journal of Cutaneous Medicine and Surgery*, vol. 22, no. 2, pp. 194–199, 2018.

[11] C. Pettit, S. Massick, and M. Bechtel, "Cannabidiol-induced acute generalized exanthematous pustulosis," *Dermatitis*, vol. 29, no. 6, pp. 345-346, 2018.

No Severe Adverse Effects from Intravitreally Injected Putative Adipose Tissue-Derived Stem Cells

Carsten Faber, Steffen Heegaard, and Jens Folke Kiilgaard

Department of Ophthalmology, University Hospital Copenhagen, Rigshospitalet, Denmark

Correspondence should be addressed to Carsten Faber; carstenfaber@gmail.com

Academic Editor: Kevin J. Blinder

This study reports findings from a 56-year-old patient, who had received bilateral intravitreal injection of putative adipose tissue-derived stem cells at a private clinic in India with the promise of treatment of NAION. During an observation period of 8, respectively, 18 months, the intravitreally injected cells remained silent in the vitreous bodies without either therapeutic effects or complications. The cells cleared with vitrectomy without evidence of integration in the optic nerve or retina. Contrary to recent reports on patients receiving intravitreal injections of similar putative stem cells with the aim of treating AMD, our patient suffered no devastating ocular consequences. *Summary.* Contrary to recent reports, this case demonstrated no devastating consequences of intravitreal injection of adipose tissue-derived stem cells during an observation period of up to 18 months. After vitrectomy, the cells cleared without evidence of either harm or integration.

1. Introduction

Stem cells have emerged as a promising therapeutic modality for multiple diseases [1–3]. Besides bone marrow and limbal transplantation, much needs to be learned before stem cell therapy can reach clinical practice. Despite this lack of knowledge about safety and efficacy, private clinics in several countries offer stem cell therapy promising treatment of multiple diseases.

Recent reports have described four cases of putative adipose tissue-derived "stem cells" injected intravitreally in patients (aged 72 to 88 years) with age-related macular degeneration in two different private clinics [4, 5]. While devastating consequences of the procedures, including retinal hemorrhage and detachment with proliferative vitreoretinopathy (PVR) in almost all injected eyes, were described in detail, the actual fate of the injected stem cells was not described.

2. Case

A 56-year-old male with vision loss from sequential nonarteritic anterior ischemic optic neuropathy (NAION) with a complete visual field defect and a visual acuity of 1/50 Snellen in each eye (Figure 1(a)) was seen acutely due to a further, painless decrease in visual acuity in both eyes. A visual acuity of light perception was noted. On examination, whitish, dense vitreal opacities partly obscuring views of deeply atrophic optic nerves and otherwise unremarkable retinas were seen. The conjunctivae were white and no anterior uveitis was seen.

The patient revealed that two months earlier he received intravitreal injections in both eyes of putative stem cells prepared from his abdominal subcutaneous adipose tissue. The full procedure from harvesting of adipose tissue to intravitreal injection had a total duration of about two hours and was carried out at a private clinic in New Delhi, India. Further details about the procedure were not known.

The patient was observed and demonstrated a stable condition for several months (Figure 1(a)). Eight months after stem cell injection, we performed vitrectomy in the left eye and—after a further 10 months—also in the right eye. The dense opacities were purely localized to the vitreous bodies and cleared completely with vitrectomy (Figure 1(b) and video, supplementary material (available here)). The hyaloids were very adherent to the retinae which probably was the

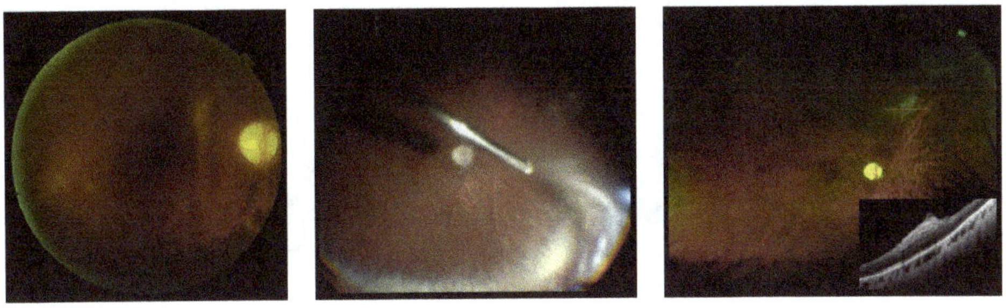

(a) (b) (c)

Figure 1: (a) Dense vitreal opacities are seen 2 months after intravitreal injection of adipose tissue-derived stem cells in the right eye. This condition remained unchanged during an 18-month observation period until vitrectomy was performed. (b) During vitrectomy, the dense opacities were seen localized to the vitreous body; no retinal integration or reaction was evident. (c) Two months after vitrectomy, the eye remained silent with unchanged epiretinal remnants from the adherent hyaloid. The left eye had similar findings before, during, and after vitrectomy.

cause of the intraoperative complications: in the left eye a localized retinal detachment was induced and in the right a retinal tear was induced, both were treated accordingly. Specimens from both eyes were examined microscopically and included few vimentin-positive cells compatible with cells of mesenchymal origin. We did not identify cells differentiated into a retinal or neuronal phenotype. Following the immediate postoperative period, no intraocular reaction was observed in either eye. Visual acuity remained poor. Epiretinal remnants from the adherent hyaloid were noted in the right eye, and these remained unchanged for several months (Figure 1(c)).

3. Discussion

This case demonstrates that cell suspensions of putative stem cells may be injected intravitreally without severe adverse effects. Whether this was due to entrapment in the vitreous body or simply lack of function of putative stem cell population is not known. The posterior hyaloid was very adherent in both eyes, which may be an effect from or a response to the intravitreally placed cell population. We did, however, not note any signs of cellular integration in the retina or the optic nerve and certainly no therapeutic effect was noted.

The cell suspensions remained intravitreally for 8-18 months. Besides unchanged vitreal clouding, no serious adverse effects were noted in the observation period. In agreement with the immune privilege of the eye including the vitreous, this demonstrates that heterogeneously transplanted cells can remain silent without inducing an inflammatory response in the vitreous. This is unlike previous reports where intravitreal injections of similar adipose tissue-derived cell populations resulted in early and serious complications in all treated eyes. This included high intraocular pressure, anterior uveitis, lens subluxation, vitreal and intraretinal hemorrhage, and retinal detachment with aggressive PVR [4, 5]. This difference may relate to different methods of harvesting and isolating adipose tissue-derived stem cells resulting in debris or toxicity inducing these reactions rather than a reaction to the cell isolate per se. We speculate that another explanation for the observed clinical difference could be the absence of posterior vitreous detachment. In the present case, cell suspensions were probably injected into the persistent vitreous bodies. In the previous cases, all patients were older than 70 years with end-stage AMD, and the cell suspensions were probably injected in close contact with the retina due to posterior vitreous detachment.

The stem cell technique holds great promise for treatment and cure of a wide range of diseases; however, more research is needed. Currently, some private clinics, with a promise of cure, are exploiting patients with untreatable diseases. This case demonstrates that patients should be discouraged from such unethical and costly treatments.

Disclosure

This case has previously been presented at the 18th Euretina Congress, September 2018, in Vienna.

References

[1] M. Mandai, A. Watanabe, Y. Kurimoto et al., "Autologous induced stem-cell-derived retinal cells for macular degeneration," *The New England Journal of Medicine*, vol. 376, no. 11, pp. 1038–1046, 2017.

[2] E. L. Feldman, N. M. Boulis, J. Hur et al., "Intraspinal neural stem cell transplantation in amyotrophic lateral sclerosis: phase 1 trial outcomes," *Annals of Neurology*, vol. 75, no. 3, pp. 363–373, 2014.

[3] E. Díez-Tejedor, M. Gutiérrez-Fernández, P. Martínez-Sánchez et al., "Reparative therapy for acute ischemic stroke with allogeneic mesenchymal stem cells from adipose tissue: a safety assessment: a phase II randomized, double- blind, placebo-controlled, single-center, pilot clinical trial," *Journal of Stroke and Cerebrovascular Diseases*, vol. 23, no. 10, pp. 2694–2700, 2014.

[4] S. S. Saraf, M. A. Cunningham, A. E. Kuriyan et al., "Bilateral retinal detachments after intravitreal injection of adipose-derived "stem cells" in a patient with exudative macular degeneration," *Ophthalmic Surgery, Lasers and Imaging Retina*, vol. 48, no. 9, pp. 772–775, 2017.

[5] A. E. Kuriyan, T. A. Albini, J. H. Townsend et al., "Vision loss after intravitreal injection of autologous "stem cells" for AMD," *The New England Journal of Medicine*, vol. 376, no. 11, pp. 1047–1053, 2017.

23

Neuroophthalmic Manifestations of Intracranial Tumours in Children

Megha Kotecha,[1] **Sarang Gotecha**,[2] **Ashish Chugh**,[2] **and Prashant Punia**[2]

[1]*Department of Ophthalmology, Dr. D.Y. Patil Medical College and Hospital, Pimpri, Pune, Maharashtra, India*
[2]*Department of Neurosurgery, Dr. D.Y. Patil Medical College and Hospital, Pimpri, Pune, Maharashtra, India*

Correspondence should be addressed to Sarang Gotecha; dr.sarangsgotecha@gmail.com

Academic Editor: Huban Atilla

Background. All children between 0 and 16 years presenting with brain tumours confirmed by Magnetic Resonance Imaging (MRI) and treated surgically in our institute were included in this study. *Objective.* The aim of this study is to evaluate the neuroophthalmic and clinical characteristics of intracranial space occupying lesions in children. *Methods.* Neuroophthalmic manifestations along with location of the tumour by contrast-enhanced MRI, type of surgical intervention, and postoperative histopathological diagnosis were evaluated. *Results.* In pediatric brain tumours, male preponderance was seen and supratentorial location was more common in general, while in older children, infratentorial tumours were more common than supratentorial tumours. Headache, vomiting, and cerebellar signs were the commonest neurological features. Diminution of vision, diplopia, and strabismus were the commonest ophthalmic symptoms. Papilledema, ophthalmoparesis, and nystagmus were the most frequent ophthalmological signs. Neurological manifestations of seizures, altered sensorium and motor deficits were more frequently seen in supratentorial tumours, while cranial nerve involvement and ataxia were seen in infratentorial tumours. Ophthalmological manifestations including diplopia, strabismus, ophthalmoparesis, and nystagmus were more frequently seen in infratentorial tumours. Astrocytoma was the most frequent histopathological diagnosis followed by medulloblastoma. *Conclusion.* Diagnosis of pediatric intracranial tumours is complex and requires a multidisciplinary approach for prompt management. An ophthalmologist should have a high index of suspicion for brain tumours especially in patients presenting with common ocular symptoms like diminution of vision, diplopia, and strabismus without any neurological symptoms.

1. Introduction

Central nervous system tumours (CNS) are the most common solid tumours in children and a leading cause of mortality and morbidity in children worldwide [1, 2]. In India, according to the Indian Council of Medical Research, National Cancer Registry data, the incidence of pediatric brain tumours is around 2% [2].

Despite advances in neuroimaging, early diagnosis of pediatric CNS tumours remains a dilemma. Contributing factors to this problem are varied presentation and rarity of these tumours in childhood [3]. The frequent presentation of brain tumours in children includes features of raised intracranial pressure like headache and vomiting. However, in about 10% of affected children, visual symptoms can be the mode of presentation [4]. A lack of awareness of the ophthalmic signs and symptoms of brain tumours can lead to a delayed diagnosis and their management.

Visual manifestations of brain tumours in children include blurring of vision, diplopia, ocular nerve palsy, papilledema, optic atrophy, ptosis, nystagmus, strabismus, proptosis, and photophobia. [5] As the visual system in children is still developing, brain tumours and their surgical management can alter the normal neuroanatomical structures of the visual system and cause permanent visual impairment [6].

The purpose of this study is to evaluate the neuroophthalmic and clinical characteristics of intracranial-space-occupying lesions in children.

2. Materials and Methods

This prospective observational study was carried out for a period of 2.5 years from June 2017 to December 2019 after Ethical Committee Clearance. All children between 0 and

16 years presenting with brain tumours confirmed by Magnetic Resonance Imaging (MRI) and treated surgically in our institute were included in this study. Patients who had received chemotherapy or radiotherapy before surgery or with coexistent primary neoplasm elsewhere were excluded from the study. Patient's age; gender; neurological symptoms which include history of headache, nausea/vomiting, seizures, and anosmia; and neurological signs which include cerebellar signs, speech involvement, motor deficits, altered sensorium, endocrine involvement, and cranial nerve palsies were evaluated by the neurosurgical team.

Ophthalmic features which include diminution of vision and visual field defects, ocular pain, red eye, proptosis, papilledema, disc pallor, shunting of vessels, ptosis, pupil abnormality, nystagmus, and strabismus were evaluated by the ophthalmologist.

Other parameters which were evaluated were the location of the tumour by contrast-enhanced MRI, type of surgical intervention, and postoperative histopathological diagnosis.

3. Results

A total of 35 patients were evaluated. Ages ranged from 8 months to 16 years, and the mean age of the patients was 8.28 years. The average duration of symptoms in our study was 6.45 weeks.

According to the location, 16 cases were infratentorial in location and 19 cases were supratentorial in location. Frequency of neurological signs and symptoms according to supra- and infratentorial locations are mentioned in Table 1.

23 patients presented with ocular symptoms at the time of presentation, whereas 31 patients were found to have abnormal findings after detailed ophthalmic evaluation. The ophthalmic manifestations of the patients according to infratentorial and supratentorial locations are illustrated in Table 2.

commonest ophthalmic symptoms were diminution of vision and diplopia, and the most common ophthalmic sign was papilledema followed by ophthalmoparesis and nystagmus.

The location of the tumours according to their age distribution is illustrated in Table 3. Cerebellar tumours were highest in number, followed by sellar region tumours. Out of the 6 sellar region tumours, 1 case was a sellar tumour, 2 cases had a suprasellar extension, 1 case had a suprasellar and parasellar extension, and 1 case was parasellar in location. Out of the 5 ventricular tumours, 3 cases were in the left lateral ventricle, and 1 case each was in the third ventricle and the 4th ventricle.

3.1. Operative Characteristics. The type of surgical interventions are mentioned in Table 4. Surgical resection of the tumours was done in 28 (80%) patients, CSF diversion procedure was done in 4 (11.4%) patients, stereotactic biopsy of the patient was done in 1 (2.9%) patient, and primary radiation therapy was advised in 2 (5.7%) patients.

The histopathological diagnosis of all the patients and their distribution according to their location are mentioned in Table 5. The most common histopathological diagnosis was astrocytoma followed by medulloblastoma.

4. Discussion

Pediatric brain tumours are a heterogenous group of neoplasms which vary in their cell of origin, mode of presentation, management protocols, and clinical outcomes [2]. Treatment of pediatric CNS neoplasms requires a multidisciplinary team which includes a neurooncologist, a neuroradiologist, a neuroophthalmologist, a neurosurgeon, and a pediatric neurologist. Survival rate in these cases have improved over the years as a result of a multidisciplinary approach, improvements in diagnostic modalities, surgical technologies, adjuvant radiotherapy and chemotherapy, and surveillance techniques for tumour recurrence [7].

This study was undertaken to observe a particular cohort of children who were clinically and radiologically diagnosed with intracranial tumours managed by the neurosurgical team along with ophthalmological examination done by the ophthalmology team.

In this study, there were 35 patients with a mean age of 8.28 years which was comparable to the study by Liu et al. [6] and Mehrazin and Yavari [8]. Fifteen patients were girls and 20 were boys. Many studies in the literature on the incidence of intracranial tumours especially studies which include adult patients show female preponderance [9, 10]. This is due to a higher incidence of meningiomas and pituitary adenomas in females among adult patients. In contrast to this observation, the literature on pediatric brain tumours suggests a higher incidence of intracranial tumours in boys similar to our study [11, 12]. In developing countries, this may also be a reflection of the prevalent gender bias of the relatives seeking treatment.

The road to diagnosis of brain tumours can be a potential challenge as many clinical symptoms can mimic other common childhood ailments. The clinical signs of the tumour can vary based on the location, age, and aggressiveness of the tumour, and a high index of suspicion followed by prompt evaluation and surgical intervention is required, the delay of which can lead to untoward complications [13]. Neurological symptoms produced by intracranial tumours can be local or general. General symptoms can result from a progressive enlargement of the tumour within the limited volume of the cranial vault causing raised intracranial pressure and related symptoms, whereas local symptoms are due to the effects of the tumour on contiguous areas of the brain [14].

The commonest neurological symptom was headache followed by nausea and vomiting which confirms the well-known predominance of symptoms of raised intracranial pressure in these cases according to the literature [2, 3, 10, 14]. The higher incidence of headache in our study can be attributed to the delay in approaching a specialist and reaching a diagnosis both of which are predominant in developing countries. In our view, as we are practicing in a tertiary care centre, more often than not, patients with complications or those requiring complex surgeries are referred to our centre which is another cause for the late presentation of cases. Intracranial tumours can cause raised intracranial pressure by various mechanisms which include increased brain volume due to the tumour itself, vasogenic edema due to the tumour, mass effect on the ventricular system leading to

TABLE 1: Frequency of neurological signs and symptoms according to supratentorial and infratentorial location of the tumour.

Clinical features	Infratentorial	Supratentorial	Total
Headache	16 (45.7%)	17(%)	33 (94.3%)
Nausea/vomiting	14 (40%)	10 (28.6%)	24 (68.6%)
Ophthalmic involvement	15 (42.9%)	15 (42.9%)	30 (85.7%)
Cerebellar signs	—	16 (45.7%)	16 (45.7%)
Ophthalmoparesis			15 (42.8%)
Cranial nerve II	14	15	29 (82.9%)
Cranial nerve III	2	1	3 (8.6%)
Cranial nerve IV	2	1	3 (8.6%)
Cranial nerve V	1	0	1 (2.9%)
Cranial nerve VI	13	2	15 (42.9%)
Cranial nerve VII	4	0	4 (11.4%)
Cranial nerve VIII	1	0	1 (2.9%)
Lower cranial nerves	2	—	2 (5.7%)
Seizures	1 (2.9%)	13 (37.1%)	14 (40%)
Altered sensorium	1 (2.9%)	4 (11.4%)	5 (14.3%)
Ataxia	4 (11.4%)	0	4 (11.4%)
Motor deficit	0	3 (8.6%)	3 (8.6%)
Endocrine involvement (stunted growth)	0	2 (5.7%)	2 (5.7%)
Increased head circumference	—	1 (2.9%)	1 (2.9%)

TABLE 2: Ophthalmic manifestations of the tumours according to infratentorial location and supratentorial location of the tumour.

	Infratentorial	Supratentorial	Total
Ophthalmic symptoms			
Visual acuity involvement	6 (17.1%)	7 (20%)	13 (37.1%)
Diplopia	11	2 (5.7%)	13 (37.1%)
Strabismus	11	1 (2.9%)	12 (34.3%)
Ptosis	2 (5.7%)	1 (2.9%)	3 (8.6%)
Ophthalmic signs			
Papilledema	9 (25.7%)	8 (22.9%)	17 (48.6%)
Ophthalmoparesis	13 (37.1%)	2 (5.7%)	15 (42.8%)
Nystagmus	13 (37.1%)	1 (2.9%)	14 (40%)
Disc pallor	5	6 (17.1%)	11 (31.4%)
Pupillary abnormality	2 (5.7%)	2 (5.7%)	4 (11.4%)

obstructive hydrocephalus, compression or invasion of the venous system by the tumour, and meningeal involvement of the tumour [1].

The other neurological signs and symptoms seen in our study were cerebellar signs (45.7%), optic nerve involvement (82.9%), other types of cranial nerve involvement (42.8%), seizures (40%), altered sensorium (14.3%), ataxia (11.4%), motor deficits (8.6%), endocrine involvement (5.7%), and increased head circumference (2.9%). These are consistent with various similar studies in the literature on pediatric intracranial tumours [2, 3, 11, 12].

Brain tumours can alter the normal neuroanatomical structures of the visual system leading to visual impairment and dysfunction which can have a lifelong impact on the quality of life of patients and their families [6]. Ophthalmological examination in these cases are not only beneficial for assessing the visual status of these patients but also helpful for prognosticating the patients and their families regarding the visual outcome which in some cases can also affect decision-making in the selection of the type of intervention in these cases.

Ophthalmic signs and symptoms are a mode of presentation in children with intracranial tumours, and the ophthalmological evaluation must be performed with greater attention as the presentation in children is less specific than that in adults [11].

Neuroophthalmologic evaluation should be done by protocol for children with brain tumours. However, early assessment of vision may not be done routinely at all hospitals due to various reasons which include (a) priority given to brain

Table 3: Tumour location according to age distribution.

Tumour location	0-5 years	6-10 years	11-16 years	Total
Cerebellar tumour	1	5	5	11 (31.4%)
Sellar region tumours	0	3	3	6 (17.14%)
Ventricular tumours	3	1	1	5 (14.3%)
Left frontal lobe tumour	0	1	2	3 (8.6%)
Pontine tumour	2	1	0	3 (8.6%)
Frontoparietal tumour	2	0	0	2 (5.7%)
Left basal ganglia tumour	0	0	1	1 (2.9%)
Multiple intracranial tumour	0	0	1	1 (2.9%)
Pineal gland tumour	1	0	0	1 (2.9%)
Prepontine tumour	1	0	0	1 (2.9%)
Right frontotemporoparietal tumour	1	0	0	1 (2.9%)
Total	11	11	13	35

Table 4: Type of surgical intervention.

Operative characteristics	Frequency	Percentage
Craniectomy with surgical resection	22	62.9%
CSF diversion	4	11.4%
Transsphenoidal gross total resection	3	8.6%
Endoscopic gross total tumour excision	2	5.7%
Primary radiotherapy	2	5.7%
Endoscopic biopsy	1	2.9%
Stereotactic biopsy	1	2.9%
Total	35	100.0%

tumours, (b) lack of apparent visual symptoms at the time of presentation, (c) inability to clearly describe symptoms which is particularly more common in young children, (d) difficulty in examining young children, and (e) difficult access to a neuroophthalmologist [1].

Out of the 35 patients in our study, 23 (65.71%) patients presented with ocular symptoms and 31 (88.57%) patients were found to have abnormal findings after detailed ophthalmological examination. Ocular symptoms at the time of presentation are higher than in some studies in the literature like the study by Liu et al. which can again be attributed to the late presentation of these cases in developing countries [6]. However, in the same study, the authors report the incidence of 90% of abnormal findings on ophthalmological examination which is similar to our study.

The visual symptoms seen in our study were diminution of vision, diplopia, strabismus, and ptosis. All these visual symptoms can be devastating and lead to long-term effects on the quality of life for the patient and the family. Visual impairment can be caused by affecting both the afferent and the efferent pathways. Direct compression of the visual pathway by the tumour can lead to diminution of vision, visual field defect, and ocular motility defects [13]. Furthermore, obstructive hydrocephalus, mass effect of the brain tumour, cerebral odema, and leptomeningeal involvement by the tumour can cause raised intracranial pressure eventually leading to papilledema, pale disc, and loss of vision. In our study, 13 (37.1%) patients presented with diminution of vision out which 6 patients of sellar region tumours had direct compression on the visual pathway, whereas in 7 patients, vision loss was secondary to raised intracranial pressure. Strabismus was present in 12 (34.3%) patients out of which 11 patients had infratentorial tumours and 1 patient had a supratentorial tumour, which is again consistent with the literature which states that strabismus is more common in posterior fossa tumours [6]. Ptosis was seen in 3 (8.6%) children which included 2 patients of pontine tumours and 1 case of sellar tumour with parasellar extension.

In their study on children diagnosed with intracranial-space-occupying lesions, Alswaina et al. have highlighted the role of an ophthalmologist in these cases. They have reported an incidence of optic atrophy in 46%, diminution of vision in 46%, papilledema in 24%, nystagmus in 24%, sixth nerve palsy in 19%, and third nerve palsy in 12% [4]. These findings were comparable to our study.

Ophthalmoparesis was seen in 15 (42%) patients in our study. Palsies of III, IV, and VI nerve were more common in children with infratentorial tumours than in children with supratentorial tumours which again correlated with the data available in the literature [15]. Acquired third nerve and fourth nerve palsies were seen in 3 cases including 2 cases of pontine tumours and one case of a sellar tumour with suprasellar and parasellar extension which were all due to direct compression on the nerves in all 3 cases. Acquired sixth nerve palsy was seen in 15 (42.9%) cases in our study out of which direct compression was seen in 6 cases and indirect compression due to posterior fossa tumours was seen in 9 cases. In patients presenting with ophthalmoparesis, after ruling out acquired palsies of the third, fourth, and sixth cranial nerves, other etiologies including myasthenia gravis, local inflammation/infection, migraine, and local infarction should be ruled out [4].

Ophthalmological signs seen in our study were papilledema, nystagmus, disc pallor, visual field defects, and pupillary abnormality. Papilledema or pale disc from pediatric brain tumours can result from tumours intrinsic to the optic nerves or optic chiasm, tumours contiguous to the optic nerve or chiasm, or tumours located elsewhere causing

Table 5: Histopathological diagnosis and their distribution according to their location.

Histopathology	Frequency	Location	Frequency
Medulloblastoma	6 (17.1%)	Cerebellum	6
		Pons	3
High-grade glioma	5 (14.3%)	Left frontal lobe	1
		Right frontoparietal lobe	1
		Cerebellum	2
Low-grade glioma	4 (11.4%)	Left frontal lobe	1
		Left lateral ventricle	1
		Bilateral frontoparietal lobe	1
Abscess	4 (11.4%)	Left frontoparietal lobe	1
		Left basal ganglia	1
		Multiple intracranial lesions	1
		4th ventricle	1
Arachnoid cyst	4 (11.4%)	Cerebellum	2
		Sellar region	1
Craniopharyngioma	4 (11.4%)	Sellar region	3
		Third ventricle	1
Choroid plexus papilloma	1 (2.9%)	Left lateral ventricle	1
Giant cell tumour	1 (2.9%)	Cerebellum	1
Infected epidermoid cyst	1 (2.9%)	Prepontine region	1
Meningioma	1 (2.9%)	Left lateral ventricle	1
Optic nerve glioma	1 (2.9%)	Sellar region	1
Pineoblastoma	1 (2.9%)	Pineal region	1
Pituitary adenoma	1 (2.9%)	Sellar region	1
Tuberculoma	1 (2.9%)	Left frontal lobe	1
Total	35		35

nonlocalizing increased intracranial pressure [4]. In our study, papilledema was seen in 17 (48.6%) cases and disc pallor was seen in 11 (31.4%) cases. Nystagmus was seen in 14 cases of which 10 cases were posterior fossa tumours, 3 cases were pontine tumours, and 1 case was pineal gland tumour.

In our study, visual field defects were present clinically and confirmed by perimetry as bitemporal hemianopia in 2 patients of sellar region tumours. However, 4 patients had clinical symptoms of field defects which could not be confirmed by perimetry due to noncompliance of the children. In a study carried out by Harbert et al., the authors reported that 15.2% of children with CNS tumours have visual field defects that go unrecognized and recommended that serial neuroophthalmological evaluation of children with brain tumours is required to diagnose a visual field defect since patient or caregiver reporting may be limited [16].

Pupillary abnormality was seen in 4 patients (11.4%) out of which 2 patients were cases of pineal region tumours, and these patients presented with features of Perinaud's syndrome which include upgaze palsy convergence-retraction nystagmus, light-near dissociation of pupils, and lid retraction [5].

After complete neurological and ophthalmic evaluation of the patient, imaging was done in all patients with suspected intracranial tumours. Contrast-enhanced MRI of the brain is the investigation of choice which was done in all our cases. Additionally, depending on the type and location of the tumour, MRI angiogram to display vasculature alongside the tumour, MR spectroscopy to assess the metabolic activity of the tumour, and functional MRI and tractography to provide additional information on the course of important white matter tracts and their relationship with the tumour were done for planning of surgery. Sedation was required in younger children or children not cooperative to undergo MRI.

In our study, 20% of the cases were located in the cerebral cortex, 31.4% of the cases were located in the cerebellum, 8.6% of the cases were located in the brainstem, 17.1% of the cases were located in the pituitary and suprasellar region, and 14.2% of the cases were intraventricular in location. According to the literature, about 25-30% are in a supratentorial location, followed by cerebellum (15-20%), brainstem (10-12%), pituitary and suprasellar regions (10-15%), and brain ventricles (5-6.4%) which is comparable to our study [17, 18].

Of the 35 tumours, 19 (54.3%) were supratentorial and 16 (45.7%) were infratentorial. This was comparable to the study carried out by Suresh . [13] Neurological and visual symptoms according to their locations are listed in Table 3. In our study, incidence of neurological features including seizures, altered sensorium, and motor deficits are higher in supratentorial tumours, whereas incidence of cranial nerve involvement and ataxia were higher in infratentorial tumours. Incidence of ophthalmological manifestations including diplopia, strabismus, ophthalmoparesis, and nystagmus are higher in infratentorial tumours. All these findings are comparable to the study on clinical presentation of supratentorial and infratentorial intracranial tumours in pediatric patients by Sánchez-Sánchez . [19]

In older children, infratentorial tumours are more common than supratentorial tumours [4, 20]. Consistent with the literature, in our series, 11 of 16 patients with posterior fossa tumours were older children. Ophthalmological signs and symptoms were present in 15 out of 16 patients (93.75%). This is higher in comparison to a study of posterior fossa tumours by Gadgil ., the reason for which can be attributed to the retrospective nature of their study and neglect of ocular presentation at initial evaluation as reported by the authors [21]. In our prospective study, detailed ophthalmological examination was done at the time of presentation by the ophthalmology team. Neurological presentation of posterior fossa tumours were as follows: headache and cerebellar signs, which were present in all the patients; nausea and vomiting, which were present in 14 (87.5%) of the cases; nystagmus, which was present in 13 (81.25%) of the cases; strabismus, which was seen in 11 (68.75%) of the cases; and papilledema, which was seen in 9 (56.25%) of the cases.

Out of the 16 cases of posterior fossa tumours in our study, medulloblastoma (6 cases) was the commonest tumour followed by astrocytoma (5 cases). This is in contrast to most studies on pediatric posterior fossa tumours which state that the incidence of astrocytoma is higher than that of medulloblastoma in these cases [22, 23]. The other posterior fossa tumours seen in our study were arachnoid cyst (3 cases), giant cell tumour (1 case), and infected epidermoid cyst (1 case).

Six cases of sellar region tumours were seen in our study, out of which 3 cases were craniopharyngiomas, one case each of pituitary adenoma, arachnoid cyst, and optic nerve glioma. This collaborates with the study of Laws and Sheehan, who have suggested that diagnosis of sellar region tumours in pediatric patients requires a multidisciplinary approach and detailed ophthalmic and neurological tests are critical in these cases [24].

Surgical resection is the main modality of treatment for most pediatric brain tumours. Depending on the tumour type, the goals of surgical management are to achieve a tissue diagnosis and reestablish normal CSF (cerebrospinal fluid) pathways, CSF diversion, tumour debulking, and complete tumour resection [25]. In accordance with these principles, craniectomy with surgical resection was done in 22 cases and CSF diversion was done in 4 cases, out of which ventriculoperitoneal shunt was done in 3 cases and cystoperitoneal shunt was done in 1 case; endoscopic procedure was done in 6 cases, out of which endoscopic transsphenoidal excision was done in 3 cases, endoscopic tumour excision was done in 2 cases, and endoscopic biopsy was done in 1 case; stereotactic biopsy was done in 1 case; and a patient was referred for primary radiotherapy in 2 cases.

Astrocytoma was the most frequent tumour seen in our study followed by medulloblastoma. This is consistent with most studies in the literature [2, 6, 15, 26–28].

The frequency of craniopharyngioma (11.4%) in the present study was high in our study but was comparable to various studies from India, Egypt, Japan, and Brazil [29–34]. Kassam et al. had a classification system for craniopharyngiomas based on the infundibulum to strategize the surgical approach. Type I tumours are preinfundibular, which are subchiasmatic tumours displacing the optic chiasm superiorly and posteriorly. Type II tumours are transinfundibular, which can extend into the third ventricle. Type III is retroinfundibular, which can either extend superiorly into the third ventricle or inferiorly into the pontine cisterns [35]. Type IV tumours are primarily located in the third ventricles. According to this classification, there was 1 case each of type I and type IV and there were 2 cases of type II.

The other tumours present in our study include pineoblastoma, meningioma, choroid plexus papilloma, pituitary adenoma, and tuberculoma which are comparable to various studies in the literature [4, 29, 33, 34, 36].

5. Limitation of the Study

Statistical significance was not evaluated because of the very small sample size of the study.

6. Conclusions

To conclude, diagnosis of pediatric intracranial tumours is complex and requires a multidisciplinary approach for prompt management. Neuroophthalmic manifestations are common but can be easily missed in children with intracranial tumours. With increased survival rates, pediatric intracranial tumours with ophthalmic involvement can cause devastating long-term consequences due to vision loss or ocular motor abnormalities eventually leading to decreased quality of life.

An ophthalmologist should have a high index of suspicion for brain tumours especially in patients presenting with common ocular symptoms like diminution of vision, diplopia, and strabismus without any neurological symptoms. Ophthalmological evaluation and monitoring can also be helpful in these cases for preoperative planning and systematic treatment monitoring and for postoperative prognostication and multidisciplinary care of the patient.

We also conclude that in any child presenting to an ophthalmologist with additional signs and symptoms that could result from a CNS tumour, a thorough neuroophthalmic examination should be done. This can help in early diagnosis and prompt management of pediatric intracranial tumours and also helps in improvement of visual prognosis. Other salient features observed and concluded in our study include the following:

(1) In pediatric brain tumours, male preponderance is seen which collaborates with many studies in the literature. Supratentorial location was more common in general, while in older children, infratentorial tumours are more common than supratentorial tumours

(2) Headache, vomiting, and cerebellar signs were the commonest neurological features; diminution of

vision, diplopia, and strabismus were the commonest ophthalmic symptoms; while papilledema, ophthalmoparesis, and nystagmus were the most frequent ophthalmological signs

(3) Neurological manifestations of seizures, altered sensorium, and motor deficits were more frequently seen in supratentorial tumours, while cranial nerve involvement and ataxia were seen in infratentorial tumours. Ophthalmological manifestations including diplopia, strabismus, ophthalmoparesis, and nystagmus were more frequently seen in infratentorial tumours

(4) Astrocytoma was the commonest histopathological diagnosis followed by medulloblastoma, which again collaborated with various studies in the literature

References

[1] S. Jariyakosol and J. Peragallo, "The effects of primary brain tumors on vision and quality of life in pediatric patients," *Seminars in Neurology*, vol. 35, no. 5, pp. 587–598, 2015.

[2] R. Madhavan, B. Kannabiran, A. Nithya, J. Kani, P. Balasubramaniam, and S. Shanmugakumar, "Pediatric brain tumors: an analysis of 5 years of data from a tertiary cancer care center, India," *Indian journal of cancer*, vol. 53, no. 4, pp. 562–565, 2016.

[3] S. Wilne, J. Collier, C. Kennedy, K. Koller, R. Grundy, and D. Walker, "Presentation of childhood CNS tumours: a systematic review and meta-analysis," *The Lancet Oncology*, vol. 8, no. 8, pp. 685–695, 2007.

[4] A. Khan, N. Alswaina, S. Elkhamary, and M. Shammari, "Ophthalmic features of outpatient children diagnosed with intracranial space-occupying lesions by ophthalmologists," *Middle East African Journal of Ophthalmology*, vol. 22, no. 3, pp. 327–330, 2015.

[5] J. H. Peragallo, "Effects of brain tumors on vision in children," *International Ophthalmology Clinics*, vol. 58, no. 4, pp. 83–95, 2018.

[6] Y. Liu, C. Abongwa, S. Ashwal, D. D. Deming, and T. W. Winter, "Referral for ophthalmology evaluation and visual sequelae in children with primary brain tumors," *JAMA Network Open*, vol. 2, no. 8, article e198273, 2019.

[7] H. R. Gittleman, Q. T. Ostrom, C. D. Rouse et al., "Trends in central nervous system tumor incidence relative to other common cancers in adults, adolescents, and children in the United States, 2000 to 2010," *Cancer*, vol. 121, no. 1, pp. 102–112, 2015.

[8] M. Mehrazin and P. Yavari, "Morphological pattern and frequency of intracranial tumors in children," *Child's Nervous System*, vol. 23, no. 2, pp. 157–162, 2007.

[9] S. Deshmukh, D. Das, H. Bhattacharjee et al., "Profile of brain tumors having ocular manifestations in a tertiary eye care institute: a retrospective study," *TNOA Journal of Ophthalmic Science and Research*, vol. 56, no. 2, p. 71, 2018.

[10] N. Tagoe, V. Essuman, G. Fordjuor, J. Akpalu, P. Bankah, and T. Ndanu, "Neuro-ophthalmic and clinical characteristics of brain tumours in a tertiary hospital in Ghana," *Ghana Medical Journal*, vol. 49, no. 3, pp. 181–186, 2015.

[11] S. H. Wilne, "The presenting features of brain tumours: a review of 200 cases," *Archives of Disease in Childhood*, vol. 91, no. 6, pp. 502–506, 2006.

[12] I. Sim Ng, J. Sales Marques, and A. Hei, "Neuro-ophthalmic and clinical characteristics of brain tumors in children in Macau," *Acta Scientific Paediatrics*, vol. 2, no. 11, pp. 19–22, 2019.

[13] S. Suresh, A. Srinivasan, J. Scott, S. Rao, B. Chidambaram, and S. Chandrasekar, "Profile and outcome of pediatric brain tumors—experience from a tertiary care pediatric oncology unit in South India," *Journal of Pediatric Neurosciences*, vol. 12, no. 3, pp. 237–244, 2017.

[14] N. Shirazi, M. Gupta, N. K. Bhat, B. P. Kalra, R. Kumar, and M. Saini, "Profile of primary pediatric brain and spinal cord tumors from North India," *Indian Journal of Medical and Paediatric Oncology*, vol. 38, no. 1, pp. 10–14, 2017.

[15] G. Mole, R. Edminson, A. Higham, C. Hopper, and D. Hildebrand, "The management of childhood intracranial tumours and the role of the ophthalmologist," *Neuroophthalmology*, vol. 43, no. 6, pp. 375–381, 2019.

[16] M. J. Harbert, L. A. Yeh-Nayre, H. S. O'Halloran, M. L. Levy, and J. R. Crawford, "Unrecognized visual field deficits in children with primary central nervous system brain tumors," *Journal of Neuro-Oncology*, vol. 107, no. 3, pp. 545–549, 2012.

[17] Q. T. Ostrom, P. M. de Blank, C. Kruchko et al., "Alex's Lemonade Stand Foundation infant and childhood primary brain and central nervous system tumors diagnosed in the United States in 2007–2011," *Neuro-Oncology*, vol. 16, suppl_10, pp. x1–x36, 2015.

[18] J. C. Chiang and D. W. Ellison, "Molecular pathology of paediatric central nervous system tumours: pediatric CNS tumors," *The Journal of Pathology*, vol. 241, no. 2, pp. 159–172, 2017.

[19] L. M. Sánchez-Sánchez, J. Vázquez-Moreno, J. A. Heredia-Delgado, and R. Sevilla-Castillo, "Clinical presentation of supratentorial and infratentorial intracranial tumors in pediatric patients," *Gaceta Médica de México*, vol. 152, no. 2, pp. 158–162, 2016.

[20] M. C. Brodsky, "Neuro-ophthalmologic manifestations of systemic and intracranial disease," in *Pediatric Neuro-Ophthalmology*, pp. 503–596, Springer New York, New York, NY, 2010.

[21] N. Gadgil, K. Stormes, V. Shah, and S. Lam, "353 comparison of ocular outcomes in pediatric posterior fossa tumors," *Neurosurgery*, vol. 65, CN_suppl_1, pp. 140-141, 2018.

[22] T. A. G. M. Huisman, "Posterior fossa tumors in children: differential diagnosis and advanced imaging techniques," *The Neuroradiology Journal*, vol. 20, no. 4, pp. 449–460, 2007.

[23] A. Poretti, A. Meoded, and T. A. G. M. Huisman, "Neuroimaging of pediatric posterior fossa tumors including review of the literature," *Journal of Magnetic Resonance Imaging*, vol. 35, no. 1, pp. 32–47, 2012.

[24] E. R. Laws Jr. and J. P. Sheehan, "Pituitary Surgery—A Modern Approach," in *Frontiers of Hormone Research*, vol. 34, pp. 83–104, Karger, Basel, 2006.

[25] G. G. Heuer, E. M. Jackson, S. N. Magge, and P. B. Storm, "Surgical management of pediatric brain tumors," *Expert Review of Anticancer Therapy*, vol. 7, no. sup1, pp. S61–S68, 2007.

[26] E. O. Uche, M. T. Shokunbi, A. O. Malomo, E. E. U. Akang, I. Lagunju, and S. D. Amanor-Boadu, "Pediatric brain tumors in Nigeria: clinical profile, management strategies, and outcome," *Child's Nervous System*, vol. 29, no. 7, pp. 1131–1135, 2013.

[27] S. Beygi, S. Saadat, S. B. Jazayeri, and V. Rahimi-Movaghar, "Epidemiology of pediatric primary malignant central nervous system tumors in Iran: a 10 year report of National Cancer

Registry," *Cancer Epidemiology*, vol. 37, no. 4, pp. 396–401, 2013.

[28] F. Bilqees, K. Samina, and T. Mohammad, "Morphological pattern and frequency of central nervous system tumours in children," *Journal of Ayub Medical College, Abbottabad*, vol. 28, no. 1, pp. 44–46, 2016.

[29] A. Govindan, R. M. Parambil, and J. P. Alapatt, "Pediatric intracranial tumors over a 5-year period in a tertiary care center of North Kerala, India: a retrospective analysis," *Asian journal of neurosurgery*, vol. 13, no. 4, pp. 1112–1117, 2018.

[30] K. Makino, H. Nakamura, S. Yano, and J. I. Kuratsu, "Population-based epidemiological study of primary intracranial tumors in childhood," *Child's Nervous System*, vol. 26, no. 8, pp. 1029–1034, 2010.

[31] C. Sarkar, A. Jain, M. Sharma et al., "Spectrum of pediatric brain tumors in India: a multi-institutional study," *Neurology India*, vol. 59, no. 2, p. 208, 2011.

[32] J. R. Asirvatham, A. N. Deepti, R. Chyne et al., "Pediatric tumors of the central nervous system: a retrospective study of 1, 043 cases from a tertiary care center in South India," *Child's Nervous System*, vol. 27, no. 8, pp. 1257–1263, 2011.

[33] M. A. El-Gaidi, "Descriptive epidemiology of pediatric intracranial neoplasms in Egypt," *Pediatric Neurosurgery*, vol. 47, no. 6, pp. 385–395, 2012.

[34] S. Rosemberg and D. Fujiwara, "Epidemiology of pediatric tumors of the nervous system according to the WHO 2000 classification: a report of 1,195 cases from a single institution," *Child's Nervous System*, vol. 21, no. 11, pp. 940–944, 2005.

[35] A. B. Kassam, P. A. Gardner, C. H. Snyderman, R. L. Carrau, A. H. Mintz, and D. M. Prevedello, "Expanded endonasal approach, a fully endoscopic transnasal approach for the resection of midline suprasellar craniopharyngiomas: a new classification based on the infundibulum," *JNS*, vol. 108, no. 4, pp. 715–728, 2008.

[36] Z. Kaderali, M. Lamberti-Pasculli, and J. T. Rutka, "The changing epidemiology of paediatric brain tumours: a review from the Hospital for Sick Children," *Child's Nervous System*, vol. 25, no. 7, pp. 787–793, 2009.

24

Atypical Focal Choroidal Excavation with Macular Hole in a Patient with Alagille Syndrome

Manami Misawa, Hironobu Tampo, and Shinji Makino

Department of Ophthalmology, Jichi Medical University, Tochigi, Shimotsuke, Japan

Correspondence should be addressed to Shinji Makino; makichan@jichi.ac.jp

Academic Editor: Cristiano Giusti

This study is aimed at reporting a rare and unusual focal choroidal excavation with a macular hole in a patient with Alagille syndrome (AGS). A 21-year-old woman with an established early-life AGS diagnosis was referred to our hospital prior to liver transplantation. Examination revealed best-corrected visual acuity of 16/20 and 20/20 in the right and left eye, respectively. Slit-lamp examination was positive for posterior embryotoxon in both eyes. Fundoscopy revealed diffuse choroidal hypopigmentation with increased visibility of the choroidal blood vessels and circumferential chorioretinal atrophy in the mid-peripheral and peripheral retina in both eyes. A full-thickness macular hole with underlying focal choroidal excavation was observed in the right eye. Optical coherence tomography through the macula confirmed choroidal excavation with a full-thickness macular hole in the right eye. To our knowledge, this is the first report describing focal choroidal excavation with a macular hole in an AGS patient.

1. Introduction

Alagille syndrome (AGS) is clinically characterized by neonatal cholestatic jaundice with intrahepatic bile duct hypoplasia [1]. AGS is an autosomal dominant multiorgan disorder caused by aberrations in the Notch signaling pathway [2, 3], with an estimated prevalence of 1 in 30,000 to 70,000 live births [2, 3]. The majority (greater than 97%) of cases result from pathogenic variants in the Jagged canonical Notch ligand 1 (*JAG1*) gene on chromosome 20p12.18 with <1% of cases resulting from mutations in the *NOTCH2* gene (1p13) [2, 3]. Ocular findings include posterior embryotoxon, iris abnormalities, optic disc anomalies, and fundus changes [1–3].

Focal choroidal excavation (FCE) is a new disease entity of unknown origin first described by Jampol et al. [4] in 2006. FCE is defined as an area of concavity in the choroid, mostly in the macula and rarely in the extramacular region. Although initially considered congenital, an increasing number of cases have been reported in association with other retinochoroidal pathologies such as central serous choroidopathy, choroidal neovascularization, polypoidal choroidal vasculopathy, choroiditis, and choroidal tumors [5].

Herein, we report an atypical FCE with macular hole in an AGS patient.

2. Case Presentation

The patient was a 21-year-old woman diagnosed with AGS in early life. She was referred to the Jichi Medical University Hospital prior to liver transplantation. She had no problems with cognitive functioning. Her medical history was significant for systemic manifestations of AGS, including tetralogy of Fallot. On ophthalmic examination, the best-corrected visual acuity was 16/20 with $-2.50D - 2.00D \times 175°$ in the right eye and 20/20 with plane in the left. There was no abnormal ocular motility in either eye. Slit-lamp examination revealed posterior embryotoxon and iris stromal atrophy in both eyes (Figure 1). Anterior-segment optical coherence tomography (OCT) confirmed posterior embryotoxon and iris stromal atrophy (Figure 2). Fundoscopy revealed diffuse choroidal hypopigmentation with increased visibility of the choroidal blood vessels in both eyes (Figure 3). A full-thickness macular hole with underlying choroidal excavation was observed in the right eye

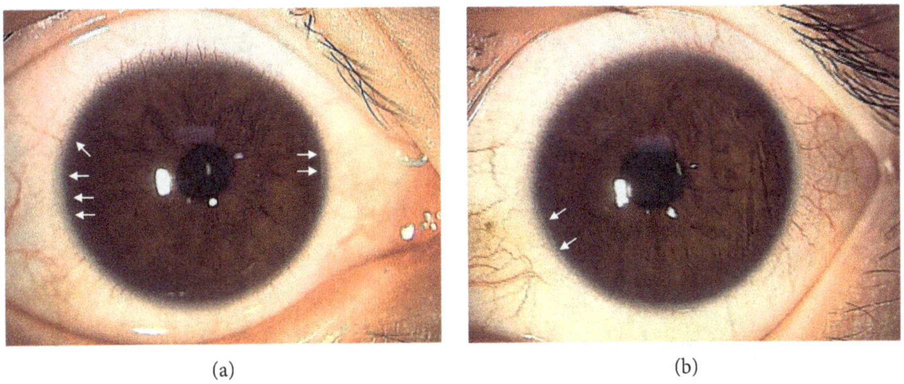

FIGURE 1: Slit-lamp photographs of the right (a) and left (b) eyes show posterior embryotoxon (arrows) and iris stromal atrophy.

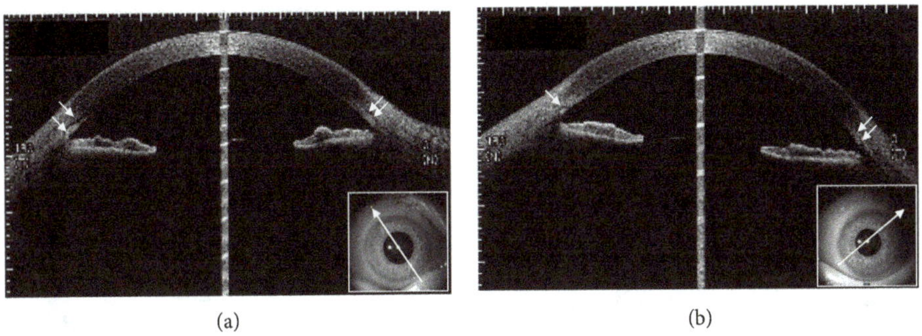

FIGURE 2: Anterior-segment optical coherence tomography images of the right (a) and left (b) eyes show posterior embryotoxon (arrows) and iris stromal atrophy.

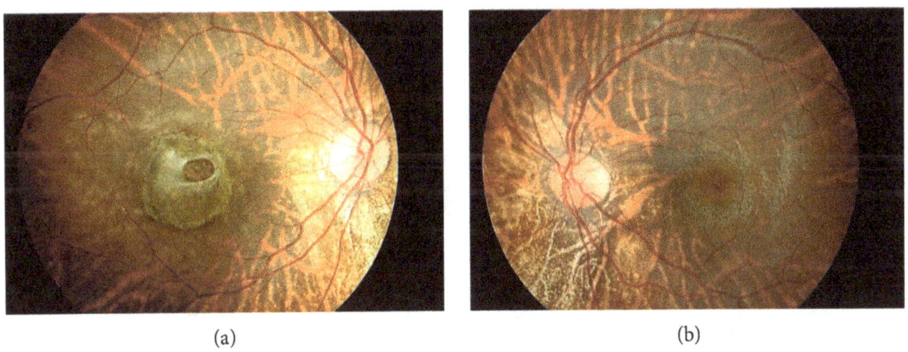

FIGURE 3: Fundus photographs of the right (a) and left (b) eyes. Note the diffuse choroidal hypopigmentation with increased visibility of the choroidal blood vessels. A full-thickness macular hole with underlying choroidal excavation observed in the right eye.

(Figure 3(a)). Moreover, circumferential chorioretinal atrophy was detected in the mid-peripheral and peripheral retina (Figure 4). Fundus autofluorescence (FAF) imaging clearly revealed the hypoautofluorescent areas corresponding to circumferential chorioretinal atrophy (Figure 5). Further, loss of autofluorescence was detected in the macular area of the right eye (Figure 5(a)). An OCT scan through the macula demonstrated FCE with a full-thickness macular hole in the right eye (Figure 6(a)). The patient was scheduled to undergo liver transplantation.

3. Discussion

Here, we report unusual ocular findings in an AGS patient.

In 1999, Hingorani et al. [1] evaluated 22 AGS patients. The most common ocular abnormalities in AGS were posterior embryotoxon (95%), iris abnormalities (45%), diffuse fundus hypopigmentation (57%), speckling of the retinal pigment epithelium (33%), and optic disc anomalies (76%). Recently, da Palma et al. [2] examined 46 eyes in 23 AGS patients, identifying anterior-segment findings were present in 74% (17/23) of them. Posterior embryotoxon was the most common anterior chamber abnormality, identified in 70% (16/23) of patients. Iris stromal hypoplasia was present in five patients (22%). Posterior segment abnormalities were reported in 96% (22/23) of patients. Abnormalities of the optic disc were observed in 12 (52%) patients. Macular appearance varied from normal (22%) to diffuse atrophy,

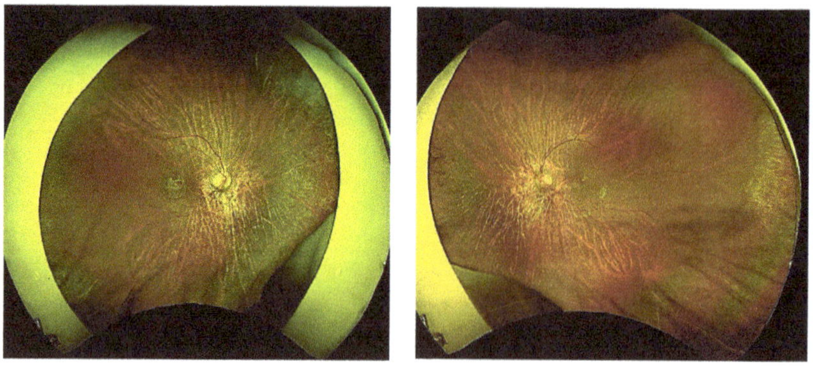

(a) (b)

Figure 4: Right (a) and left (b) wide-field fundus photographs. Note a circumferential chorioretinal atrophy in the mid-peripheral and peripheral retina.

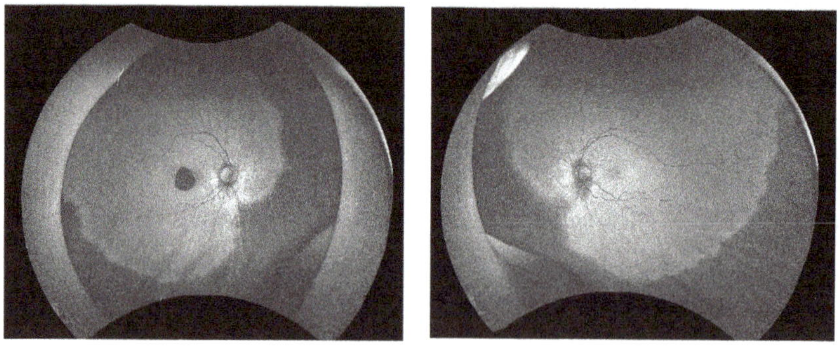

(a) (b)

Figure 5: Right (a) and left (b) wide-field fundus autofluorescence images. Note the hypoautofluorescent areas corresponding with a circumferential chorioretinal atrophy in the mid-peripheral and peripheral retina. Autofluorescence loss is detected in the macular area in the right eye.

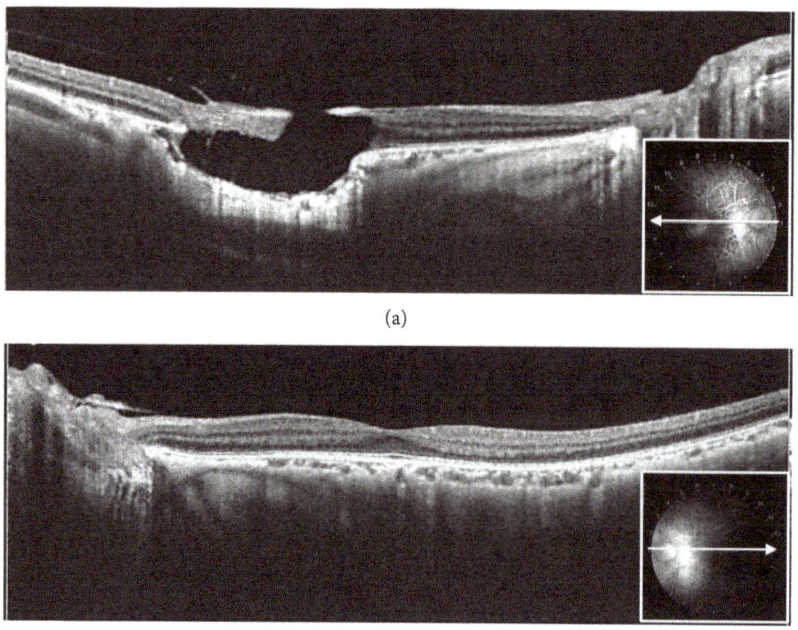

(a)

(b)

Figure 6: Right (a) and left (b) optical coherence tomography images. Note a full-thickness macular hole with underlying choroidal excavation in the right eye.

and 78% of all patients exhibited macular changes, including atrophy, pigmentation mottling, and granular changes. Peripheral chorioretinal abnormalities, reported in 22 (96%) patients, were the most frequent ocular findings in their series. This circumferential chorioretinal atrophy in the peripheral retina, assessed via wide-field FAF imaging, was first documented by Esmaili [6].

Interestingly, FCE with a full-thickness macular hole was observed in the present case. To our knowledge, this is the first report describing FCE with a macular hole in AGS patient. Few cases of FCE with a full-thickness macular hole have been reported in the literature. Hirawat et al. [7] reported FCE with a macular hole in a case of advanced retinitis pigmentosa. They speculated that inflammation due to retinitis pigmentosa could have caused disruption of the choroidal stroma, leading to atrophy and excavation. Although it is uncertain whether the development of FCE with a macular hole was consequential or coincidental, we speculate that in this patient, chorioretinal atrophy produced damage at the level of photoreceptors, the retinal pigment epithelium, and choriocapillaris, and then, the macular hole formed through the above mechanisms. The etiology of FCE remains unclear, and careful observation of fellow eyes with chorioretinal atrophy is required in such cases. Additional cases need to be examined to characterize these rare and unusual FCEs with macular holes in AGS. Ophthalmological evaluation with multimodal imaging should be pursued for all AGS patients.

References

[1] M. Hingorani, K. K. Nischal, A. Davies et al., "Ocular abnormalities in Alagille syndrome[1]," *Ophthalmology*, vol. 106, no. 2, pp. 330–337, 1999.

[2] M. M. da Palma, A. D. Igelman, C. Ku et al., "Characterization of the spectrum of ophthalmic changes in patients with Alagille syndrome," *Investigative Ophthalmology & Visual Science*, vol. 62, no. 7, p. 27, 2021.

[3] M. R. Cheema, L. G. Stone, P. W. Sellar et al., "Long-term follow-up of a patient with JAG1-associated retinopathy," *Documenta Ophthalmologica*, vol. 143, no. 2, pp. 237–247, 2021.

[4] L. M. Jampol, J. Shankle, R. Schroeder, P. Tornambe, R. F. Spaide, and M. R. Hee, "Diagnostic and therapeutic challenges," *Retina*, vol. 26, no. 9, pp. 1072–1076, 2006.

[5] S. Verma, V. Kumar, S. Azad et al., "Focal choroidal excavation: review of literature," *The British Journal of Ophthalmology*, vol. 105, no. 8, pp. 1043–1048, 2021.

[6] D. D. Esmaili, "Chorioretinal atrophy in Alagille syndrome," *Retinal Cases and Brief Reports*, vol. 9, no. 4, pp. 330–332, 2015.

[7] R. S. Hirawat, C. K. Nagesha, and C. Poddar, "Focal choroidal excavation with macular hole in a case of advanced retinitis pigmentosa," *Indian Journal of Ophthalmology*, vol. 68, no. 10, p. 2262, 2020.

25

Posterior Microphthalmia, Peripheral Pigmentary Retinal Changes, Yellow Lesions and Cleft Lip: A Case Report and Literature Review

Nasser G. Alsaedi[1,2] **and Khalid Alrubaie**[1]

[1]*King Khaled Eye Specialist Hospital, Riyadh, Saudi Arabia*
[2]*King Abdullah Medical City, Makkah, Saudi Arabia*

Correspondence should be addressed to Nasser G. Alsaedi; alsaaadi9@hotmail.com

Academic Editor: Stephen G. Schwartz

Purpose. Posterior microphthalmia is a sporadic or inherited developmental ocular anomaly that may occur isolated or in association with multiple ocular and systemic anomalies. This report documents a case of posterior microphthalmia with atypical presentation including white dots in the posterior pole in addition to systemic anomalies including facial defect that can represent an underlying genetic mutation. *Method.* Case report. *Results.* A 29-year-old male with high hyperopia and history of bilateral clear lens presented with pigmentary changes and white-yellow dots in the posterior pole in both eyes. Patient had a history of cleft lip repair. A complete ocular evaluation including A/B scan and optical coherence tomography confirmed the diagnosis of posterior microphthalmia with a retinitis pigmentosa like fundus and drusen deposits in the subretinal pigment epithelium. *Conclusion.* The white-yellow drusenoid deposits in the posterior pole in association with posterior microphthalmia are poorly documented in the literature. Cases of craniofacial developmental defects in association with posterior microphthalmia may represent a genetic defect.

1. Introduction

Posterior microphthalmia is a sporadic or inherited developmental ocular anomaly that may occur isolated or in association with multiple ocular and systemic anomalies. Ocular association including retinitis pigmentosa and optic disc drusen were first published by Buys et al. in 1999 [1]. In 2017, Plaza et al. documented white dots in the posterior pole as a new ocular finding associated with posterior microphthalmia [2]. Microphthalmia has been reported to be associated with multiple systemic anomalies including, mental retardation, craniofacial malformations (e.g., cleft lip/palate), and anomalies of the hands and feet and can be a finding in other congenital syndromes [3]. We document a rare case of posterior microphthalmia with other ocular and extraocular anomalies.

2. Case Report

A 29-year-old Saudi male presented to our institution (King Khaled Eye Specialist Hospital, KKESH) on 2007 seeking a refractive procedure. The patient had a history of cleft lip repair and had no systemic illness at presentation. The patient denied ocular trauma, ocular surgery or a family history of visual dysfunction. On ocular examination, the visual acuity in the right eye (OD) was 20/50 with a subjective cycloplegic refraction of +15.25 - 0.75 x 140° and 20/30 in the left eye (OS) with a subjective cycloplegic refraction of +15.00 -0.50 x 30°. The interpupillary distance was 63 mm. Intraocular pressure in both eyes (OU) was 19 mmHg. Slit lamp examination was unremarkable OU. White-to-white corneal measurements were 12.2 mm OD and 11.5 mm OS as measured with the slit lamp. The steepest keratometry (K) was 48.3 D at 31° OD and 48.8 D at 116° OS. The corneal thickness measurements were

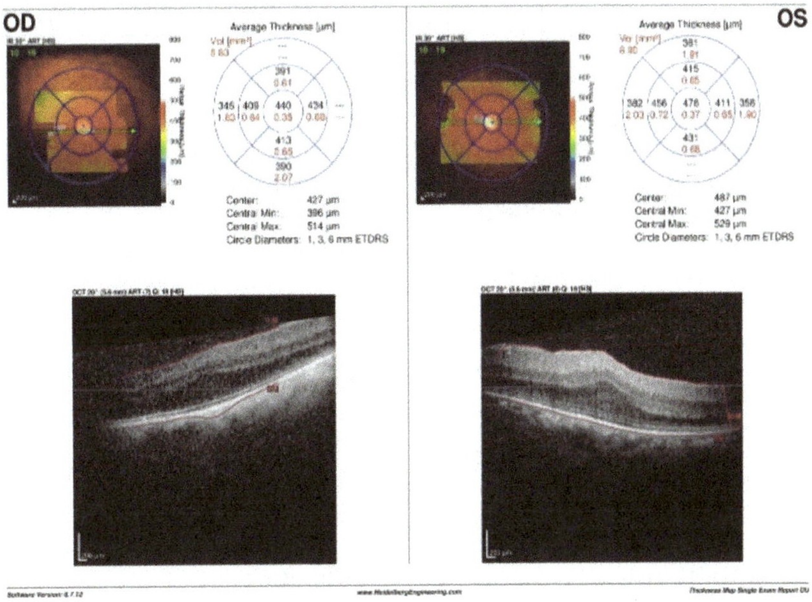

FIGURE 1: Spectral domain optical coherence tomography of both maculae and horizontal cut, depicting an inverted U-shaped papillomacular folds of the neurosensory retina, greater in the left eye with preservation of the majority of outer retinal layers.

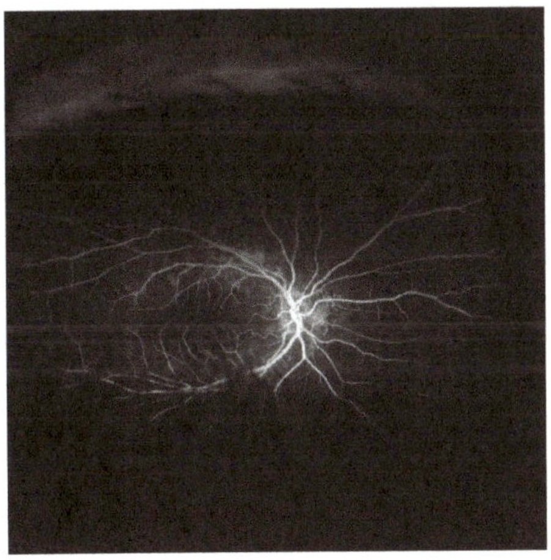

FIGURE 2: Fundus fluorescein angiography in later phases showing hyperfluorescent deposits in the posterior pole without leakage.

512 μm OD and 511 μm OS. The biometric measurements as measured by (Orbscan IIz, Bausch and Lomb, Rochester, NY, USA) of the anterior chamber depth revealed 3.32 mm OD and 3.49 mm OS. Iris examination indicated patent peripheral YAG laser iridotomies bilaterally without correctopia OU Piggyback intraocular lenses were present OU.

Indirect ophthalmoscopy was remarkable for crowded optic discs and subretinal drusenoid yellow-white dots symmetrically distributed in the posterior pole OU. Bilaterally, the retinal blood vessels appeared normal, with no clinically obvious papillomacular folds and peripheral pigmentary bone spicule pigmentation.

Macular spectral-domain optical coherence tomography (SD-OCT) revealed inverted U-shaped papillomacular folds OU (Figure 1). Posterior microphthalmia was then suspected and A-scan axial length measurements were 16.40 mm OD and 16.65 mm OS. Fluorescein angiography showed no optic nerve head staining or leakage. Staining of the yellowish subretinal drusenoids deposits was seen in the later frames OU (Figure 2). The diagnosis of posterior microphthalmia was confirmed with the given findings and no further intervention was recommended.

3. Discussion

Posterior microphthalmia is a rare developmental anomaly and is defined as a normal eye with multiple ocular findings that includes high hyperopia, normal or subnormal anterior segment structures, short axial length that may vary from 12.30 mm to 20.36 mm, papillomacular folds, pseudo-papilledema, thick choroid, and sclera [4]. Posterior microphthalmia is considered a rare subtype of microphthalmia in which there is total axial length reduction with a normal or near normal cornea. Microphthalmos is defined as a structural defect with total axial length at least two standard deviations below age-matched controls or an anteroposterior diameter less than 20 mm in adults [5, 6]. Microphthalmia is categorized generally into pure and complex, pure if there are no associated ocular defects and complex if there are other associated major ocular defects [7]. Our case report presented with ocular and systemic associations.

The association of microphthalmia with pigmentary retinal changes has been previously reported. In 1958, Hermann described 13 patients of 4 generations in a family that showed autosomal dominant transmission of microphthalmia with a variety of retinal pigmentary changes. Hermann also documented two cases reported by Catsch that had microphthalmia with retinitis pigmentosa [8].

In 1965, Franceschetti et al. described a nonconsanguineous family comprised of four individuals with microphthalmia, retinal degeneration, and dental anomalies. They postulated a probable autosomal recessive pattern of inheritance in this association (MIM 251700) [9]. In 1999, Buys et al. published the first combination of nanophthalmos, retinitis pigmentosa, and optic disc drusen that was observed in a 68-year-old male and they proposed that a retinitis pigmentosa-like presentation in such patients may be due to chronic choroidal effusion and serous retinal detachments [1]. These associations described by Buys et al. were subsequently shown to be associated with a frameshift mutation of MFRP (Membrane-type Frizzled-Related Protein) confirming the syndrome of posterior microphthalmos, retinitis pigmentosa, foveoschisis, and optic disc drusen [10]. Interestingly, the association of optic disc drusen with retinitis pigmentosa is well known in the literature. Grover et al. reviewed 262 patients with retinitis pigmentosa and found that 9.2% had optic disc drusen [11]. Another ocular finding in our case is the white/yellow dots in the posterior pole. These white dots in the posterior pole in association with posterior microphthalmia are similar to a case first reported by Plaza et al. in 2017 with posterior microphthalmia, retinitis pigmentosa, optic disc drusen syndrome, and additional findings of yellow macular dots that were not included as criteria for this syndrome [2].

Ayala-Ramires et al. described the criteria for the syndrome as follows: posterior microphthalmos with anteroposterior diameter between 13 mm and 18.5 mm; normal corneal and anterior chamber diameters; high hyperopia, between +8.00 and +25.00 D; optic nerve head drusen with campimetric defects similar to those caused by simple chronic glaucoma; retinal dystrophy compatible with pigment retinosis confirmed by electroretinogram in association with foveoschisis, cystoid macular edema, or foveolar thickening [12]. The yellow dots reported by Plaza et al. were located at the level of retinal pigmented epithelium and the fluorescein angiography indicated a broad window defect with hyperfluorescence of these dots in the later phases [2]. These yellow dots behave like drusen and we postulate that the association of this syndrome with drusen can be found in the disc or the retina.

Papillomacular fold is an ocular finding in posterior microphthalmia and is considered one of the causes of reduced vision. It is confined only to the neurosensory layer sparing the retinal pigment epithelium, choroid, and sclera [13]. It is important for the ophthalmologist to be aware of this finding as this can be confused or mistaken as cystoid macular edema [14]. Additionally, we recommend axial length measurements in patients with hyperopia over +8.00 D and similar posterior segment findings. The SD-OCT finding in our case indicates absence of the normal foveal pit or *fovea plana* that is also associated with microphthalmos, ocular albinism, retinopathy of prematurity, and aniridia [15, 16]. The term fovea plana instead of foveal hypoplasia

Table 1: A Practical Classification of Microphthalmia/Coloboma.

Isolated
Microphthalmia
Colobomatous
Isolated uveoretinal coloboma
Microphthalmia with cyst
Non-colobomatous
Microphthalmia with Ocular Anomalies
Cataract
Myopia and corectopia
Ectopia lentis
congenital retinal detachment
Persistent Hyperplastic Primary Vitreous
Aicardi syndrome
Microphthalmia with Mental Retardation
Mental retardation
Mental retardation and congenital spastic diplegia (Sjogren-Larsson)
Microphthalmia with Craniofacial Malformations
Facio-Auriculo-Vertebral sequence
Hallermann-Streiff syndrome
Amniotic band syndrome
Transverse facial cleft
Cleft lip/palate
Microcephaly
Microcephaly and retinal folds
Hydrocephalus and congenital retinal non-attachment (Warburg syndrome)
Microphthalmia with Malformations of the Hands and Feet
Polydactyly
Waardenburg's recessive anophthalmia syndrome
Microphthalmia with Multiple Congenital Anomalies (Syndromes)
CHARGE association
Duker syndrome
Lenz microphthalmia syndrome
Oculo-Dento-Osseous Dysplasia
Cryptophthalmos syndrome
Cerebro-Oculo-Facial Syndrome
Goltz syndrome or focal dermal hypoplasia
Lowe syndrome
Meckel-Gruber syndrome
Basal cell nevus syndrome of Gorlin-Goltz
Cross syndrome
Microphthalmia with linear skin defects
Microphthalmia in Chromosomal Anomalies
T-13 (Patau)
4p- (Wolf-Hirschorn)
18q-
18r
T-18 (Edward)
Cat-eye syndrome (marker 22)
Other chromosomal aberrations

TABLE 1: Continued.

Microphthalmia and Intrauterine Insults
Maternal drug intake: thalidomide, alcohol, isotretinoin, others
Maternal vitamin A deficiency
Maternal fever or radiation exposure
Maternal uncontrolled phenylketonuria
Intrauterine infections: CMV, EBV, Varicella, Herpes simplex, Rubella, Toxoplasmosis

Adopted from [3].

was suggested by Marmor when the cone is preserved both anatomically and functionally despite the absence of the foveal pit [17]. Fovea plana can be found in normal eyes and up to a 3% incidence had been reported in children with clinically normal eyes [18].

The extraocular manifestation of patients with microphthalmia spectrum includes multisystemic malformations of the heart, renal, face, and central nervous system [19]. A systemic work-up should be performed in patients with multiple malformations and a chromosomal microarray study or exome sequencing may be required in those with multiple malformations (Table 1) [3].

4. Conclusion

Posterior microphthalmia should be suspected in cases with high hyperopia. The occurrence of posterior microphthalmia with other ocular and systemic associations has been reported in the literature. The white-yellow dots in the posterior pole in posterior microphthalmia are an atypical finding and poorly described in the literature. Cases of craniofacial developmental defects in association with ocular anomalies including posterior microphthalmia may represent genetic/chromosomal defects. We recommend evaluating such cases to establish a distinct pattern of inheritance.

References

[1] Y. M. Buys and C. J. Pavlin, "Retinitis pigmentosa, nanophthalmos, and optic disc drusen: A case report," *Ophthalmology*, vol. 106, no. 3, pp. 619–622, 1999.

[2] P. Plaza, O. Iturralde, and C. Abascal, "Posterior microphthalmos, retinitis pigmentosa and optic disc drusen with white dots. A case report," *Archivos de la Sociedad Espanola de Oftalmologia*, vol. 92, no. 11, pp. 555–558, 2017.

[3] O. Arif, M. D. Khan, and M. D. Elias Traboulsi, "Microphthalmia, anophthalmia, coloboma and nanophthalmos (includes Charge association)," 2016, https://www.aao.org.

[4] S. R. Nowilaty, A. O. Khan, M. A. Aldahmesh, K. F. Tabbara, A. Al-Amri, and F. S. Alkuraya, "Biometric and molecular characterization of clinically diagnosed posterior microphthalmos," *American Journal of Ophthalmology*, vol. 155, no. 2, pp. 361–372, 2013.

[5] R. Ayala-Ramirez, F. Graue-Wiechers, V. Robredo, M. Amato-Almanza, I. Horta-Diez, and J. C. Zenteno, "A new autosomal recessive syndrome consisting of pasterior microphthalmos, retinitis pigmentosa, foveoschisis, and optic disc drusen is caused by a MFRP gene mutation," *Molecular Vision*, vol. 12, pp. 1483–1489, 2006.

[6] M. J. Elder, "Aetiology of severe visual impairment and blindness in microphthalmos," *British Journal of Ophthalmology*, vol. 78, no. 5, pp. 332–334, 1994.

[7] E. I. Traboulsi, "Colobomatou smicrophthalmia, anophthalmia, and associated malformation syndromes," in *Genetic Diseases of the Eye*, E. I. Traboulsi, Ed., pp. 51–80, Oxford University Press, New York, NY, USA, 1998.

[8] P. Hermann, "Le syndrome microphtalmie-rétinite pigmentaireglaucome," *Archives of Ophthalmology*, vol. 18, pp. 17–24, 1958.

[9] A. Franceschetti and H. Gernet, "Ultrasonics diagnosis of microphthalmia without microcornea, with macrophakia, high hypermetropia associated with tapeto-retinal degeneration, a glaucomatous predisposition and dental anomalies (new familial syndrome)," *Archives d'Ophtalmologie et Revue Générale d'Ophtalmologie*, vol. 25, pp. 105–116, 1965.

[10] J. Crespi, J. A. Buil, and F. Bassaganyas, "A novel mutation confirms MFRP as the gene causing the syndrome of nanophthalmos-renititis pigmentosa-foveoschisis-optic disk drusen," *American Journal of Ophthalmology*, vol. 146, no. 2, pp. 323–328, 2008.

[11] S. Grover, G. A. Fishman, and J. Brown Jr., "Frequency of optic disc or parapapillary nerve fiber layer drusen in retinitis pigmentosa," *Ophthalmology*, vol. 104, no. 2, pp. 295–298, 1997.

[12] R. Ayala-Ramirez, F. Graue-Wiechers, V. Roberdo, M. Amato-Almanza, I. Horta-Diez, and J. C. Zenteno, "A new autosomalrecessive syndrome consisting of posterior microphthalmos,retinitis pigmentosa, foveoschisis, and optic disc drusen iscaused by a MFRP gene mutation," *Molecular Vision*, vol. 4, pp. 1483–1489, 2006.

[13] T. E. Jackson, Y. C. Yang, and G. A. Shun-Shin, "Spectral domain optical coherence tomography findings in retinal folds associated with posterior microphthalmos," *Journal of American Association for Pediatric Ophthalmology and Strabismus*, vol. 16, no. 4, pp. 389–391, 2012.

[14] A. A. Albar, S. R. Nowilaty, and N. G. Ghazi, "Posterior microphthalmos and papillomacular fold-associated cystic changes misdiagnosed as cystoid macular edema following cataract extraction," *Clinical Ophthalmology*, vol. 9, pp. 73–76, 2015.

[15] A. Vincent, V. Kemmanu, R. Shetty, V. Anandula, B. Madhavarao, and B. Shetty, "Variable expressivity of ocular associations of foveal hypoplasia in a family," *Eye*, vol. 23, no. 8, pp. 1735–1739, 2009.

[16] V. M. Villegas, S. G. Schwartz, T. D. Hamet, C. A. McKeown, H. Capó, and H. W. Flynn, "Variable clinical profile of fovea plana in normal children," *Ophthalmic Surgery, Lasers and Imaging Retina*, vol. 49, no. 4, pp. 251–257, 2018.

[17] M. F. Marmor, S. S. Choi, R. J. Zawadzki, and J. S. Werner, "Visual insignificance of the foveal pit: Reassessment of foveal hypoplasia as fovea plana," *JAMA Ophtalmology*, vol. 126, no. 7, pp. 907–913, 2008.

[18] S. Noval, S. F. Freedman, S. Asrani, and M. A. El-Dairi, "Incidence of fovea plana in normal children," *Journal of American Association for Pediatric Ophthalmology and Strabismus*, vol. 18, no. 5, pp. 471–475, 2014.

[19] E. Raveh, B. C. Papsin, and V. Forte, "Branchio-oculo-facial syndrome," *International Journal of Pediatric Otorhinolaryngology*, vol. 53, no. 2, pp. 149–156, 2000.

26

Optic Coherence Tomography Angiography Findings of Bilateral Choroidal Neovascularization Associated with Optic Disc Drusen Treated with Intravitreal Aflibercept Injection

Melih Akıdan,[1] **Mehmet Bulut**,[2] **Lütfiye Yaprak**,[2] **Muhammet Kazım Erol**,[2] **and Elcin Suren**[2]

[1]*Department of Ophthalmology, Antalya Kepez State Hospital, Antalya, Turkey*
[2]*Department of Ophtalmology, Antalya Education and Research Hospital, Antalya, Turkey*

Correspondence should be addressed to Melih Akıdan; melcihhh@yahoo.com

Academic Editor: Alexander A. Bialasiewicz

Purpose. The purpose of this case report is to present the findings of optical coherence tomography angiography (OCTA) of a patient with bilateral choroidal neovascularization (CNV) associated with optic disc drusen (ODD), who was treated with intravitreal aflibercept injection. *Case presentation.* A 14-year-old girl presented with a complaint of visual loss and metamorphopsia in her both eyes. Best-corrected visual acuity (BCVA) was 20/32 and 20/25, respectively, in the right and left eyes. Intraocular pressure and anterior segment examination were normal. Dilated fundus examination revealed elevated optic discs with blurred margins in both eyes. In addition, slightly elevated yellow lesion extending from optic nerve head to the macula was observed bilaterally. The patient underwent imaging with colour fundus photography, fundus autofluorescence (FAF), fundus fluorescein angiography (FFA), spectral-domain optic coherence tomography (SD-OCT), OCTA, orbital ultrasonography (USG), and computed tomography (CT). In particular, OCTA demonstrated clearly the large circular CNV complex in the right eye and the CNV structure in the left eye containing slightly activated main trunk and minimal vessel loops in the papillomacular region. CNV secondary to bilateral ODD was suspected. Intravitreal aflibercept injections were performed in 3 doses to the right eye and a single dose to the left eye. After the injections, BCVA reached its complete level in both eyes. SD-OCT revealed irregularity of RPE in the temporal region of the optic disc and complete regression of the subretinal fluid. Interestingly, the entire CNV complex including the main trunk completely disappeared in OCTA. CNV complex was not observed in OCTA during 1-year follow-up, and peripapillary and macular vascular density measurements did not show any significant change. BCVA was preserved, and no additional injections were needed. *Conclusion.* It is possible that OCTA can be used for detailed evaluation of CNV associated with ODD, response to anti-VEGF treatment, and peripapillary and macular vascular density. There is a need for further studies to confirm the changes such as disappearance of CNV in OCTA after injection as we observed in our patient.

1. Introduction

Optic disc drusen (ODD) are calcified hyaline-like deposits in the optic nerve head that are mainly located in front of the lamina cribrosa. They are often bilateral (67%-91%), and their incidence is 0.4%-20.4% in general population while there is female preponderance in their prevalence. They are usually benign and vision sparing; however, they may rarely complicate with visual field defects, haemorrhages, choroidal neovascularization (CNV), serous maculopathy, vascular occlusion, and nonarteritic ischemic optic neuropathy (NAION) [1].

Various imaging methods have been used in order to detect ODD accurately and reliably, which include ultrasonography (USG), enhanced depth imaging-OCT (EDI-OCT), fluorescein fundus angiography (FFA), and fundus autofluorescence (FAF), and the newest application is optical coherence tomography angiography (OCTA, Optovue, Inc., Fremont, CA, USA) [2].

Noninvasive imaging of the retina, choroidal, and disc microvasculature is now possible with OCTA and without the use of exogenous intravenous dye injection. It can provide information for the evaluation of both structure and blood flow. It particularly allows the assessment of CNV morphology and features activity as well as the timing of and response to anti-VEGF treatment of CNV [3, 4]. It has been increasingly used for the diagnosis and imaging of paediatric retinal vascular disease and especially CNV as it is both reliable and noninvasive [5].

The OCTA studies in the literature mainly focus on microvascular changes associated with optic disc drusen. To the best of our knowledge, only Ong et al. demonstrated inactivate CNV associated with ODD in 1 case with OCTA in a series of 8 paediatric patients with CNV. However, this is the first time to report an interesting change in CNV after injection and long-term follow-up findings.

2. Case Report

A 14-year-old girl was referred to us with complaints of visual loss and metamorphopsia in both eyes that had persisted for 1 week. Her best-corrected visual acuity (BCVA) was 20/32 in the right eye and 20/25 in the left eye. Her ocular and systemic history was unremarkable. Her intraocular pressure and anterior segment examination were normal. Dilated fundus examination revealed elevated optic discs with blurred margins in both eyes. In addition, slightly elevated yellow lesion extending from optic nerve head to the macula was observed bilaterally (Figures 1(a) and 1(d)). The patient underwent imaging with colour fundus photography, FAF, FFA, spectral-domain optic coherence tomography (SD-OCT, Cirrus HD OCT 5000, Carl Zeiss Meditec Inc., Dublin, CA, USA), OCTA, orbital USG, and computed tomography (CT). FAF showed bilateral aspect of white refractile and hyperautofluorescence bodies on the surface of the optic nerve linked with the drusen and a hypoautofluorescent and hyperautofluorescent lesion in the papillomacular region (Figures 1(b) and 1(e)). FFA showed no hyperfluorescence or leakage with blurred borders of the optic disc, and early hyperfluorescence and intense leakage that might be associated with CNV were observed in both eyes with the right eye predominance (Figures 1(c) and 1(f)). The peripheral retina was normal. B-mode USG showed hyperechogenic appearance, and orbital CT revealed papilla as bright spots which might be associated with optic disc drusen (Figure 1(g)). SD-OCT showed retinal thickening, subretinal hyperreflectivity in the papillomacular region bilaterally, and subfoveal fluid in the right eye (Figures 1(h) and 1(i)). Furthermore, macular and retinal nerve fiber layer (RNFL) thickness measurements were recorded (Table 1).

OCTA revealed superficial and deep capillary density, foveal avascular zone, flow, and en face images in the macula (Table 2). A large circular CNV complex with main trunk, multiple dense thin capillaries branching from the main trunk in a tree-like manner, and frequent anastomoses was observed in the papillomacular region of the right eye in the outer retina and choriocapillaris cross-sections (Figures 2(a) and 2(b)). In the left eye, CNV with main trunk, minimal vessel loops, and capillaries was observed, which was considered as slightly activated (Figures 2(c) and 2(d)). Moreover, radial papillary capillary density was measured with OCTA (Table 2). Density was lower in the areas associated with nasal quadrant compared to the other quadrants.

All evaluations suggested CNV secondary to ODD, and intravitreal aflibercept was injected in 3 doses to the right eye and a single dose to the left eye. Three doses were injected to the right eye every other month. After the first injection, BCVA remained as 20/32 and increased to 20/25 after the second one. After the third dose of injection to the right eye and the first one to the left eye, BCVA was 20/20 in both eyes. After the injections in both eyes, SD-OCT revealed RPE irregularity in the temporal region of the optic disc and complete regression of the subretinal fluid. OCTA interestingly showed that the entire CNV compete including the main trunk disappeared (Figures 3(a) to 3(d)). CNV complex was not observed with OCTA, and no significant change was observed in the peripapillary and macular vascular density measurements, and findings which might be correlated with RNFL measurements were not detected in 1-year follow-up. BCVA was preserved, and no additional injections were needed.

3. Discussion

CNV associated with ODD is a very rare complication, which has been reported in both adults and children [6]. In most of the patients, CNV membranes associated with ODD occur nasally; however, they may also occur temporally resulting in serous haemorrhagic maculopathy, cystoid macular edema, and macular scarring [7]. Its pathogenesis is unknown. Possible mechanisms involved in this complication include the compressive effect of drusen on the surrounding blood vessels, which leads to mechanical impairment of peripapillary vascular integrity, vascular congestion, or ischemia. Retinal ischemia and the release of VEGF may be the factors that trigger the development of CNV [8, 9]. Treatment must be provided if vision is jeopardized. The modern antivascular endothelial growth factor (VEGF) medications, photodynamic therapy, and surgical removal have each been demonstrated to be successful [10]. Anti-VEGF agents have been increasingly preferred as the first-line treatment because they ensure high visual acuity and disease stabilization usually with fewer intravitreal injections especially in paediatric cases, and recurrence is almost never observed. Gan and Long reported complete resolution after 3 doses of injection in cases for whom aflibercept was injected for the first time [11]. Knape et al. reported rapid and atraumatic resolution with the combination of bevacizumab and focal laser photocoagulation [12]. Alkın et al. emphasized that CNV secondary to ODD might be more sensitive than CNV secondary to age-related macular degeneration (AMD) in cases injected with a single dose of ranibizumab [13]. We achieved rapid response and did not observe recurrence in cases injected with 3 doses of aflibercept in the right eye and a single dose

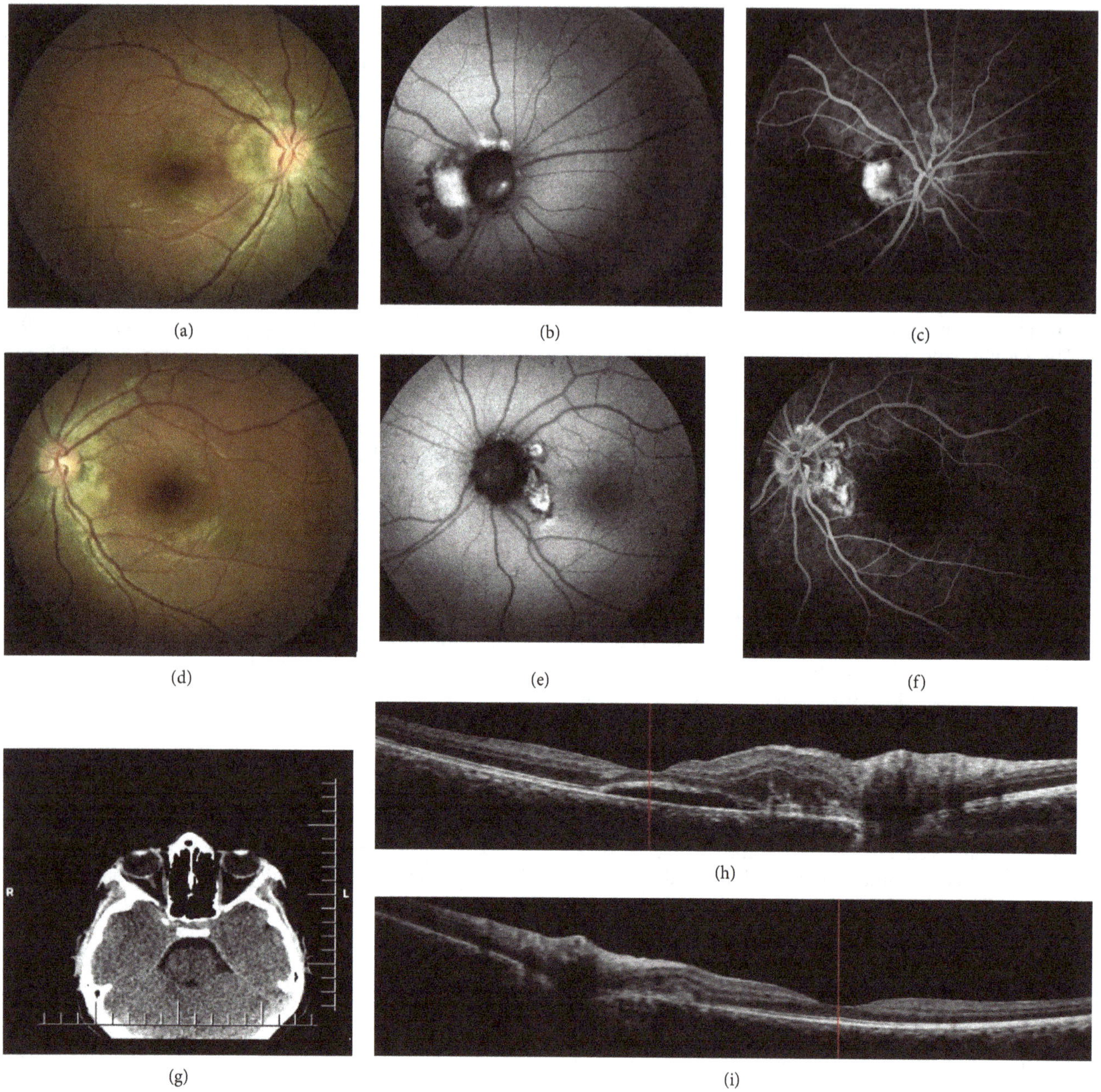

Figure 1: On the first day. (a and d) Fundus image of the right and left eyes; elevated optic disc with blurred margin and slightly elevated yellow lesion extending from optic nerve head to the macula. (b and e) FAF image of the right and left eyes; hyperautofluorescence bodies on the surface of the optic nerve linked with the drusen and hyperautofluorescent lesion in the papillomacular region. (c and f) FFA image of the right and left eyes; hyperfluorescence and intense leakage that might be associated with CNV. (g) Orbital CT image of the right and left eyes; bright spot on papilla associated with optic disc drusen. (h) SD-OCT image of the right eye; retinal thickening, subretinal hyperreflectivity, and subfoveal fluid in the papillomacular region. (i) SD-OCT image of the left eye; retinal thickening and subretinal hyperreflectivity in the papillomacular region.

of aflibercept in the left eye and whom we followed for 12 months with OCTA.

4 different CNV patterns associated with exudative age-related macular degeneration can be detected with OCTA: Medusa pattern: central feeder vessel, circular peripheral anastomosis, thin branches, and hypointense halo; seafan pattern: eccentric feeder vessel, thin branches, and hypointense halo; indistinct network pattern: thin branches and hypointense halo; and pruned vascular tree pattern: persistence of main vascular trunks [14]. Pruned vascular tree pattern is considered as inactivate and usually followed up. The morphology of CNV and structural response to anti-VEGF treatment are strongly correlated. Anti-VEGF is ineffective for the vascular trunk while it is effective for especially the newly formed capillaries from preexisting vascular trunks while there is a correlation between better functional outcomes an increased vascularity of the CNV [15]. Spaide demonstrates reprofileration 20-50 days after the injection [16].

Table 1: On the first day, 3rd month, and 12th month; OCT and RNFL thickness measurements.

Thickness (μm)	Day 1		Month 3		Month 12	
Macular						
Fovea	232	250	236	248	239	251
Parafovea	337	340	339	335	338	348
Superior-hemi	339	342	340	338	339	350
Inferior-hemi	335	337	337	333	336	345
Temporal	323	319	328	316	327	328
Superior	348	349	349	344	349	358
Nasal	335	350	335	347	332	354
Inferior	343	340	344	334	343	350
Perifovea	318	322	316	316	316	325
Superior-hemi	322	328	317	322	315	330
Inferior-hemi	315	316	314	310	316	320
Temporal	293	296	299	292	297	302
Superior	322	330	320	323	318	333
Nasal	341	349	330	342	329	346
Inferior	317	313	314	307	318	320
Retinal nerve fiber layer						
Whole	129	126	126	125	129	134
Superior-hemi	123	130	121	129	122	142
Inferior-hemi	137	122	131	121	136	126
Nasal superior	111	107	116	102	117	110
Nasal inferior	107	97	100	91	108	98
Inferior nasal	145	146	142	141	149	147
Inferior temporal	195	173	202	182	211	184
Temporal inferior	108	74	87	78	82	80
Temporal superior	100	97	88	100	91	107
Superior temporal	176	179	173	185	174	201
Superior nasal	118	157	119	150	117	174

Cells are divided into two to show the results of the right and left eyes separately.

However, long-term inactivation can be ensured with fewer anti-VEGF injections in cases of CNV associated with high myopia, punctate inner choroidopathy (PIC), choroidal osteoma, optic nerve drusen like our patient, and idiopathic with lower activity than AMD [17–20]. The literature does not contain wide range of data which can be used to assess why stabilization can be achieved with fewer injections and make comparisons with CNV patterns of AMD with OCTA as highlighted above and assess reproliferation.

The most striking finding after injection in our case was the absence of CNV visualization in OCTA. The absence of CNV visualization in OCTA was associated with clinical and SD-OCT exudative inactivity [14]. In fact, inactive lesions are visualized as pruned vascular tree pattern, presence of large linear vessel with no or minimal anastomosis in OCTA. This may be due to other reasons such as the masking effect generated by a high PED, media opacities, or the presence of haemorrhages [21]. However, they were not observed in the follow-up of our patient. Hua and Ning demonstrated the development of atrophy in the CNV complex after 3 doses of anti-VEGF injections in PIC cases with high myopia and round dark region visualization due to no-perfusion/hypopefusion zone in the choriocapillaris [22]. This situation which was also observed in our case can be interpreted as decreased signal due to inactivity, but the absence of pruned vascular tree pattern may at least contribute to explaining why atrophy/shrinkage can develop in the main vascular trunk and why non-AMD CNV causes are more benign and can be stabilized longer with fewer injections.

In the literature, only Ong et al. demonstrated inactive CNV associated with ODD in 1 case with OCTA in a series of 8 paediatric patients with CNV. A 12-year-old female patient first underwent injection and photodynamic therapy in the left eye; however, OCTA revealed two large calibre vessels and a lack of fine capillaries, anastomoses, and vessel loops, which was considered as inactive sub-RPE CNV lesion [23]. This is the first paper to report a case with an interesting change in CNV visualization after injection and followed up for a long term for both CNV and vascular density. On the other hand, studies on OCTA for ODD mainly focus on microvascular changes. Biçer and Atilla showed that macular vascular density located in different regions decreased both at

Table 2: On the first day, 3rd month, and 12th month; OCTA macula and disc vascular density, FAZ, and flow measurements.

	Day 1		Month 3		Month 12	
Disc-capillary density						
Radial peripapillary (%)						
Whole	49.1	48.6	49.2	48.1	48.2	48.5
Inside disc	46.9	45.3	45.9	43.3	40.6	45.9
Peripapillary	51.7	51.0	51.1	49.5	50.7	50.4
Superior-hemi	50.7	50.8	51.2	49.9	50.7	50.5
Inferior-hemi	52.8	51.2	50.9	49	50.7	50.2
Nasal superior	45.8	47.8	46	47.1	46.1	46.3
Nasal inferior	49.1	46.6	48.4	46.6	49.6	46.3
Inferior nasal	53.1	50.9	52.3	45.4	51.8	48.3
Inferior temporal	53.8	57.2	52.3	53.1	49.7	57.2
Temporal inferior	56	51.5	51.4	52.2	51.7	51.1
Temporal superior	57.3	55.3	57.1	56	56.7	58.2
Superior temporal	56.1	53.2	55.9	53.3	52.4	50.9
Superior nasal	45.7	47.9	47.2	43.9	48.2	47.7
Macula-capillary density						
Superficial (%)						
Whole	52.4	53.2	54.5	54.1	53.5	51.9
Superior-hemi	53.5	53	54.8	53.7	53.3	51.9
Inferior-hemi	54.6	50.8	54.2	54.5	53.6	51.9
Fovea	15.2	17.1	14.6	17.7	15.7	15.3
Parafovea	55.3	53.6	58.2	58.1	56.8	55
Superior-hemi	57.1	53.5	57.8	56.6	55.9	54.1
Inferior-hemi	56.8	56.8	58.6	59.6	57.7	56
Temporal	56.2	52.8	55.5	56.5	56.1	54.1
Superior	58.5	55.6	58.8	57.4	57.2	53.6
Nasal	56.7	59.3	57.5	57.9	55.4	55.6
Inferior	60	55.9	61	60.5	58.4	56.8
Perifovea	52.8	51.8	54.3	54.5	53.3	52.9
Superior-hemi	53.1	53.5	54.7	54.3	52.9	53.2
Inferior-hemi	53.6	54.1	53.9	54.7	53.6	52.7
Temporal	50.3	52	51.8	52.2	50.8	52.5
Superior	54.2	54.7	54.7	53.9	52.4	53.1
Nasal	57.5	53.4	57.7	58.2	57.4	55.2
Inferior	53.4	52.4	52.6	53.8	52.2	50.9
Deep (%)						
Whole	48.1	47.6	48.3	48.4	48	46.9
Superior-hemi	49.9	47.9	50.3	47.9	49.7	47.4
Inferior-hemi	46.4	48.5	46.4	49	46	46.4
Fovea	32.3	30.1	30.6	29.1	32.7	29.2
Parafovea	55.8	53.9	56.4	55.1	55.5	55.7
Superior-hemi	56.7	55.7	56.7	55.2	56.2	55.9
Inferior-hemi	55.6	56.2	56	54.9	54.8	55.5
Temporal	55.8	57.5	55	57.4	55.6	57.8
Superior	56.5	53.4	57.8	53.7	55.5	55.3
Nasal	57.9	55.2	58.3	55.9	58.1	55.8
Inferior	52.3	51.8	54.4	53.4	52.8	53.9

TABLE 2: Continued.

	Day 1		Month 3		Month 12	
Perifovea	50.1	48.3	50.7	50.1	48.1	46.3
Superior-hemi	50.2	48.6	52.8	49.8	49	46.7
Inferior-hemi	48.5	47.4	48.6	50.4	47.2	45.8
Temporal	54.8	54.3	56.1	54.6	55.5	49.5
Superior	49.4	49.2	53.3	49.4	47.3	47.4
Nasal	43.9	43.4	46.4	46.5	44.6	42.8
Inferior	46.7	48.1	47.8	50	45.8	45.3
Foveal avascular zone (mm^2)						
Retina	352	376	347	389	358	386
Foveal flow						
Outer retina	0.558	0.732	0.346	0.846	0.602	0.665
Choriocapillaris	2.101	2.068	2.087	2.091	2.195	2.058

Cells are divided into two to show the results of the right and left eyes separately.

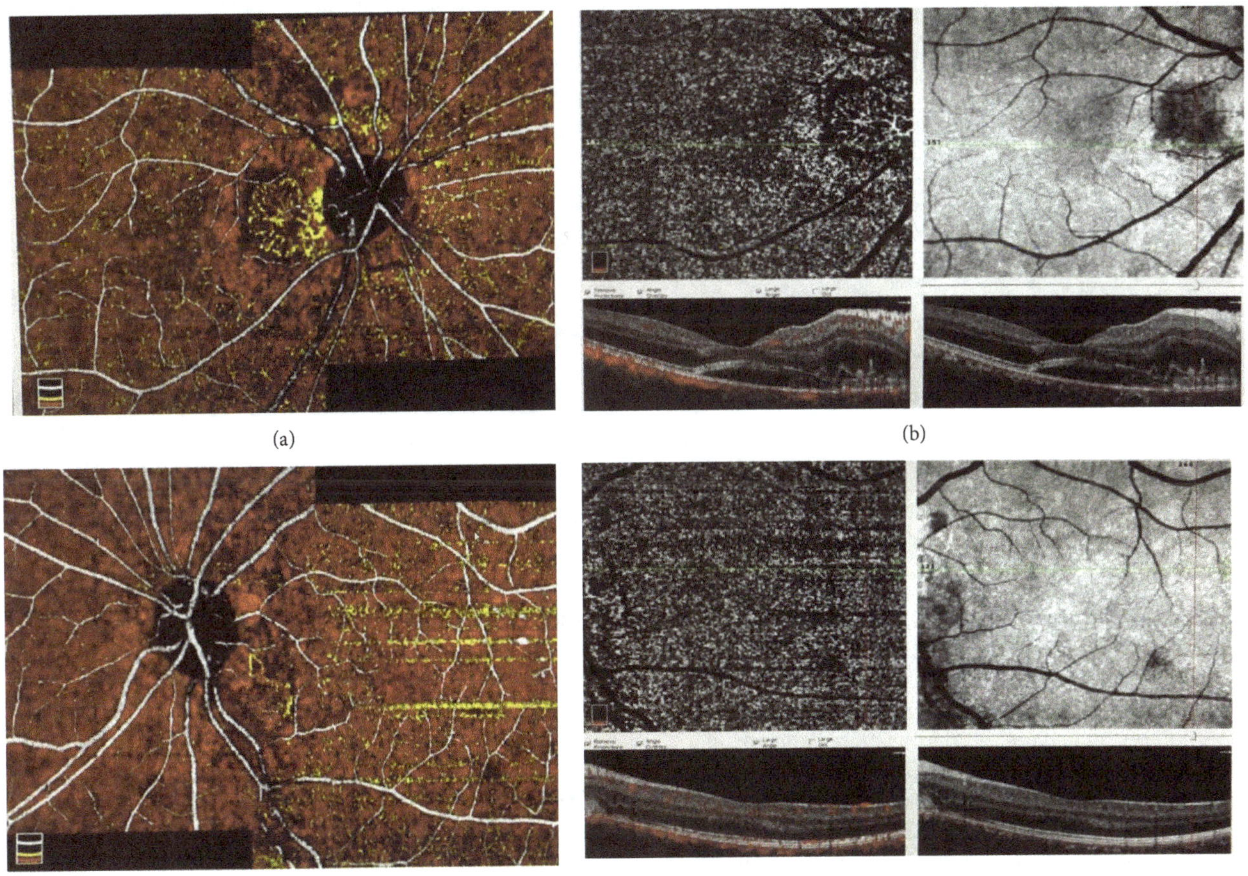

(a) (b) (c) (d)

FIGURE 2: On the first day. (a) Unified and coloured OCTA image of the right eye; circular CNV complex with main trunk, multiple dense thin capillaries branching from the main trunk and frequent anastomoses (yellow). (b) Outer retina cross-section and en face OCTA image of the right eye. (c) Unified and coloured OCTA image of the left eye; CNV with main trunk, minimal vessel loops, and capillaries (yellow). (d) Outer retina cross-section and en face OCTA image of the left eye.

the superficial and deep capillary layer in cases with bilateral ODD, and there was a density loss in the peripapillary area especially the nasal region. They reported that ODD findings could be used to demonstrate that enlarged ODD might cause acute or chronic ischemia by compressing nerve fibers or surrounding vessel [24]. Aghdam et al. compared patients with ODD, NAION, and normal individuals and reported that optic nerve head vessel density was lower in the NAION

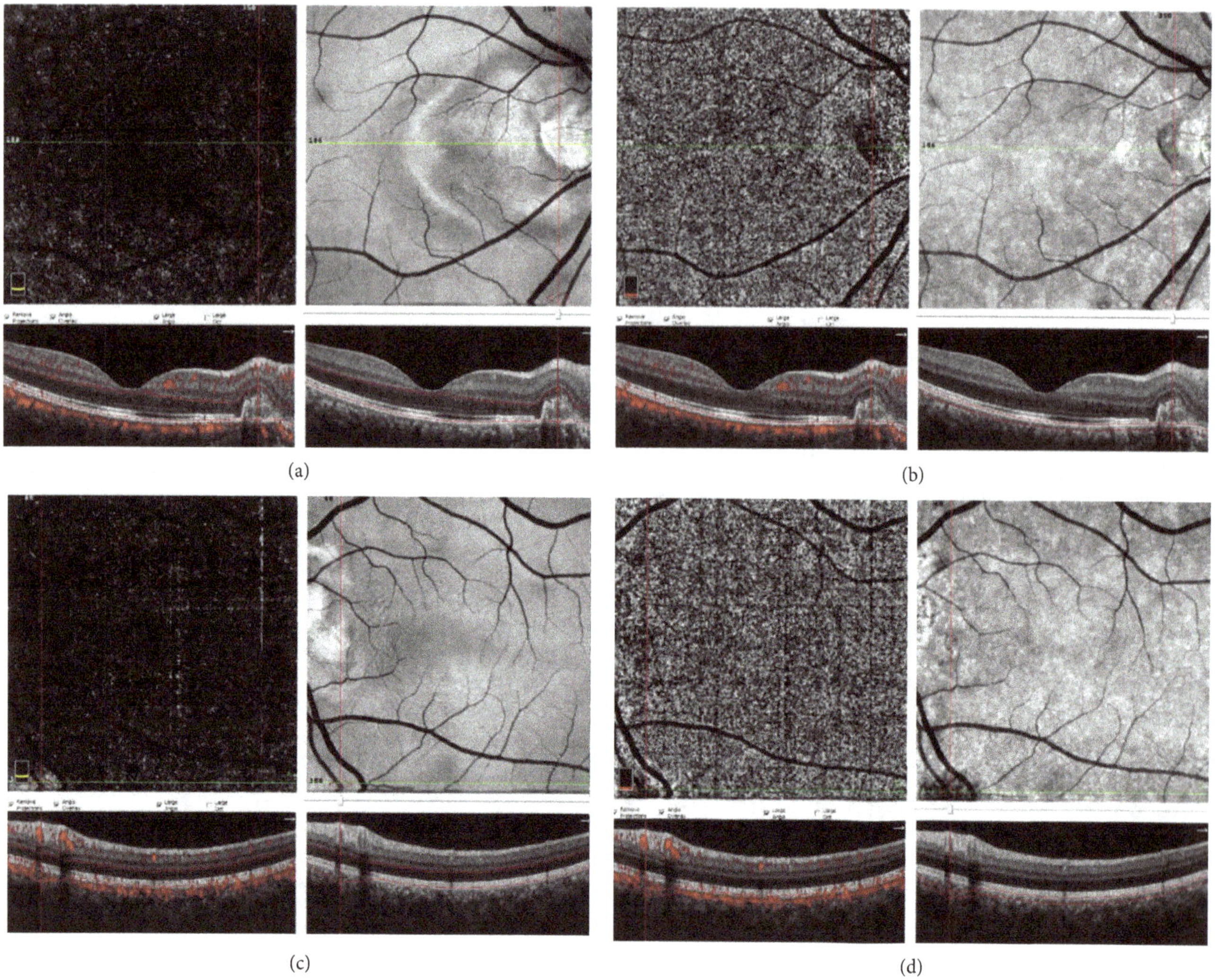

Figure 3: At 3 months. (a and b) Outer retina, choriocapillaris cross-sections, and en face OCTA image of the right eye; CNV complex including the main trunk disappearance. (c and d) Outer retina, choriocapillaris cross-sections, and en face OCTA image of the left eye; entire CNV compete of including the main trunk disappearance.

group than in the other groups [25]. Cennamo et al. reported that flow rate measurements were correlated with ganglion cell layer thickness and OCTA examination can be an early marker to show the axonal damage in patients with ODD [26]. Similarly, Engelke et al. demonstrated the correlation between vascular density and RNFL and ganglion cell complex (GCC) and peripapillary capillary density loss compared to the normal group [27]. In our case, however, peripapillary capillary density evaluation revealed that the vascular density in the nasal quadrants was lower than those in the other quadrants, which was an interesting finding. However, changes that might be correlated in both RNFL and disc and macular vascular density measurements were not detected contrary to the abovementioned reports.

In conclusion, it is possible to evaluate vascular density, presence of associated CNV, and response to injection with OCTA in patients with optic nerve diseases such as ODD. Nonetheless, there is a need for further studies to confirm the changes in CNV visualization like in our case with OCTA that has been increasingly used.

Disclosure

The authors have no proprietary or commercial interest in any materials discussed in this article.

Authors' Contributions

Melih Akıdan, Mehmet Bulut, and Lütfiye Yaprak did the surgical and medical practice. Melih Akıdan, Mehmet Bulut, Lütfiye Yaprak, and Elcin Suren developed the concept. Melih Akıdan, Mehmet Bulut, Muhammet Kazım Erol, and Elcin Suren designed the study. Melih Akıdan, Mehmet Bulut, Lütfiye Yaprak, and Muhammet Kazım Erol are responsible for the data collection or processing. Melih Akıdan, Mehmet Bulut, Lütfiye Yaprak, and Elcin Suren analyzed and interpreted the data. Melih Akıdan, Mehmet Bulut, and Muhammet Kazım Erol performed the literature search. Melih Akıdan, Mehmet Bulut, Lütfiye Yaprak, Muhammet Kazım Erol, and Elcin Suren wrote the manuscript.

References

[1] K. S. Padhy and U. C. Behera, "Optic disc drusen precipitating central retinal vein occlusion in young," *BMJ Case Reports*, vol. 8, no. 7, pp. 1–3, 2019.

[2] R. Gise, E. D. Gaier, and G. Heidary, "Diagnosis and imaging of optic nerve head drusen," *Seminars in Ophthalmology*, vol. 34, no. 4, pp. 256–263, 2019.

[3] B. Lumbroso, M. Rispoli, M. C. Savastano, Y. Jia, O. Tan, and D. Huang, "Optical coherence tomography angiography study of choroidal neovascularization early response after treatment," *Developments in Ophthalmology*, vol. 56, pp. 77–85, 2016.

[4] R. Wang, Z. Liang, and X. Liu, "Diagnostic accuracy of optical coherence tomography angiography for choroidal neovascularization: a systematic review and meta-analysis," *BMC Ophthalmology*, vol. 19, no. 1, article 162, 2019.

[5] C. Veronese, C. Maiolo, D. Huang et al., "Optical coherence tomography angiography in pediatric choroidal neovascularization," *American Journal of Ophthalmology Case Reports*, vol. 2, pp. 37–40, 2016.

[6] N. A. Saffra and B. J. Reinherz, "Peripapillary choroidal neovascularization associated with optic nerve head drusen treated with anti-vegf agents," *Case Reports in Ophthalmology*, vol. 10, no. 1, pp. 51–55, 2015.

[7] J. Rotruck, "A review of optic disc drusen in children," *International Ophthalmology Clinics*, vol. 58, no. 4, pp. 67–82, 2018.

[8] B. Delas, L. Almudi, and M. Asaad, "Bilateral choroidal neovascularization associated with optic nerve head drusen treated by antivascular endothelial growth factor therapy," *Clinical Ophthalmology*, vol. 2012, pp. 225–230, 2012.

[9] D. Z. Law, F. P. Yang, and S. C. Teoh, "Case report of optic disc drusen with simultaneous peripapillary subretinal hemorrhage and central retinal vein occlusion," *Case Reports in Ophthalmological Medicine*, vol. 2014, Article ID 156178, 4 pages, 2014.

[10] E. Palmer, J. Gale, J. G. Crowston, and A. P. Wells, "Optic nerve head drusen: an update," *Neuro-Ophthalmology*, vol. 42, no. 6, pp. 367–384, 2018.

[11] W. L. Gan and V. W. Long, "Paediatric case of peripapillary choroidal neovascularisation associated with optic disc drusen treated with aflibercept," *BMJ Case Reports*, vol. 14, no. 1, 2019.

[12] R. M. Knape, E. M. Zavaleta, C. L. Clark, N. Khuddus, and M. C. Peden, "Intravitreal bevacizumab treatment of bilateral peripapillary choroidal neovascularization from optic nerve head drusen," *Journal of American Association for Pediatric Ophthalmology and Strabismus*, vol. 15, no. 1, pp. 87–90, 2011.

[13] Z. Alkın, A. Ozkaya, I. Yılmaz, and A. T. Yazici, "A single injection of intravitreal ranibizumab in the treatment of choroidal neovascularisation secondary to optic nerve head drusen in a child," *Case Reports*, vol. 2014, 2014.

[14] A. Miere, P. Butori, S. Y. Cohen et al., "Vascular remodeling of choroidal neovascularization after anti-vascular endothelial growth factor therapy visualized on optical coherence tomography angiography," *Retina*, vol. 39, no. 3, pp. 548–557, 2019.

[15] Y. Ichiyama, T. Sawada, Y. Ito, M. Kakinoki, and M. Ohji, "Optical coherence tomography angiography reveals blood flow in choroidal neovascular membrane in remission phase of neovascular age-related macular degeneration," *Retina*, vol. 37, no. 4, pp. 724–730, 2017.

[16] R. F. Spaide, "Optical coherence tomography angiography signs of vascular abnormalization with antiangiogenic therapy for choroidal neovascularization," *American Journal of Ophthalmology*, vol. 160, no. 1, pp. 6–16, 2015.

[17] C. Traversi, E. Nuti, D. Marigliani et al., "Forty-two-month outcome of intravitreal bevacizumab in myopic choroidal neovascularization," *Graefe's Archive for Clinical and Experimental Ophthalmology*, vol. 253, no. 4, article 2721, pp. 511–517, 2015.

[18] L. Arrevola, M. A. Acero, and M. J. Peral, "Two-year outcome of aflibercept for the treatment of choroidal neovascularization in punctate inner choroidopathy," *Case Reports in Ophthalmological Medicine*, vol. 10, no. 1, pp. 24–31, 2019.

[19] Q. Chen, X. Yu, Z. Sun, and H. Dai, "The application of OCTA in assessment of anti-VEGF therapy for idiopathic choroidal neovascularization," *Journal of Ophthalmology*, vol. 2016, Article ID 5608250, 8 pages, 2016.

[20] J. T. Szelog, M. A. Bonini Filho, D. R. Lally, T. E. de Carlo, and J. S. Duker, "Optical coherence tomography angiography for detecting choroidal neovascularization secondary to choroidal osteoma," *Ophthalmic Surgery, Lasers and Imaging Retina*, vol. 47, no. 1, pp. 69–72, 2016.

[21] R. F. Spaide, J. G. Fujimoto, and N. K. Waheed, "Image artifacts in optical coherence tomography angiography," *Retina*, vol. 35, no. 11, pp. 2163–2180, 2015.

[22] R. Hua and H. Ning, "Using optical coherence tomography angiography to guide the treatment of pathological myopic patients with submacular haemorrhage," *Photodiagnosis and Photodynamic Therapy*, vol. 28, pp. 105–109, 2019.

[23] S. S. Ong, S. T. Hsu, D. Grewal et al., "Appearance of pediatric choroidal neovascular membranes on optical coherence tomography angiography," *Graefe's Archive for Clinical and Experimental Ophthalmology*, vol. 258, no. 1, pp. 89–98, 2020.

[24] O. Biçer and H. Atilla, "Microvascular changes associated with optic disc drusen: case report," *Turkish Journal of Ophthalmology*, vol. 49, no. 5, pp. 300–304, 2019.

[25] K. A. Aghdam, M. A. Khorasani, M. S. Sanjari et al., "Optical coherence tomography angiography features of optic nerve head drusen and nonarteritic anterior ischemic optic neuropathy," *Canadian Journal of Ophthalmology*, vol. 54, no. 4, pp. 495–500, 2019.

[26] G. Cennamo, S. Tebaldi, F. Amoroso, D. Arvanitis, M. Breve, and G. Cennamo, "Optical coherence tomography angiography in optic nerve drusen," *Ophthalmic Research*, vol. 59, no. 2, pp. 76–80, 2018.

[27] H. Engelke, M. Shajari, J. Riedel, N. Mohr, S. G. Priglinger, and M. J. Mackert, "OCT angiography in optic disc drusen: comparison with structural and functional parameters," *British Journal Ophthalmology*, 2019.

27

Nodular Scleritis Revealing Metastasis of Breast Cancer: Diagnosis not to be Neglected

Belghmaidi Sarah[1], **Ghazza Ahmed**[1], **Boutgayout Saloua**[1], **Hajji Ibtissam**[1], **Moutaouakil Abdeljalil**[1], **Dref Maria**[2], **Fakhri Anass**[2], **and Raiss Hanane**[2]

[1]*Ophthalmology Department, Mohammed VI University Hospital, Marrakech, Morocco*
[2]*Histopathology Department, Mohammed VI University Hospital, Marrakech, Morocco*

Correspondence should be addressed to Belghmaidi Sarah; sarahhhbelgh@gmail.com

Academic Editor: Cristiano Giusti

We report the case of ocular metastasis in a 48-year-old woman presenting left eye redness and pain. The patient was followed in another health institution for nodular scleritis and received systemic corticosteroids with moderate improvement. Medical history revealed that she was diagnosed three years ago with invasive ductal carcinoma of the left breast treated by tumorectomy with ganglion dissection. An ophthalmological examination found a hard scleral nodule with vascular architectural disorganization. A biopsy was performed, and the histopathological study revealed the presence of secondary tumor proliferation of poorly differentiated carcinoma of mammary cancer. This case report shows the fact that any unusual ocular presentation, even one simulating anterior scleritis, in a patient with a history of breast cancer should raise suspicion of metastasis.

1. Introduction

Breast cancer is the most common neoplastic disease diagnosed in women. Metastatic tumor accounts for the most common ocular malignancy [1]. Despite recent developments in early diagnosis and active treatment, it is estimated that up to one-third of patients diagnosed with breast cancer will develop metastasis [2].

Metastasis can be found in almost any part of the eye and orbit; the incidence of ocular metastasis in breast cancer presents variable rates between 5 and 30% [3].

The most common location is the choroid; the choroid is predominantly affected with an incidence of nearly 80% of total ocular metastasis [4]. However, the scleral localization is exceptional.

The purpose of this work is to describe a case of metastatic involvement of the sclera in breast carcinoma and to discuss related literature on ocular metastasis in breast carcinoma.

2. Case Presentation

A 48-year-old single woman was admitted to the ophthalmic emergency department for pain and redness in the left eye. The patient was followed in another health institution for nodular scleritis and received systemic corticosteroids with moderate improvement of the symptomatology.

On ophthalmological examination, the best corrected visual acuity in her left eye was 0.1 LogMAR. A slit lamp examination revealed a hard scleral nodule with vascular architectural disorganization next to the nodule and dilatation of the scleral vessels (Figure 1), with a juxtanodular Dellen effect without infiltration (Figure 2). A phenylephrine test was negative. Fundus evaluation under mydriasis was unremarkable.

Medical history revealed that she was diagnosed three years ago with invasive ductal carcinoma of the left breast, and she underwent a left-side tumorectomy with ganglion dissection afterward. Postoperatively, she started

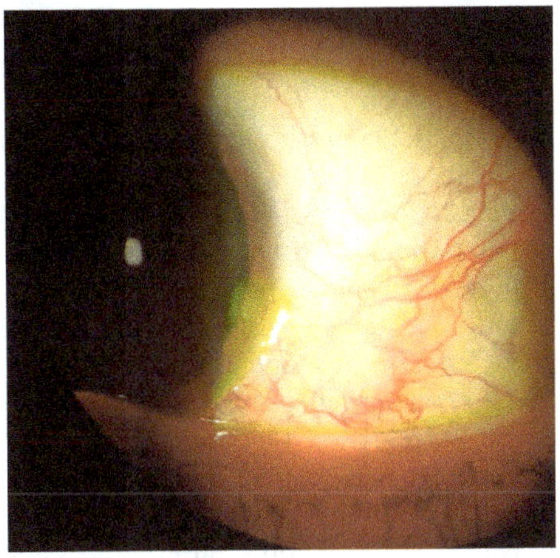

Figure 1: Aspect of nodular scleritis with dilatation of scleral vessels with peripheral corneal thinning.

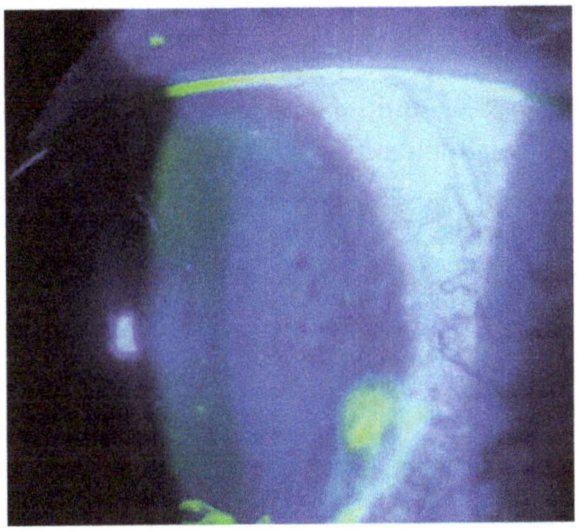

Figure 2: Dellen effect near the scleral nodule.

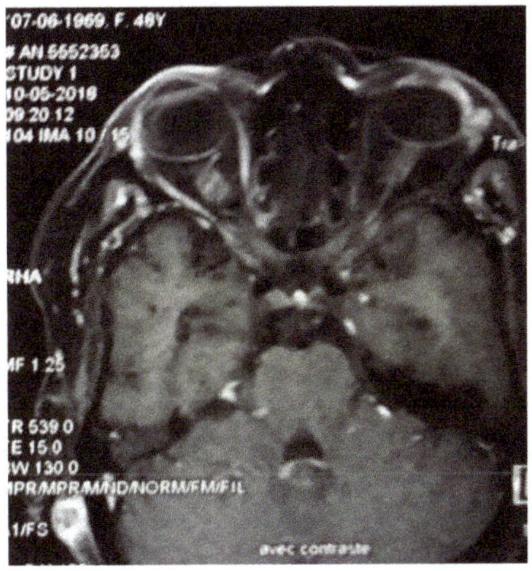

Figure 3: MRI objectifying a voluminous cerebellar lesion enhanced after gadolinium injection with temporal left scleral thickening.

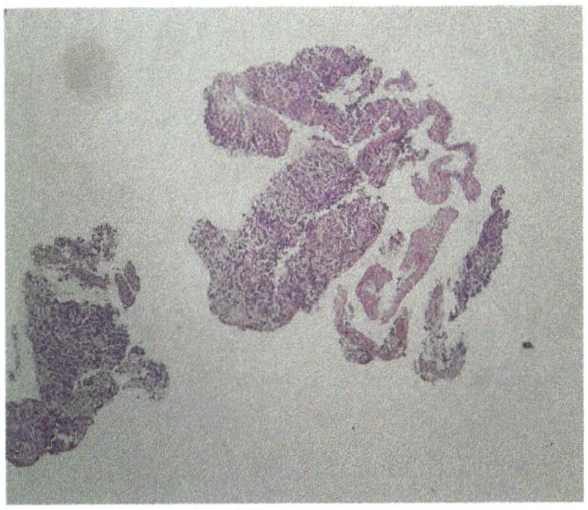

Figure 4: HE × 40. A conjunctival mucosa whose chorion is largely dissociated by an invasive carcinomatous proliferation.

treatment with adriamycin, cyclophosphamide, and docetotaxel. After the completion of 3 cycles of chemotherapy, external beam therapy of her thoracic wall was performed once a week for 8 weeks.

The clinical examination found multiple dermal cutaneous nodular lesions and an axillary lymphadenopathy of 1 cm/1 cm.

Oculocerebral MRI showed subtentorial and supratentorial lesions: the largest of them is cerebellar and enhances after gadolinium injection, with temporal left scleral thickening (Figure 3).

Retinography with ocular ultrasound, looking for secondary choroidal localization, was performed and did not reveal abnormalities.

In addition, thoracoabdominopelvic CT showed multiple secondary-level pulmonary lesions with moderate-grade pleurisy and right intra-atrial thrombus.

Biopsy of the temporal left sclera was performed to establish a positive diagnosis and initiate appropriate treatment.

The histopathological study revealed the presence of secondary tumor proliferation of poorly differentiated carcinoma of mammary cancer (Figures 4, 5, 6, and 7).

The final diagnosis was a scleral metastasis of breast cancer, so the patient was admitted to the oncology department for management and treatment. Unfortunately, the patient presented later respiratory distress with cardiocirculatory arrest. The resuscitation measures were in vain.

3. Discussion

The majority of ocular and orbital metastases are caused by breast cancer [5]. The reported incidence of breast cancer metastasis in ocular structures in clinical series varies between 8 and 10%. However, its incidence may be underestimated because of the concurrent involvement of major organs like lungs, liver, or bone which may have more serious consequences dominating the patient's clinical situation.

The ocular manifestations observed during cancers are related either to the invasion or compression of the structures of the eye or the orbit, or to a paraneoplastic syndrome secondary to autoantibodies directed against structures of the eye, or to systemic complications of cancers or their treatments [6, 7].

The uveal tissue, especially the choroid, is the primary ocular site of breast cancer metastasis accounting for 81% of total ocular metastasis [4].

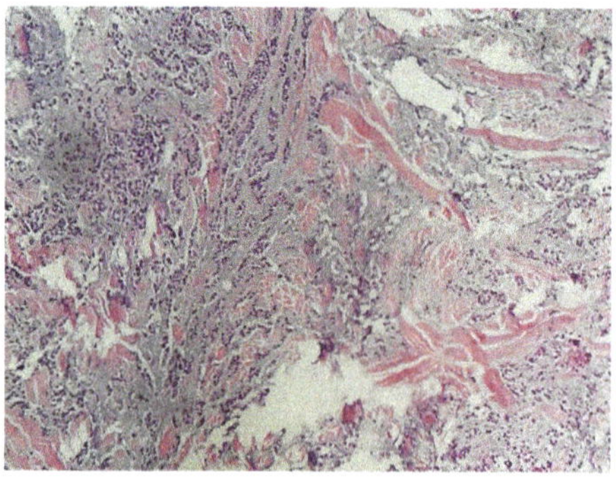

FIGURE 5: HE × 200. Carcinomatous proliferation arranged in lobules, spans, and cords. The stroma is fibroinflammatory hyalinized in places. The cells are of medium size, with anisokaryotic, hyperchromic nuclei, with irregular contours with rare mitotic figures. The eosinophilic cytoplasm is scarce.

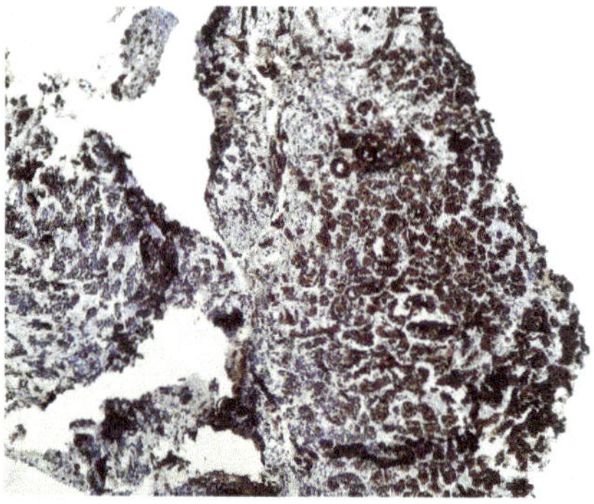

FIGURE 6: HE × 400. Intense and diffuse cytoplasmic expression of carcinomatous cells of the anti-CK7 antibody.

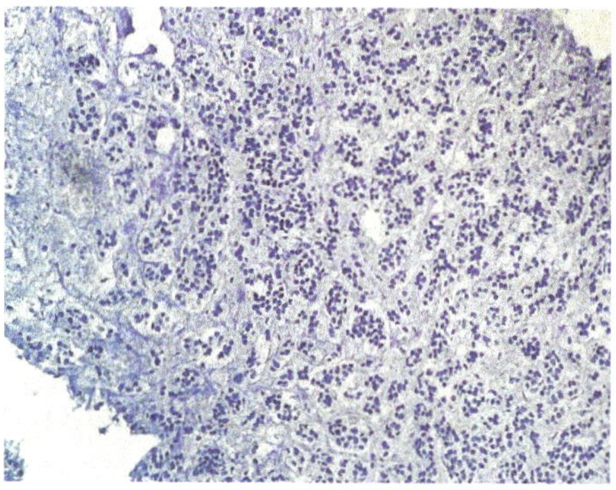

FIGURE 7: ×400. Absence of expression of the carcinomatous cells of the anti-CK20 antibody.

Sclerotic involvement is an extremely rare form and may be revealed by a scleral nodule that may simulate anterior nodular scleritis, decreased visual acuity, ocular redness, eye pain, or watery eyes [8].

The diagnosis of an oculoorbital secondary lesion is first clinical then radiological by oculoorbital MRI in search of scleral thickening and local extension to other locoregional oculoorbital structures including invasion of the ethmoidal sinus cells or intracranial extension threatening the patient's vital prognosis in the short term (ICHT and risk of cerebral involvement).

Laboratory studies should be carried out to exclude other conditions that may cause scleral redness and thickness like granulomatous, vasculitis, endocrine, and immunologic diseases. Biopsy of the involved tissue is necessary for positive diagnosis.

Ocular metastasis usually presents in patients with breast cancer 20 to 40 months after initial diagnosis [9].

At the time of diagnosis of ocular metastasis, 85% of patients already had lung metastasis [9]. Therefore, treatment of ocular metastasis is almost always palliative.

Secondary oculoorbital lesions are of poor prognosis regardless the histological type of the primary tumor. Recent studies have shown that the 2-year survival rate was 1.3 and 27%. Another more recent study showed a mean survival of 7.4 months after the discovery of oculoorbital metastasis regardless of the histological type of the primary tumor [8].

4. Conclusion

Breast cancer is a common source of ocular metastasis. This case report highlights the fact that any unusual ocular presentation, even one simulating anterior scleritis, in a patient with a history of breast cancer should raise suspicion of metastasis.

References

[1] I. Georgalas, T. Paraskevopoulos, C. Koutsandrea et al., "Ophthalmic metastasis of breast cancer and ocular side effects from breast cancer treatment and management: mini review," *BioMed Research International*, vol. 2015, Article ID 574086, 8 pages, 2015.

[2] S. Dogan, F. Andre, and M. Arnedos, "Issues in clinical research for metastatic breast cancer," *Current Opinion in Oncology*, vol. 25, no. 6, pp. 625–629, 2013.

[3] K.-M. Kreusel, T. Wiegel, M. Stange, N. Bornfeld, and M. H. Foerster, "Intraocular metastases of metastatic breast carcinoma in the woman. Incidence, risk factors and therapy," *Der Ophthalmologe*, vol. 97, no. 5, pp. 342–346, 2000.

[4] J. A. Shields and C. L. Shields, "Metastatic tumors to the intraocular structures," in *Intraocular Tumors*, J. A. Shields and C. L. Shields, Eds., pp. 207–238, Saunders, Philadelphia, 1992.

[5] R. L. Font and A. P. Ferry, "Carcinoma metastatic to the eye and orbit. III. A clinicopathologic study of 28 cases metastatic to the orbit," *Cancer*, vol. 38, no. 3, pp. 1326–1335, 1976.

[6] C. Bachmeyer, A. Frazier, A. Meftah, J. Cadranel, and G. Grateau, "Ocular metastases heralding non-small cell lung cancer: two cases," *La Revue de Médecine Interne*, vol. 27, no. 11, pp. 865–868, 2006.

[7] P. De Potter, D. Disneur, L. Levecq, and B. Snyers, "Ocular Manifestations of cancer," *Journal français d'ophtalmologie*, vol. 25, no. 2, pp. 194–202, 2002.

[8] R. Mahmodlou, F. A. Amoli, A. Abbasi, S. A. S. Mokhtari, and S. Pourasghary, "Case report: scleral metastasis of esophageal squamous cell carcinoma," *Ophthalmology and Therapy*, vol. 7, no. 1, article 118, pp. 185–189, 2018.

[9] A. P. Ferry, "Metastatic carcinoma of the eye and ocular adnexa," *International Ophthalmology Clinics*, vol. 7, no. 3, pp. 615–658, 1967.

28

Contralateral Posterior Chamber Phakic Intraocular Lens Implantation as Rehabilitation of Refractive Lens Exchange with a Monofocal Intraocular Lens in a Young, Nonpresbyopic, Bilateral Highly-Myopic Patient

Kepa Balparda [1] **Claudia Marcela Vanegas-Ramírez** [2] **Laura Segura-Muñoz** [3] **and Manuela Gómez-Londoño** [3]

[1] *Department of Cornea and Refractive Surgery, Clínica de Oftalmología Sandiego, Medellín, Colombia*
[2] *Department of Ophthalmology, Universidad Pontificia Bolivariana, Medellín, Colombia*
[3] *School of Medicine, Universidad Pontificia Bolivariana, Medellín, Colombia*

Correspondence should be addressed to Kepa Balparda; kb@kepabalparda.com

Academic Editor: Stephen G. Schwartz

Background. Refractive errors are widespread in the human population; nowadays, numerous surgical options allow for efficient and safe correction them. One of the main elements to ensure success in this kind of intervention will depend on the careful patient and surgical approach selection. Excimer laser corneal surgery is considered by most for low to moderate ametropias. Another option, which has been suggested may be safer, is to cut a small corneal lenticule with femtosecond laser, and then extracting it through a small incision. Nevertheless, in some specific cases, such as patients with high refractive error or those with some corneal abnormality, laser corneal ablations are considered unsafe from either a biomechanical or refractive standpoint. In this kind of particular cases, Phakic Intraocular Lens (P-IOL) implantation constitutes attractive, highly predictable and safe option. *Objective.* The authors want to show the case of a young high-myopic woman, already pseudophakic in one eye, where the P-IOL implantation in the fellow eye yielded excellent short-term visual results, and high patient's satisfaction, is presented. *Materials.* The authors present the case of a 32-years-old, highly myopic female patient underwent a Refractive Lens Exchange (RLE) with a monofocal Intraocular Lens (IOL) implantation in her left eye elsewhere, and developed severe visual issues, especially regarding near-work. Symptoms resolved through the implantation of a posterior chamber P-IOL in the contralateral eye. *Results.* The postoperative course was unremarkable, inflammation was mild, and visual recovery was quick. There was no need to perform any procedure on her left eye or to use any reading glasses, as unilateral effective near vision through her right eye was enough for all her daily tasks. *Conclusions.* RLE in young pre-presbyopic highly myopic patients may not be an advisable alternative in most cases, because of the high risks of retinal complications observed. In addition, eliminating accommodation will cause significant limitations, and multifocal IOLs currently available are far from the quality of vision that a young human crystalline lens yields. On the other hand, implantation of a P-IOL is a good option if eye conditions are optimal, as it preserves natural accommodation. In this case an EyeCryl Phakic Toric® IOL showed excellent short-term refractive predictability and safety.

1. Introduction

Refractive errors are widespread in the human population. According to Holden and collaborators [1], 22.9% of the world population (1.406 million people) have myopia [defined as a refractive error ≤ -0.50 Diopters (D)], while 163 million (2.7% of the world population) have high myopia (refractive error ≤ -5.0 D). Among some populations in Southeast Asia, the prevalence of myopia reaches much higher levels in young adults, being up to 80–90%, while high myopia prevalence could reach 20% and they have increased during the last decades, conforming a true epidemic of myopia [2]. In Colombia data are still not so high. Recently it was found that 11.6% of children (8–17 years old) and 14.4% of adults (35–55 years old) were myopic [3].

Uncorrected ametropia may significantly decrease quality of life, and surgical correction may have the advantage of setting patients free from external refractive elements for most situations. Nowadays, numerous surgical options allow for efficient and safe correction of refractive errors. One of the main elements to ensure success in this kind of intervention will depend on the careful patient and surgical approach selection, depending on each case. Excimer laser corneal surgery (including LASIK, PRK, and other similar surgeries) is considered by most as the go-to surgical technique for low to moderate ametropias [4]. Another option, which has been suggested may be safer, is to cut a small corneal lenticule with femtosecond laser, and then extracting it through a small incision (Relex SMILE).

Nevertheless, in some specific cases, such as patients with high refractive error or those with some corneal abnormality (thin pachymetry or ectasias), laser corneal ablations are considered unsafe from either a biomechanical (risk of ectasia) or refractive (excessive corneal flattening) standpoint. In this kind of particular cases, Phakic Intraocular Lens (P-IOL) implantation constitutes an attractive, highly predictable and safe option. The advantages of P-IOLs over pseudophakic IOLs include that the former allow for keeping the accommodation potential of the crystalline lens in young patients, while the use of pseudophakic IOLs eliminates it, and also that they are not associated with retinal complications in high myopes. On the other hand, phacoemulsication has been related with significant increased risk of retinal detachment in such patients [5–7].

In this article, the authors present the case of a 32-years-old, highly myopic female patient, who underwent Refractive Lens Exchange (RLE) with a monofocal IOL implantation in her left eye at another clinic. The patient then developed severe visual issues, especially regarding near-work vision. Symptoms resolved through the implantation of a P-IOL in the contralateral eye.

2. Case Presentation

A 32-years-old female patient concurred to the main author's private practice in the search for a second opinion regarding her ocular state. The patient had undergone RLE with the implantation of a monofocal IOL (AcrySof SA60AT; Alcon Surgical, Forth Worth, United States) in her left eye seven months before. From the moment of surgery, the patient developed severe asthenopia, headache, and dizziness, especially for near vision. Due to her job as a secretary, she was an avid computer user during at least 9 hours per day. The patient did not tolerate the use of contact lenses, and she was also unable to use glasses comfortably. The patient ended up resigning her job due to her inability to work comfortably on the computer.

Upon questioning about this medical decision, she claimed that she had been referred to a Comprehensive Ophthalmology specialist through her public health insurance because of high bilateral myopia. She also claimed that the original Surgeon explained that the Colombian public health system did not include P-IOL implantation, so he advised to patient to undergo RLE in both eyes and then use reading glasses. Reviewing previous clinical records, she was found to have original myopia of −18.00 D/+1.50 D × 140° in her left eye, with no history of congenital nor juvenile cataract. She also referred that the Surgeon never suggested using any high-technology IOL (trifocal, multifocal, etc.). Prior to her original surgery, she used glasses, as she did not tolerate contact lens use.

Upon clinical evaluation, the patient had an uncorrected distance visual acuity of 20/2000 and 20/40 in her right and left eyes, respectively. Her manifest refraction and distance corrected visual acuity were −22.00 D/+4.75 D × 105° (20/20) on her right eye and −0.75 D/+1.00 D × 137° (20/25) on her left eye. Near uncorrected vision on her right eye was 20/20 while it was 20/400 on the left one.

The physical examination of the anterior segment of her right eye was unremarkable. Her retina was thin upon examination, but not predisposing lesions were detected. Her left eye had a clear cornea, with a Monofocal IOL well-placed inside the capsular bag and no posterior capsular opacification. The rest of the clinical evaluation was completely normal.

Ocular biometry of the right eye (IOLMaster 500; Carl Zeiss Meditec AG; Jena, Alemania) reflected a flat keratometry of 41.9 D × 17°, and a steep keratometry of 45.1 D × 107°; her white to white distance was 11.2 mm, and her anterior chamber depth was 3.06 mm. Her endothelial cell count of the right eye was 2565 cells/mm^2 with all parameters being normal. In an effort to normalize her vision and diminish her near-vision symptoms, especially since she was unable to tolerate either glasses or contact lenses, we suggested the patient undergo posterior chamber P-IOL implantation in her right eye and leave the left eye untouched. She accepted and a −21.50 D/+3.50 D × 90° (size 12.0 mm) posterior chamber Toric P-IOL (EyeCryl Phakic IOL, Biotech Vision Care; Ahmedabad, India) was implanted in her right eye. The refractive target was +0.50 D.

Surgical implantation was performed under peribulbar anesthesia by the main author (K.B.) as follows: the patient was draped and the eye cleaned; then a paracenthesis and a 2.8 mm main incision were created, and the anterior chamber was filled with 1% Sodium Hyaluronate Ophthalmic Viscosurgical Device (Provisc®; Alcon Surgical; Forth Worth, United States). The P-IOL was mounted and injected inside the anterior chamber. Afterward, the lens was positioned in the correct toric markings, and all four haptics were positioned behind the iris in the ciliary sulcus. Then, the Ophthalmic Viscosurgical Device was removed, and 1% Acetylcholine was injected intracamerally to achieve proper pupillary miosis. Post-surgical regimen included 0.5% Moxifloxacin (Moxipharm®; Opharm; Bogotá, Colombia) and 1% Prednisolone (Predilab®; iLab Colombia; Bogotá, Colombia).

The postoperative course was unremarkable, inflammation was mild, and visual recovery was quick. On the first day after surgery, her uncorrected distance visual acuity of 20/25 and uncorrected near visual acuity of 20/20 in her right eye. On the first month after surgery, her uncorrected distance visual acuity was 20/15 in her right eye, with a manifest refraction of +0.75 D/−0.25 D × 74°. The patient claimed that starting at two days after surgery, her visual symptoms resolved about

100%, and she was able to use computed and write normally. Headaches subsided, and she was able to return to her job. Her endothelial cell count in the right eye, one month after surgery was 2511 cells/mm^2 and no significant change on cellular size or form could be detected.

So far, the patient has been observed for four months after surgery. On last evaluation, her uncorrected distance and near vision have remained unchanged, and her last manifest refraction was +0.75 D/−0.25 D × 78°.

There was no need to perform any procedure on her left eye or to use any reading glasses, as unilateral effective near vision through her right eye was enough for all her daily tasks.

3. Discussion

High myopia, usually defined as a spherical equivalent ≤−5.00 D or ≤−6.00 D is a relatively common condition worldwide, with wide geographical variance [1, 2, 8]. As these patients frequently look for refractive corrective procedures, it is the responsibility of the Refractive Surgeon to determine the best option for them, and this decision must be based on several elements that are both clinical and anatomical. Patients with low to moderate myopia and suitable cornea may be good candidates for laser approach, either excimer one (LASIK, PRK, etc.) or Femtosecond-based one (SMILE) [9]. Those patients with relatively low refractive error and some corneal irregularity, such as those with mild keratoconus may undergo combined surgery with topography-guided PRK and Corneal Collagen Crosslinking (CXL); technique known as Athen's Protocol [10, 11].

Nevertheless, patients with high myopia or those with abnormally thin cornea represent a complex clinical scenario, as corneal-based surgery would create undesirably unstable anterior segment with potential complications such as laser-related ectasia. In these patients, IOL implantation may be considered, this will provide mean to correct almost any value of refractive error while preserving full corneal stability. The decision on whether to maintain or extract the crystalline lens will reside many elements, including the patient's age and lens status, whether it is clear or clouded by cataract.

Patients with visually-significant cataract do well with crystalline lens extraction via phacoemulsification coupled with a pseudophakic IOL implantation, either monofocal or multifocal/trifocal/EDOF, keeping in mind that the former group will need the help of reading glasses for most near-vision activities [12]. Presbyopic patients with clear lens, especially those over 55 years old could be good candidates for RLE with implantation of pseudophakic IOL, most probably a multifocal/trifocal/EDOF. In some of them, it may be acceptable to implant a monofocal IOL keeping in mind that these will not completely compensate for presbyopia unless some monovision is attempted and achieved.

All these options are applicable in patients who are already presbyopic, especially those over 50–55 years old.

Nevertheless, nonpresbyopic patients represent exceptional group that demands different approach. Patients under the age of 40–45 still have useful accommodative potential, their near-vision will be clear as long as the eye is emmetrope, or near so. Therefore, in young patients, preserving the integrity of the crystalline lens is of paramount importance, and proper technique should be sought, as long as it is viable according to the clinical scenario.

Furthermore, lens extraction has been related with increased risk of retinal detachment in young highly myopic patients. In a classic study was related with late medium-term (7 years) prevalence of retinal detachment of 8.1% in pre-presbyopic patients [5]. In a more recent study conducted by Alio et al. [6], patients were divided into 2 groups according to age (group 1 ≤ 50 years and group 2 > 50 years) and axial length (≤ 28.0 mm and > 28.0 mm). Eyes with longer axial lengths showed greater incidences of retinal detachment. This complication was also more frequent in younger patients (3.65% in group 1 compared to 2.52% in group 2, $p < 0.05$). Risk factors for retinal detachment included: increase in axial length, age less than 50 years, males, sex, Caucasian race, peripheral retinal degenerations, intraoperative rupture of the posterior capsule, and Nd: YAG capsulotomy. Therefore, currently it is considered that RLE should not be performed in young eyes with no posterior vitreous detachment [7].

Some authors have suggested that an RLE with a multifocal IOL implantation may be a viable option for young, nonpresbyopic patients not good candidates for any other kind of approach [13]. Frings et al. [14] described their experience with 16 patients (5 myopic and 11 hyperopic) with mean age of 31 ± 6 years old who were implanted with a multifocal IOL. Both objective and subjective results were excellent, and only one of the patients "would not have chosen this surgery again" [14]. This may be viable option in highly hyperopic young patients with shallow anterior chamber depth that contraindicates P-IOL implantation, but this usually is not the case for highly myopic patients (such as the one we report here) whose eyes (including anterior chamber depth) tend to be bigger than average.

As has been mentioned, for most young pre-presbyopic patients, preserving natural accommodation is much better than pursuing multifocality, not only from a medical standpoint but also from refractive one. For this, both laser vision correction (in suitable patients) and P-IOL implantation are excellent alternatives much better than multifocal pseudophakia. Pop and Payette [15] compared visual results and satisfaction of young patients implanted with Artisan phakic IOL (OPHTEC BV; Groningen, The Netherlands) with patients undergoing RLE finding that the former group had a better refractive prediction (were closer to emmetropia) and that P-IOL implantation "provided a better overall outcome for young patients with high hyperopia whose accommodation was preserved" [15]. It is crucial to keep in mind that this study included hyperopic patients, who have a decreased visual acuity not only for far vision but also for near vision. Highly myopic patients, tend to have excellent near vision (although their focal distance is short), so it is probable that satisfaction rates, especially for near vision, would be poor in case of multifocal IOL implantation.

Currently, most studies concerning pseudophakic IOL implantation in young pre-presbyopic patients include highly hyperopic cases. Nevertheless, for myopic patients, there is consensus that P-IOL implantation is way better alternative, as accommodation is preserved. The patient in this article was instructed to undergo RLE with a monofocal IOL implantation, allegedly to comply with Colombian social security laws, which cover phacoemulsification for cataracts, but do not cover P-IOL implantation. The patient claimed that the original idea of the prior surgeon was to perform the same surgery in the other eye and then proceed with, reading glasses for both eyes. This approach is, according to current knowledge, wrong and should be avoided if other options are available. As already discussed, performing phacoemulsification in young myopic patients has been linked to a higher likelihood of retinal detachment. Besides, if pseudophakia were necessary, as would be the case if the patient had a congenital cataract (which she did not have), it would have been better to implant a multifocal IOL to preserve some near vision which could help decrease symptoms, especially in the meantime before surgery of the other eye. When we met the patient, she had a great anisometropia and was highly symptomatic, especially for near vision. She did not tolerate her contact lens on her right eye and using glasses with a highly myopic prescription in only one eye was not tolerated and increased her visual strain.

Upon carefully discussing the case with the patient and her mother, we decided to perform P-IOL implantation in the contralateral eye. With this approach, we sought to correct her high myopia and anisometropia, while preserving accommodation so she could have usable vision for her near tasks. Implantation of posterior chamber P-IOL corrected myopia, and left the patient emmetrope, with excellent near and far vision, and complete resolution of her symptoms.

This case highlights the fact that correct decision making is of paramount importance when the surgeon is planning to correct ametropic patient, taking into account previous refractive state and age. Obviously, decisions should be based on the best clinical experience, and not solely on bureaucratic issues as seems to have been the case in the first surgery of the patient. In case of doubt, sound clinical judgment should guide decisions, and it should be kept in mind that the first obligation of the physician is to cause no harm to the patient, so sometimes it may be wiser to choose not to operate on patient if they cannot pay for the right surgical approach in their individual case.

This case also showed that, just as has been reported by Yasa et al. [16], implantation of a new posterior chamber P-IOL (EyeCryl Phakic Toric) is predictable and safe option for refractive correction in highly myopic eyes. Nevertheless, to date there are no published long term studies on this specific kind of lenses, so results, specially regarding endothelial cell stability and cataract formation, are currently lacking. It should be noted that both endothelial cell loss and cataract formation are among the described potential complications related to both anterior chamber and posterior chamber P-IOLs. In order to decrease the possibility of these complications, implantation of this kind of IOLs should be reserved for patients with a correctly-sized anterior chamber depth (of at least 2.8 mm as measured from corneal endothelium).

4. Conclusion

In the absence of clinically significant cataract, phacoemulsification in young pre-presbyopic high myopic patients may not be the best option in most scenarios. If it is to be done, implanting a multifocal IOL will probably be the best selection for most patients (if the macula is not compromised with myopic changes). Whenever it is possible, implantation of a P-IOL is a much better option, as it preserves natural accommodation, which is unparalleled by current pseudophakic IOLs, and in addition is not related with an increased risk of retinal detachment. This case also supports the excellent short-term refractive predictability and safety of Toric EyeCryl Phakic IOL, however long- term follow-up examinations of these patients are necessary in order to evaluate endothelial cells density and the transparency of the crystalline lens.

References

[1] B. A. Holden, T. R. Fricke, D. A. Wilson et al., "Global prevalence of myopia and high myopia and temporal trends from 2000 through 2050," *Ophthalmology*, vol. 123, no. 5, pp. 1036–1042, 2016.

[2] I. G. Morgan, A. N. French, R. S. Ashby et al., "The epidemics of myopia: aetiology and prevention," *Progress in Retinal and Eye Research*, vol. 62, pp. 134–149, 2018.

[3] V. Galvis, A. Tello, J. Otero et al., "Prevalence of refractive errors in Colombia: MIOPUR study," *British Journal of Ophthalmology*, vol. 102, no. 10, pp. 1320–1323, 2018.

[4] K. Balparda, A. M. Diaz, and A. M. Londono, "Refractive surgery training during residency – do not be afraid of the dark," *Clinical Ophthalmology*, vol. 8, pp. 2297–2300, 2014.

[5] J. Colin, A. Robinet, and B. Cochener, "Retinal detachment after clear lens extraction for high myopia: seven-year follow-up," *Ophthalmology*, vol. 106, no. 12, pp. 2281–2285, 1999.

[6] J. L. Alio, "Lens surgery (cataract and refractive lens exchange) and retinal detachment risk in myopes: still an issue?" *British Journal of Ophthalmology*, vol. 95, no. 3, pp. 301–303, 2011.

[7] J. L. Alio, A. Grzybowski, and D. Romaniuk, "Refractive lens exchange in modern practice: when and when not to do it?" *Eye and Vision*, vol. 1, no. 1, p. 10, 2014.

[8] O. Parssinen and M. Kauppinen, "Risk factors for high myopia: a 22-year follow-up study from childhood to adulthood," *Acta Ophthalmologica*, vol. 97, no. 5, pp. 510–518, 2018.

[9] L. Y. Chen and E. E. Manche, "Comparison of femtosecond and excimer laser platforms available for corneal refractive surgery," *Current Opinion in Ophthalmology*, vol. 27, no. 4, pp. 316–322, 2016.

[10] A. J. Kanellopoulos and G. Asimellis, "Keratoconus management: long-term stability of topography-guided normalization combined with high-fluence CXL stabilization (the Athens Protocol)," *Journal of Refractive Surgery*, vol. 30, no. 2, pp. 88–93, 2014.

[11] A. J. Kanellopoulos and P. S. Binder, "Management of corneal ectasia after LASIK with combined, same-day, topography-guided partial transepithelial PRK and collagen cross-linking: the athens protocol," *Journal of Refractive Surgery*, vol. 27, no. 5, pp. 323–331, 2011.

[12] S. Shah, C. Peris-Martinez, T. Reinhard, and P. Vinciguerra, "Visual outcomes after cataract surgery: multifocal versus monofocal intraocular lenses," *Journal of Refractive Surgery*, vol. 31, no. 10, pp. 658–666, 2015.

[13] R. H. Trivedi and M. E. Wilson, "Refractive lens exchange with intraocular lens implantation in hyperopic eyes of a patient

with Angelman syndrome," *Journal of Cataract and Refractive Surgery*, vol. 36, no. 8, pp. 1432–1434, 2010.

[14] A. Frings, J. Steinberg, S. Linke, J. V. Druchkiv, and T. Katz, "Multifocal intraocular lens (MIOL) surgery in young nonpresbyopic ametropes: reasonable and safe?" *Der Ophthalmologe*, vol. 114, no. 8, pp. 722–727, 2017.

[15] M. Pop and Y. Payette, "Refractive lens exchange versus iris-claw artisan phakic intraocular lens for hyperopia," *Journal of Refractive Surgery*, vol. 20, no. 1, pp. 20–24, 2004.

[16] D. Yasa, U. Urdem, A. Agca et al., "Early results with a new posterior chamber phakic intraocular lens in patients with high myopia," *Journal of Ophthalmology*, vol. 2018, Article ID 1329874, 8 pages, 2018.

A Rare Coexistence of Isolated Unilateral Conjunctival Telangiectasia and Retinal Vascular Tortuosity

Hilal Kilinç Hekimsoy and Mehmet Ali Şekeroğlu

University of Health Sciences, Ulucanlar Eye Training and Research Hospital, Ophthalmology Clinic, Ankara, Turkey

Correspondence should be addressed to Hilal Kilinç Hekimsoy; hilal_kilinc_@hotmail.com

Academic Editor: Stephen G. Schwartz

A 55-year-old woman with no known systemic disorder and without any history of ocular disease, trauma, and surgery presented with a nonremitting conjunctival redness on her left eye that was existing since her childhood. On ophthalmological examination, an extremely rare coexistence of isolated unilateral bulbar conjunctival telangiectasia and ipsilateral retinal vascular tortuosity without any systemic and neuroradiological association was detected. We aimed to demonstrate this rare vascular coexistence and discuss differential diagnosis of the underlying causes.

1. Introduction

Conjunctival telangiectasia is a rarely encountered ocular finding which can be described as the presence of tiny dilatations of conjunctival blood vessels. It can be congenital and can accompany some systemic syndromes such as hereditary hemorrhagic telangiectasia (Rendu-Osler-Weber disease), ataxia telangiectasia, Fabry's disease, Alport syndrome, and Bloom syndrome or can be acquired especially secondary to some chronic ocular surface disorders such as ocular rosacea [1–4]. Conjunctival telangiectasia may involve one or both of the arterial and venous systems; it can occur unilaterally or bilaterally, and it can be localized or generalized.

Herein, we report an extremely rare coexistence of isolated unilateral bulbar conjunctival telangiectasia and ipsilateral retinal vascular tortuosity without any systemic or neuroradiological association and aim to discuss the differential diagnosis of the possible underlying diseases.

2. Case Report

A 55-year-old woman with no known systemic disorder and without any history of ocular disease, trauma, and surgery presented with a nonremitting conjunctival redness on her left eye that was existing since her childhood. Since she has never reported none of the ocular symptoms such as burning and foreign body sensation accompanying to redness in her eye, she had received several topical treatments including artificial tear drops, steroids, antibiotics, and nonsteroidal anti-inflammatory eye drops with poor response. She denied any family history and accompanying dermatological disorder or any systemic diseases such as hypertension, diabetes, and hyperlipidemia.

Static and dynamic assessment of both eyelids were normal without any port-wine stain, hemangioma, or facial abnormality. There was no exophthalmos or globe deviation. On ophthalmological examination, the best-corrected visual acuity was 20/20 in both eyes; intraocular pressure was 16 mmHg in the right and 17 mmHg in the left eye. Slit-lamp anterior segment examination of the right eye was normal; however, left eye revealed conjunctival and episcleral vascular dilation and tortuosity with an accompanying bulbar conjunctival telangiectasia most prominent in the lower conjunctiva near to limbus (Figures 1(a)–1(c)). The dilated examination of the fundus and fluorescein angiography was normal in the right eye; contrary, the retinal vessels were strikingly tortuous and slightly dilated in all four quadrants of the left eye without any other accompanying retinal findings such as exudation or hemorrhage (Figures 2(a)–2(d)). The optic disc and macula were normal bilaterally. There

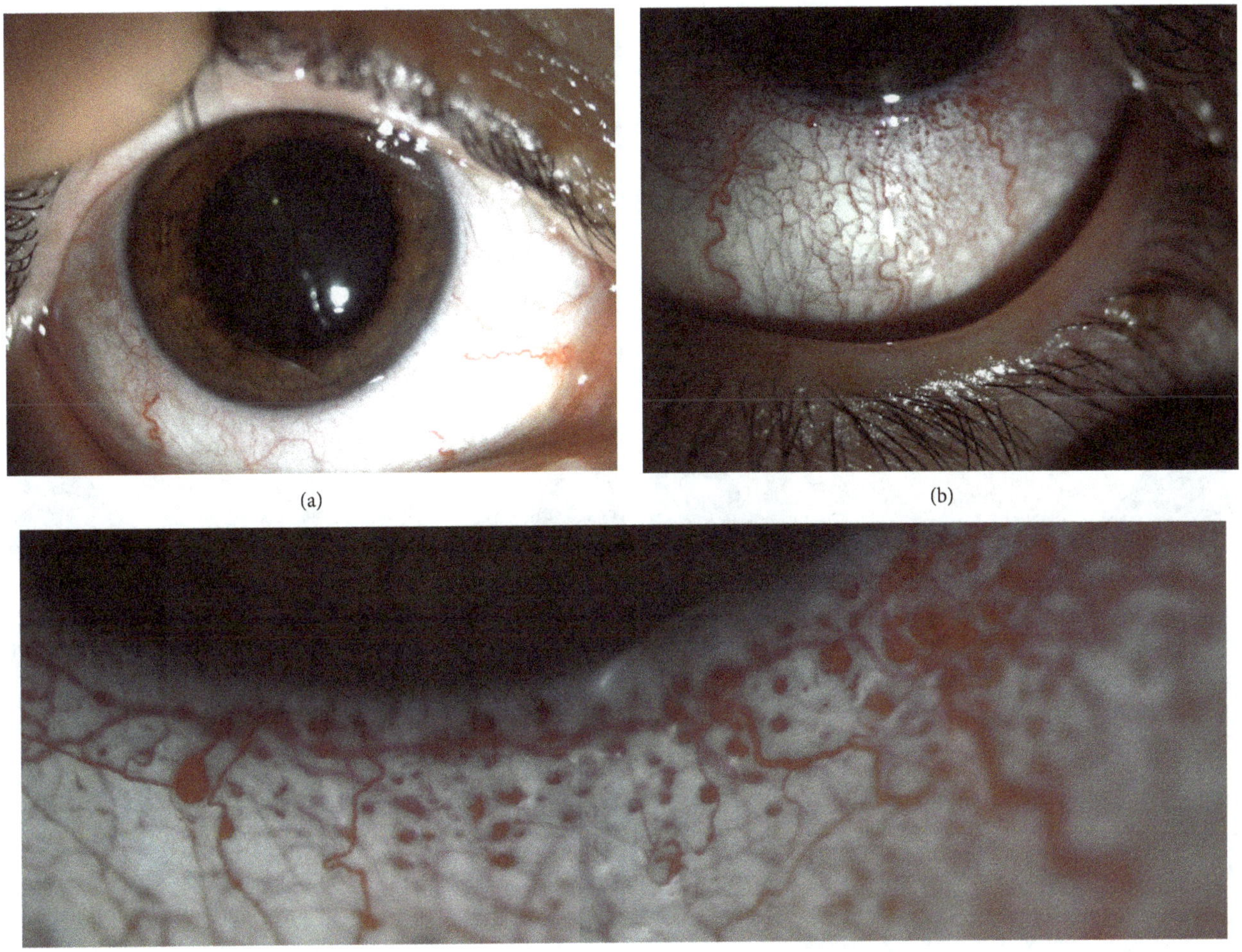

(a) (b) (c)

Figure 1: (a) Anterior segment picture of the right eye depicting normal conjunctival and episcleral vessels. (b, c) Anterior segment picture of the left eye depicting the conjunctival and episcleral vascular dilation, tortuosity, and conjunctival telangiectasia.

was no mass lesion, retinal capillary haemangioma, choroidal haemangioma, or racemose angioma in the retinal periphery on indirect ophthalmoscopy. Fundus autofluorescence imaging and optical coherence tomography angiography of the left eye revealed a striking retinal vascular tortuosity; optical coherence tomography imaging scans were normal for both eyes (Figures 3(a)–3(c)). Schirmer I and tear break-up time tests were within normal limits bilaterally.

The patient was referred to internal medicine, cardiology, dermatology, and neurology departments in order to exclude some systemic syndromes that can accompany conjunctival telangiectasia such as hereditary hemorrhagic telangiectasia (Rendu-Osler-Weber disease), ataxia telangiectasia, Fabry's disease, Alport syndrome, and Bloom syndrome and some systemic diseases that can accompany retinal vascular tortuosity such as systemic hypertension, pulmonary arterial hypertension, atherosclerosis, polycythemia vera, and sickle cell anemia. Neuroradiological assessment including brain and orbital magnetic resonance imaging with magnetic resonance angiography was performed in order to exclude any accompanying retroorbital or cranial vascular abnormality and caroticocavernous fistula. After all those aforementioned evaluations, no systemic coexistence was identified.

The patient was monitored for visual acuity, intraocular pressure, slit-lamp anterior segment, and fundus examinations during follow-up visits. The clinical findings were stable without any symptoms, and there was no change in the appearance and shape of the conjunctival, episcleral, and retinal vessels 12 months after initial examination.

3. Discussion

We herein report an extremely rare ocular abnormality of isolated unilateral bulbar conjunctival telangiectasia and ipsilateral retinal vascular tortuosity. Despite thorough systemic evaluation and imaging, we could not able to demonstrate any systemic or neuroradiological association, and ocular findings were stable during a 1-year follow-up duration.

The most commonly encountered and well-defined systemic syndromes that can accompany conjunctival telangiectasia are hereditary hemorrhagic telangiectasia (Rendu-Osler-Weber disease) and ataxia telangiectasia, and rarely Alport syndrome, Fabry's disease, and Bloom syndrome.

Hereditary hemorrhagic telangiectasia (Rendu-Osler-Weber disease) is characterized by bleeding telangiectasias throughout various vascular beds in the body. Eye

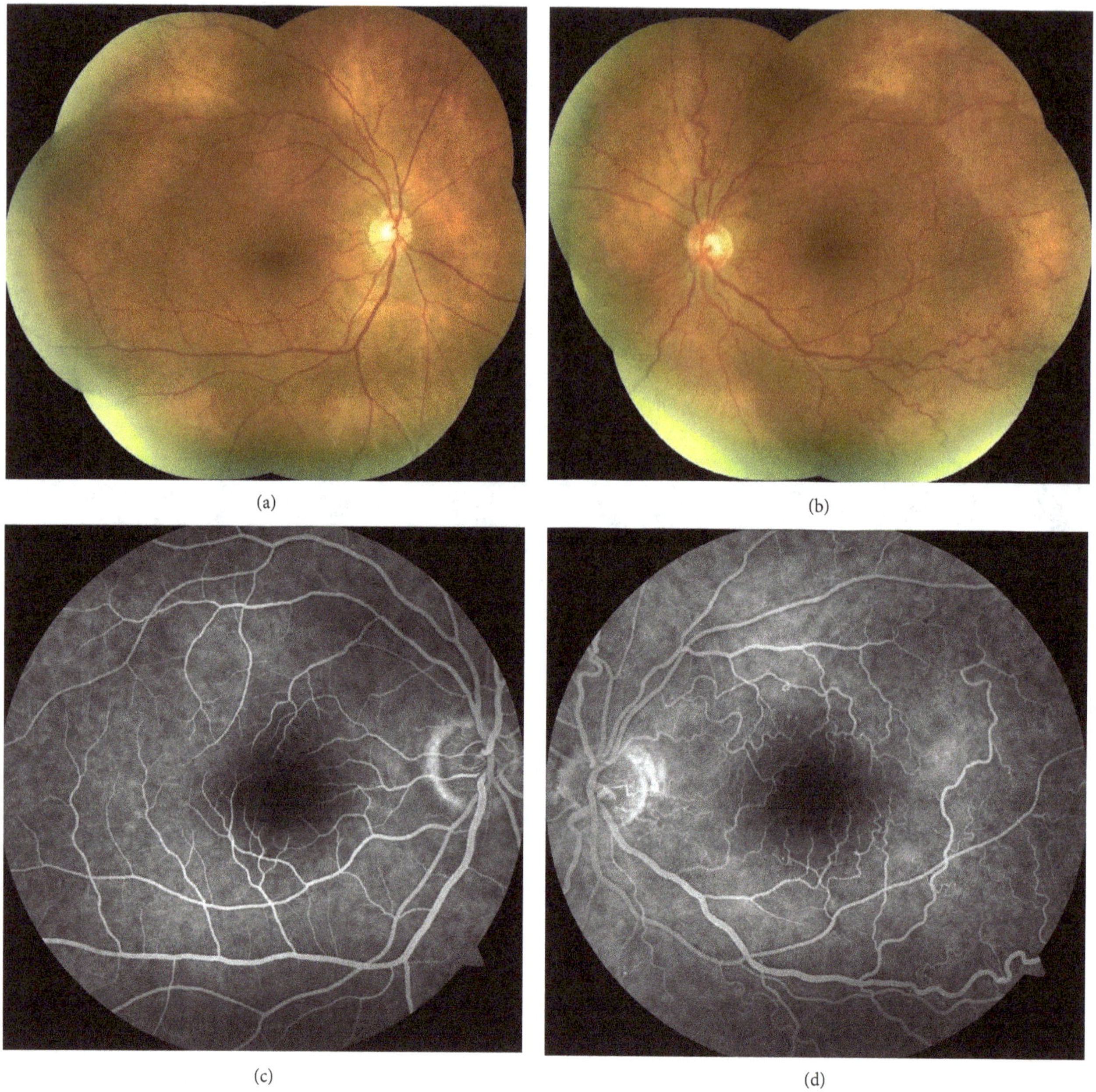

FIGURE 2: Colour fundus photograph of the right (a) and the left (b) eyes. Fundus fluorescein angiography of the right (c) and the left (d) eyes, showing normal retinal vasculature on the right and the convoluted and slightly dilated arteries and veins on the left eye.

involvement occurs in 45-65% of patients, and the most common lesions are conjunctival telangiectasias in the palpebral conjunctiva [4]. There are also some reports in the literature defining hemolacria as a finding of hereditary hemorrhagic telangiectasia [4–6]. Unilateral and bilateral conjunctival involvement has been reported in the literature. Dilatation of retinal vessels due to retinal arteriovenous malformation has been rarely seen [4, 5]. So, it was also considered in the differential diagnosis of our patient. Diagnosis of the disease is based on clinical findings of mucosal and/or skin lesions and bleeding from the lesions, and a family history [4]. However, the patient in this case had no recurrent epistaxis, hemolacria, muco-cutaneous telangiectasias, or family history of the disease. Choroidal telangiectasia was also reported in a patient with hereditary hemorrhagic telangiectasia by using indocyanine green (ICG) angiography [7]. Although retinal arteriovenous malformation was excluded by using fundus fluorescein angiography, we could not completely exclude the possibility of the presence of choroidal telangiectasia, since we did not perform ICG angiography.

Ataxia telangiectasia is an autosomal recessive disorder primarily characterized by immunodeficiency, radiation sensitivity, and cancer susceptibility along with some neurological findings such as cerebellar degeneration [8]. In ataxia telangiectasia, conjunctival-cutaneous telangiectasia are the main ocular findings. However, retinal telangiectasia or

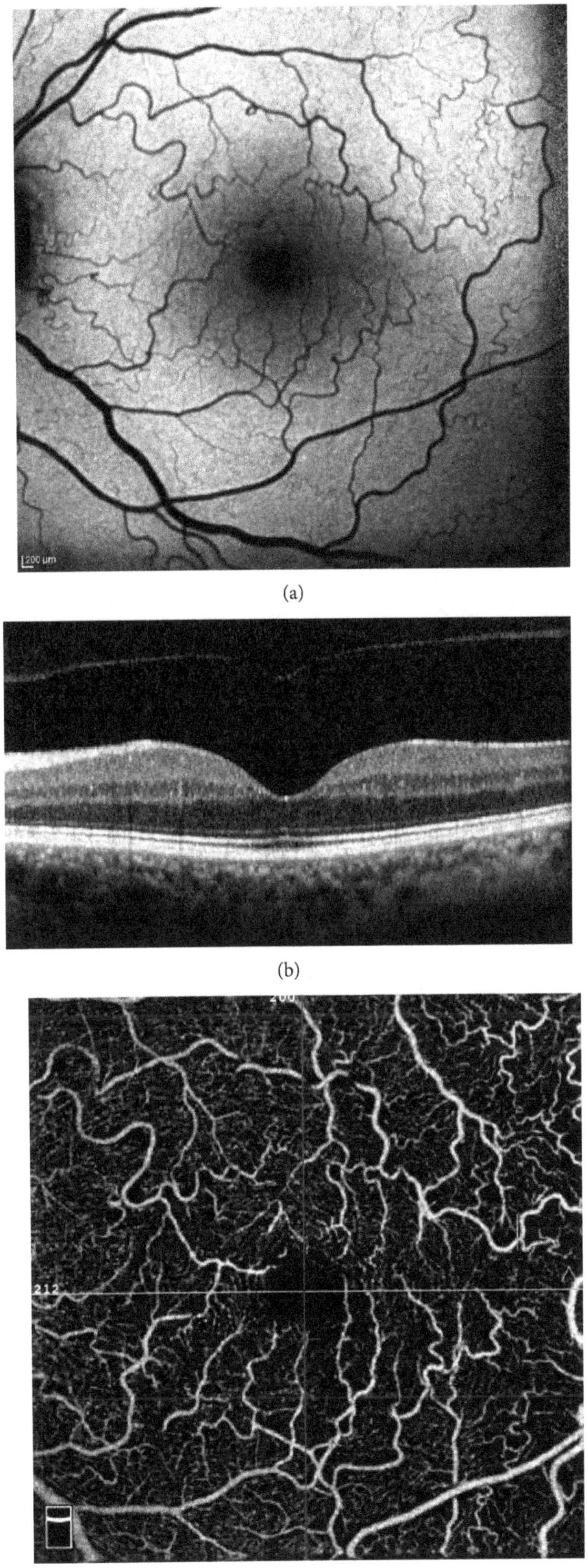

FIGURE 3: Fundus autofluorescence (a), optical coherence tomography (b), and optical coherence tomography angiography (c) imaging of the left eye.

retinal vascular changes are not evident [9]. Our patient is an otherwise healthy adult which also excludes the possibility of this diagnosis.

Conjunctival and retinal vascular tortuosity and dilatation are common in Fabry's disease. However, these often present bilaterally and vascular involvement that is mostly combined with vortex keratopathy (cornea verticillata) and lens opacity with a "spoke-like" pattern at the posterior capsule in Fabry disease [10]. These findings correlate with progressive deposition of glycosphingolipids in the ocular structures.

Caroticocavernous fistula should also be kept in mind in a patient with unilateral conjunctival and retinal vascular dilatation and tortuosity, which is an abnormal connection between the cavernous sinus and the carotid artery system and usually occurs unilaterally. These patients may have signs and symptoms such as corkscrew episcleral blood vessels in association with conjunctival chemosis and dilated, tortuous retinal veins with retinal hemorrhage, as well as proptosis, pulsating exophthalmos, diplopia, ophthalmoplegia, elevated intraocular pressure, and audible bruits [11, 12]. The patient was referred to a neuroradiology unit in order to exclude caroticocavernous fistula in the process of differential diagnosis; however, brain and orbital magnetic resonance imaging along with magnetic resonance angiography scans, all were normal.

Familial retinal arterial tortuosity is another rare disease that should be kept in mind in differential diagnosis of retinal vascular tortuosity, which is an autosomal dominant disorder affecting the retinal arterioles rather than the venous system [13]. In some cases, it has been reported that the retinal arteriolar tortuosity is accompanied by bulbar conjunctival telangiectasia [14]. Retinal arterioles typically appear in corkscrew and spiral shapes and can lead to recurrent visual symptoms complicated by preretinal and intraretinal hemorrhages [15]. Systemic involvement of nonocular vascular beds has been demonstrated in a few cases [16]. However, the diagnosis is mainly based on clinical findings of bilateral tortuosity of small and medium-sized arterioles in the peripapillary and macular regions contrary to our patient which has unilateral involvement.

Impending retinal vein occlusion can also be considered in differential diagnosis of unilateral retinal venous dilatation and tortuosity. However, both retinal and venous systems were involved in our patient. There is also no defined association of impending vein occlusion with conjunctival telangiectasia.

Last but not least, some acquired causes such as chronic phases of some ocular surface disorders should also be considered in the differential diagnosis of conjunctival telangiectasia [3, 17, 18]. Of these, ocular rosacea is the mostly encountered one. However, unilateral involvement in our patient and absence of symptoms such as foreign body sensation and burning; absence of ocular findings such as meibomian gland dysfunction, blepharitis, lid margin erythema and irregularities, and tarsal conjunctival telangiectasia helped us to exclude acquired causes in differential diagnosis.

In conclusion, isolated unilateral bulbar conjunctival telangiectasia and ipsilateral retinal vascular tortuosity without any systemic or neuroradiological association is an extremely rare coexistence. A detailed and thorough systemic evaluation is necessary to exclude some severe diseases as the underlying cause in these patients.

Consent

A written informed consent was obtained from the patient to publish medical data and figures described in this case report.

References

[1] C. Decock, J. J. De Laey, B. P. Leroy, and P. H. Kestelyn, "Alport syndrome and conjunctival telangiectasia," *Bulletin de la Société Belge d'Ophtalmologie*, vol. 290, pp. 29–31, 2003.

[2] E. E. Sahn, R. H. Hussey, and L. M. Christmann, "A Case of Bloom Syndrome with Conjunctival Telangiectasia," *Pediatric Dermatology*, vol. 14, no. 2, pp. 120–124, 1997.

[3] İ. K. Müftüoğlu and Y. A. Akova, "Clinical Findings, Follow-up and Treatment Results in Patients with Ocular Rosacea," *Türk Oftalmoloji Dergisi*, vol. 46, no. 1, pp. 1–6, 2016.

[4] F. A. Knox and D. G. Frazer, "Ophthalmic presentation of hereditary haemorrhagic telangiectasia," *Eye (London, England)*, vol. 18, no. 9, pp. 947–949, 2004.

[5] A. M. Brant, A. P. Schachat, and R. I. White, "Ocular manifestations in hereditary hemorrhagic telangiectasia (Rendu-Osler-Weber disease)," *American Journal of Ophthalmology*, vol. 107, no. 6, pp. 642–646, 1989.

[6] M. Rinaldi, E. Buscarini, C. Danesino et al., "Ocular manifestations in hereditary hemorrhagic telangiectasia (Rendu-Osler-Weber disease): A case-series," *Ophthalmic Genetics*, vol. 32, no. 1, pp. 12–17, 2010.

[7] D. C. Tsai, A. G. Wang, A. F. Lee, W. M. Hsu, J. H. Liu, and M. Y. Yen, "Choroidal telangiectasia in a patient with hereditary hemorrhagic telangiectasia," *Eye (London, England)*, vol. 16, no. 1, pp. 92–94, 2002.

[8] M. F. Lavin, "Erratum: Ataxia-telangiectasia: from a rare disorder to a paradigm for cell signalling and cancer," *Nature Reviews Molecular Cell Biology*, vol. 9, no. 12, p. 927, 2008.

[9] A. K. Farr, B. Shalev, T. O. Crawford, H. M. Lederman, J. A. Winkelstein, and M. X. Repka, "Ocular manifestations of ataxia-telangiectasia," *American Journal of Ophthalmology*, vol. 134, no. 6, pp. 891–896, 2002.

[10] A. M. Morier, J. Minteer, R. Tyszko, R. McCann, M. V. Clarke, and M. F. Browning, "Ocular manifestations of Fabry disease within in a single kindred," *Optometry*, vol. 81, no. 9, pp. 437–449, 2010.

[11] L. Zhu, B. Liu, and J. Zhong, "Post-traumatic right carotid-cavernous fistula resulting in symptoms in the contralateral eye: a case report and literature review," *BMC Ophthalmology*, vol. 18, no. 1, p. 183, 2018.

[12] I. A. Chaudhry, S. M. Elkhamry, W. Al-Rashed, and T. M. Bosley, "Carotid cavernous fistula: ophthalmological implications," *Middle East African Journal of Ophthalmology*, vol. 16, no. 2, pp. 57–63, 2009.

[13] F. K. P. Sutter and H. Helbig, "Familial Retinal Arteriolar Tortuosity: A Review," *Survey of Ophthalmology*, vol. 48, no. 3, pp. 245–255, 2003.

[14] J. H. Seo, I. Kim, and H. G. Yu, "A case of carotid aneurysm in familial retinal arterial tortuosity," *Korean Journal of Ophthalmology*, vol. 23, no. 1, pp. 57-58, 2009.

[15] F. Gekeler, K. Shinoda, M. Jünger, K. U. Bartz-Schmidt, and F. Gelisken, "Familial retinal arterial tortuosity associated with tortuosity in nail bed capillaries," *Archives of Ophthalmology*, vol. 124, no. 10, pp. 1492–1494, 2006.

[16] S. S. Saraf, A. J. Tyring, C. L. Chen et al., "Familial retinal arteriolar tortuosity and quantification of vascular tortuosity using swept-source optical coherence tomography angiography," *Am J Ophthalmol Case Rep.*, vol. 14, pp. 74–78, 2019.

[17] E. K. Akpek, A. Merchant, V. Pinar, and C. S. Foster, "Ocular Rosacea," *Ophthalmology*, vol. 104, no. 11, pp. 1863–1867, 1997.

[18] S. U. De Marchi, E. Cecchin, and S. De Marchi, "Ocular rosacea: an underdiagnosed cause of relapsing conjunctivitis-blepharitis in the elderly," *Case Reports*, vol. 2014, no. sep19 1, article bcr2014205146, 2014.

30

Impurities in Drug Vials Intended for Intravitreal Medication

Lisa Pohl, Lisa Strudel, Spyridon Dimopoulos, and Focke Ziemssen

Center for Ophthalmology, Eberhard Karl University, Tuebingen, Germany

Correspondence should be addressed to Focke Ziemssen; focke.ziemssen@med.uni-tuebingen.de

Academic Editor: Claudio Campa

Sterility is an important prerequisite for minimizing the risk of severe vision loss due to endophthalmitis after intravitreal injections. We describe three cases series of incidents where an unclear contamination of the drug solution or syringe caused the injection process to stop and continue with a new preparation. During a period of 12 months with 30,502 intravitreal injections at a tertiary center, wherein 7,076 were of the drug Aflibercept drawn up from a glass vial, three cases of the critical incident reporting system relating to intravitreal injections were identified: (1) After a typical contact with the filter cannula, the glass of an Aflibercept vial was no longer intact. (2) In the course of another injection, there was a clear deposition of debris on the outer edge of the syringe when removing the attached filter cannula. (3) After inserting the syringe into the rubber top of the vial, a whitish particle of unclear origin was identified within the drug solution. Later, this contamination/particle was identified as part of the greyish rubber that was punched out with the cannula, according to the analyses of the material sent in and the manufacturer's investigations. Thus, even in busy clinics, visual inspection of the injection solution and materials used for impurities, preferably before and after pulling them out of a vial, must be an essential part of the injection process. Even when using ready-to-use prefilled syringes (PFS), vigilance must be kept high, knowing the risk of potential contamination.

1. Introduction

Many cases of endophthalmitis occur as clustered events, because contamination of the drug solution or pathogen sources in the environment of the intravitreal injection increases the probability of a larger number of affected eyes [1–3]. High volume clinics could potentially make the intravitreal administration of drugs more prone to errors in terms of confusion between patients and eyes but also in relation to injuries to the lens and cornea.

After possible problems such as an increase in eye pressure or toxic posterior segment syndromes due to oil bubbles remaining in the eye have been described [4, 5], the awareness of residues and contamination, e.g., of the syringe stamp, has increased again. Here, we report three different findings of our critical incident reporting system, which have occurred during a calendar year and over 30,502 intravitreal injections at a tertiary center.

2. Case Presentation

In the first case, the injecting physician noticed fine break lines in the glass while drawing Aflibercept solution out of the vial (Figure 1). Previously, there were no issued reported during transport or preparation. The glass fragment was not dislocated; nevertheless, the sterility could not be regarded as assured. The manufacturer suspected a quality problem in the glass but stated that it had received no other reports of glass vials breaking or losing their integrity.

For the second case, the attentive surgeon noticed a small contamination on the outside of the syringe tip while she was replacing the filter cannula with the injection needle (Figure 2). The suspicion arose that the particle/fibres came from the inner surface of the attached filter cannula, because it had not been noticed before. That was the reason why the drug manufacturers did not think they were responsible, as they purchased the enclosed filter cannula from a third-

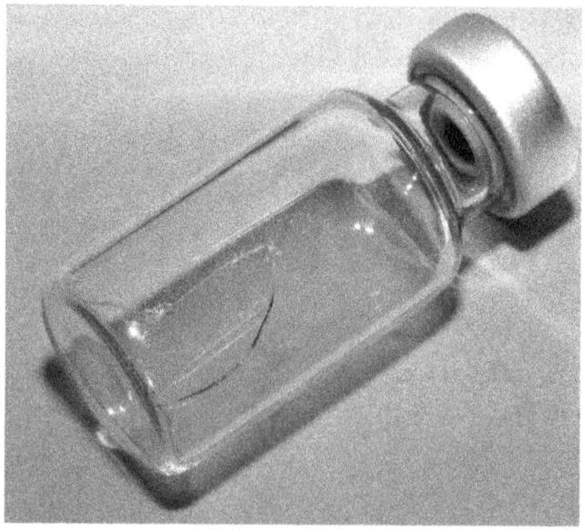

Figure 1: After a light and short contact with the filter cannula, fine continuous cracks on the glass vial were seen. Although no Aflibercept solution had escaped, the active ingredient—possibly no longer free of contamination—was not used.

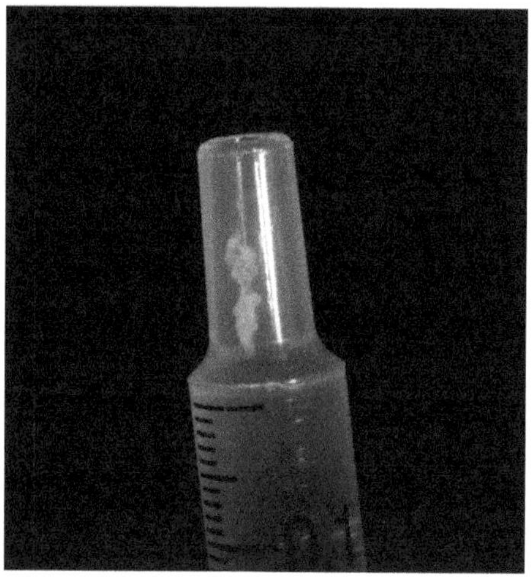

Figure 2: After removing the filter cannula, a kind of clot was observed that had not previously been seen on the syringe supplied.

party supplier. Therefore, it was not further investigated what exactly the bearing material consisted of.

During the third injection, a whitish mass was observed which had an irregular surface structure and small air bubbles on the surface (Figure 3). The manufacturer's analysis showed that it was not a bacterial contamination but part of the greyish rubber stopper that was presumably pushed into the solution with the filter cannula when it entered ("coring"). To prevent this coring, from now on the bevel tip was inserted first and pressed downward and toward the bevel so that the bevelled tip and heel enter at the same point, when the needle is inserted into the rubber top of the vial. In addition, henceforth, an inspecting look into the glass vial was introduced regularly as part of the standardized procedures.

In all three cases, the medication of the initial vial was no longer used. In accordance with professional obligations, a notification was made to the competent authority (Federal Institute and Drugs and Medical Devices). The product was sent to the pharmaceutical manufacturer (contact: bv-complaint@bayer.com), who provided a replacement in one of the three cases.

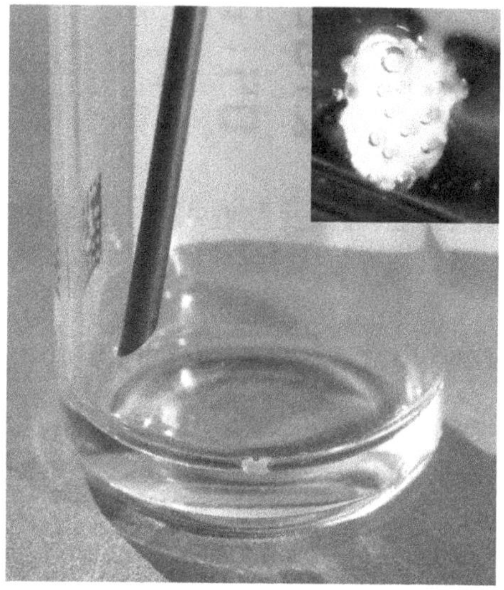

Figure 3: During the mounting process, the injector saw a larger particle of whitish colour (insert), so the process was aborted and the drug could not be used.

3. Discussion

In this case series, three different incidents were identified as possible sources of contamination before an intravitreal injection. Intravitreal injections are indeed one of the most common procedures performed in Ophthalmology. We recommend caution during every step involved in the process. Physicians should be aware that the original solutions or their accessories may contain impurities—even in labelled drugs. These may be due to production and material defects during manufacturing or may have occurred during packaging and shipping. Even if vigilance against volatile particles and aerosols is increased during these days of the COVID-19 pandemic [6], smooth surfaces or inorganic materials may contain bacterial deposits and contamination [7, 8]. It was shown that by no means must the patients' own conjunctiva be regarded as the only source of potential contamination but also the material used [9, 10] and the oral flora of the staff [11].

In all three cases reported, standard procedure was followed in the preparation or unpacking of the vial. Although we follow and adhere to very strict aseptic rules in Germany (surgery room, overgarments for patients, eye coverage after disinfection, masks, and sterile gloves), these provide little protection against impurities or potential contamination of the drug. For the very commonly repeated procedure of an intravitreal injection, we consider it sensible and necessary not only to plan for team time-out (examination of the indication and correct eye, four-eye principle) but also to maintain an open error culture and to remain vigilant against possible contamination.

The uncertainty in the latter case was mainly due to the fact that the colour of the dislocated rubber fragment differed significantly from the grey tone above. This ambiguity could have been excluded if a careful inspection of the cuvette had become an integral part of the preparation (e.g., when unpacking the materials). We also hope that the picture presented here will facilitate an assessment and differentiation for the future. It is unlikely that material problems or contamination are limited to one drug or manufacturer only [12, 13]. A prefilled syringe can also fall down or become contaminated when unpacked; however, compared to the rate of events seen with glass vials (3/7,076 ≙ 0.4‰) during 12 months, we did not observe any such events (0/23,426) during the same period.

Although users can usually rely on the high quality of the materials used and the corresponding quality controls in the manufacturing and filling process, a high degree of vigilance should be maintained at all times. A recent review covered comprehensively the wide range of different materials used in the syringes [14]: even small measures such as tapping against the syringe can lead to an increased release of foreign impurities and silicon oil. Even if prefilled syringes (PFS) will reduce the risk of contamination during preparation and speed up the actual injection process [15], a visual inspection is still helpful: no potential sources of bacteria and thus a serious threat to vision should be overlooked. Routine and organisational efficiency must not be accompanied by a loss of the individual injector's attention, while the most frequent intervention in ophthalmology is carried out.

Acknowledgments

We thank Susanne Schweyer, Michael Breuninger, and Sara Schall for the photo documentation.

References

[1] R. A. Goldberg, H. W. Flynn Jr., D. Miller, S. Gonzalez, and R. F. Isom, "Streptococcus endophthalmitis outbreak after intravitreal injection of bevacizumab: one-year outcomes and investigative results," *Ophthalmology*, vol. 120, no. 7, pp. 1448–1453, 2013.

[2] K. Xu, E. K. Chin, S. R. Bennett et al., "Endophthalmitis after Intravitreal injection of vascular endothelial growth factor Inhibitors," *Ophthalmology*, vol. 125, no. 8, pp. 1279–1286, 2018.

[3] C. Busch, M. Iglicki, M. Okada et al., "Causative pathogens of endophthalmitis after intravitreal anti-VEGF injection: an international multicenter study," *Ophthalmologica*, vol. 241, no. 4, pp. 211–219, 2019.

[4] I. U. Scott, N. L. Oden, P. C. VanVeldhuisen, M. S. Ip, B. A. Blodi, and A. N. Antoszyk, "SCORE study report 7: incidence of intravitreal silicone oil droplets associated with staked-on vs luer cone syringe design," *American Journal of Ophthalmology*, vol. 148, no. 5, pp. 725–732.e7, 2009.

[5] J. H. Yu, E. Gallemore, J. K. Kim, R. Patel, J. Calderon, and R. P. Gallemore, "Silicone oil droplets following intravitreal bevacizumab injections," *American Journal of Ophthalmology Case Reports*, vol. 10, pp. 142–144, 2018.

[6] T. H. T. Lai, E. W. H. Tang, S. K. Y. Chau, K. S. C. Fung, and K. K. W. Li, "Stepping up infection control measures in ophthalmology during the novel coronavirus outbreak: an experience from Hong Kong," *Graefe's Archive for Clinical and Experimental Ophthalmology*, vol. 258, no. 5, pp. 1049–1055, 2020.

[7] B. Sobolewska, M. Buhl, J. Liese, and F. Ziemssen, "Slit lamps and lenses: a potential source of nosocomial infections?," *Eye (London, England)*, vol. 32, no. 6, pp. 1021–1027, 2018.

[8] B. Fritz, M. März, S. Weis, S. Wahl, F. Ziemssen, and M. Egert, "Site-specific molecular analysis of the bacteriota on worn spectacles," *Scientific Reports*, vol. 10, no. 1, 2020.

[9] J. M. Stewart, S. K. Srivastava, A. E. Fung et al., "Bacterial contamination of needles used for intravitreal injections: a prospective, multicenter study," *Ocular Immunology and Inflammation*, vol. 19, no. 1, pp. 32–38, 2011.

[10] M. M. Nentwich, Y. Yactayo-Miranda, S. Weimann et al., "Bacterial contamination of needle points after intravitreal injection," *European Journal of Ophthalmology*, vol. 19, no. 2, pp. 268–272, 2018.

[11] S. J. Garg, M. Dollin, J. Hsu, P. Storey, and J. F. Vander, "Effect of a strict 'no-talking' policy during intravitreal injection on post-injection endophthalmitis," *Ophthalmic Surgery, Lasers & Imaging Retina*, vol. 46, no. 10, pp. 1028–1034, 2015.

[12] F. Forooghian, D. A. Albiani, A. W. Kirker, and A. B. Merkur, "Comparison of endophthalmitis rates following intravitreal injection of compounded bevacizumab, ranibizumab, and aflibercept," *Canadian Journal of Ophthalmology*, vol. 52, no. 6, pp. 616–619, 2017.

[13] J. M. Smith, M. T. Mathias, S. C. Oliver et al., "The influence of needle gauge and infection source on vitreous aspirate cultures," *The British Journal of Ophthalmology*, vol. 100, no. 4, pp. 453–455, 2016.

[14] G. B. Melo, N. F. S. da Cruz, G. G. Emerson et al., "Critical analysis of techniques and materials used in devices, syringes, and needles used for intravitreal injections," *Progress in Retinal and Eye Research*, no. article 100862, p. 100862, 2020.

[15] P. P. Storey, Z. Tauqeer, Y. Yonekawa et al., "The impact of prefilled syringes on endophthalmitis following intravitreal injection of ranibizumab," *American Journal of Ophthalmology*, vol. 199, pp. 200–208, 2019.

31

Isolated Superior Oblique Muscle Swelling Causing Acute Vertical Strabismus in Graves' Disease

Keiichi Aomatsu[1] **and Shunji Kusaka**[2]

[1]*Department of Ophthalmology, Nara Hospital, Kindai University Faculty of Medicine, Nara, Japan*
[2]*Department of Ophthalmology, Kindai University Faculty of Medicine, Osaka, Japan*

Correspondence should be addressed to Keiichi Aomatsu; 114731@med.kindai.ac.jp

Academic Editor: Claudio Campa

Purpose. To report a case of isolated superior oblique muscle swelling causing acute vertical strabismus in Graves' disease. *Case.* A 26-year-old woman with a 1-month history of misalignment of the right eye and diplopia was referred to us. Her visual acuity and intraocular pressures were normal in both eyes, but eye movement tests showed clear misalignment of her right eye. Antibody tests for myasthenia gravis were negative. However, blood tests revealed abnormal levels of thyroid-related factors, such as decreased thyroid-stimulating hormone, elevated free T3 and T4, and elevated anti-thyroid-stimulating hormone receptor antibody. We performed magnetic resonance imaging (MRI), which showed slight enlargement of the left superior oblique muscle. The patient was eventually diagnosed with Graves' disease with superior oblique muscle involvement and underwent a thyroidectomy. Three months postoperatively, her diplopia and abnormal eye movements had substantially resolved. *Conclusion.* Isolated superior oblique muscle involvement may be a presenting symptom of Graves' disease. It should be taken into consideration that, in the early stages of thyroid-associated ophthalmopathy (TAO) in adults, only the superior oblique muscle may be enlarged.

1. Introduction

Thyroid-associated ophthalmopathy (TAO) is an autoimmune disease often encountered in daily clinical practice that can be accompanied by unique ocular findings such as exophthalmos and eyelid abnormalities. It is not difficult to diagnose TAO if hyperthyroidism is known or exophthalmos is apparent. However, when there is no obvious exophthalmos and the patient develops acute vertical strabismus, it is difficult to distinguish it from cranial nerve palsy. There have been some reports of patients with TAO whose diagnosis was difficult due to eye movement disorders similar to superior oblique muscle paralysis [1, 2]. In TAO, the inferior rectus and medial rectus muscles are commonly involved, and the superior oblique muscle is rarely involved, but that complicates eye movement disorders [3, 4]. In this report, we diagnosed TAO, but it was difficult to distinguish it from acute strabismus due to superior oblique muscle paralysis, and it was atypical for TAO because the oblique muscle was the only affected muscle on magnetic resonance imaging (MRI). As far as we know, there have been few reports in which only the superior oblique muscle was involved in cases of hyperthyroidism.

2. Case Report

A 26-year-old woman with a 1-month history of misalignment of the right eye and diplopia was referred to the Department of Ophthalmology, Kindai University Faculty of Medicine. Starting 2 years and 4 months prior to her referral to our clinic, she underwent local steroid injections

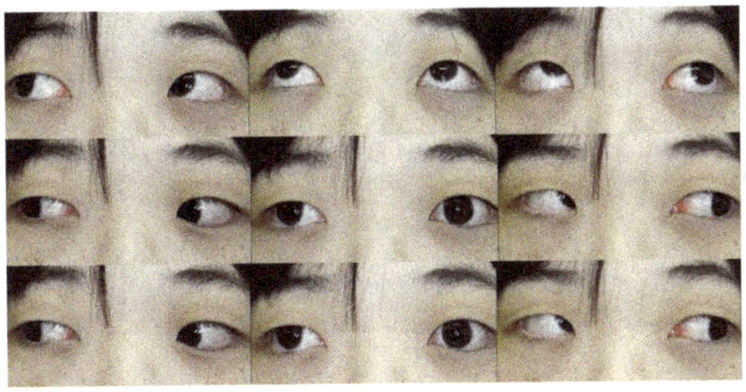

Figure 1: The patient's eye movement examination. The examination revealed overelevation of the right eye in adduction and restriction in the superior oblique muscle direction of the right eye, whereas movements of the left eye were almost normal.

for approximately 1 year, in the Department of Dermatology for alopecia areata. Her decimal visual acuity was 1.2 in each eye. Her intraocular pressure was 19 mmHg in the right eye and 20 mmHg in the left. The anterior ocular segment examination showed hypertropia of the right eye, but no conjunctival hyperemia or eyelid swelling was observed. Measurement of proptosis with a Hertel exophthalmometer showed 16 mm in each eye. Fundus examination showed no abnormalities. The misalignment of the right eye measured by an alternate prism cover test was 25-prism diopter (PD) hypertropia and 40 PD exotropia in the primary gaze position with fixation on a distant target. Eye movement examination revealed overelevation of the right eye in adduction and restriction in the superior oblique muscle direction of the right eye, with almost normal movements in the left eye (Figure 1). A dominant-eye test using a telescope showed that her left eye was dominant. In the first step of the Bielschowsky head-tilt test (BHTT), hypertropia of the right eye was observed. The second step of BHTT revealed an increase in right eye hypertropia with left gaze. The third step of BHTT was positive on right head tilts. The results of the BHTT measurements of vertical deviation were 35 PD and 14 PD on head tilts to the right and left, respectively. MRI showed a slight enlargement of the superior oblique muscle of the left eye, but neither enlargement nor abnormal signal of the four extraocular rectus muscles was seen in either eye (Figure 2). Since the patient was also aware of ptosis of the right eye, an antibody test for myasthenia gravis was performed. However, both antiacetylcholine receptor and anti-muscle-specific kinase antibodies were negative, and the Tensilon test was also negative.

A blood test, performed in the dermatology department three months earlier, showed abnormal thyroid-related values as follows. Thyroid studies revealed a decreased thyroid-stimulating hormone level of <0.01 (normal, 0.5–5 μIU/mL), an elevated free T3 level of 16.9 (normal, 2.3–4 pg/mL), an elevated free T4 level of 4.8 (normal, 0.9–1.7 ng/dL), and an elevated anti-thyroid-stimulating hormone receptor antibody level of 9.2 (normal, 0–2 U/L). From these findings, the patient was diagnosed with ophthalmopathy associated with Graves' disease, with superior oblique muscle involvement.

For detailed investigation and treatment of Graves' disease, the patient was also referred to an endocrinologist and metabolic physician. Thyrotoxicosis, such as increased sweating and diffuse thyromegaly, was confirmed, and a high uptake rate was confirmed by a thyroid isotope test. Oral treatment with thiamazole was started, but it was changed to potassium iodide due to side effects such as fever and joint pain; no remission was achieved. Therefore, a total thyroidectomy was performed by her otorhinolaryngologist, about 3 months after her first visit to our clinic. Within a few weeks after the operation, her subjective symptoms, such as hand tremors and increased sweating, improved and diplopia gradually decreased. Four months after the operation, the patient transferred from our hospital to a hospital outside the prefecture, because of relocation, but diplopia and abnormal eye position had improved at the final visit (Figure 3).

3. Discussion

TAO is relatively often identified based on characteristic eyelid findings such as eyelid edema, eyelid retraction, and lid lag or exophthalmos. However, this case differed from typical TAO in that it caused acute-onset vertical strabismus due to isolated superior oblique muscle enlargement. TAO should have been raised to the differential diagnosis at an early stage, but there were some other points that made it difficult to reach the final diagnosis. One of the difficulties in this case was determining whether the abnormal eye position was due to a neurological disease or a muscle disease. At first, the patient's chief complaint was the right eye deviation, as shown in Figure 1, so we regarded this as ocular motor dysfunction in the right eye and suspected superior oblique palsy (consistent with the BHTT results). However, based on the findings on MRI and the patient's hyperthyroidism, we forced her to fixate with her right eye. When we did so, the original abnormality of the eye position was confirmed, as shown in Figure 4(b). Because the affected eye was the dominant eye, it was suspected that the fixation effort to correct the abnormal position of the left eye induced upward and outward deviation of the right eye. There have been some reports that patients with thyroid eye disease sometimes exhibit eye movement disorders such as superior oblique palsy [1, 2]. Additionally, Chen and Dagi and Kushner pointed out that BHTT may be positive in Graves' disease which may be erroneously diagnosed as superior oblique muscle paralysis [2, 5]. In our case, no neurological abnormalities other than acute strabismus were observed, and enlargement of the left superior oblique muscle was revealed on MRI. Therefore, we diagnosed the symptoms as due to a muscle abnormality rather than nerve palsy.

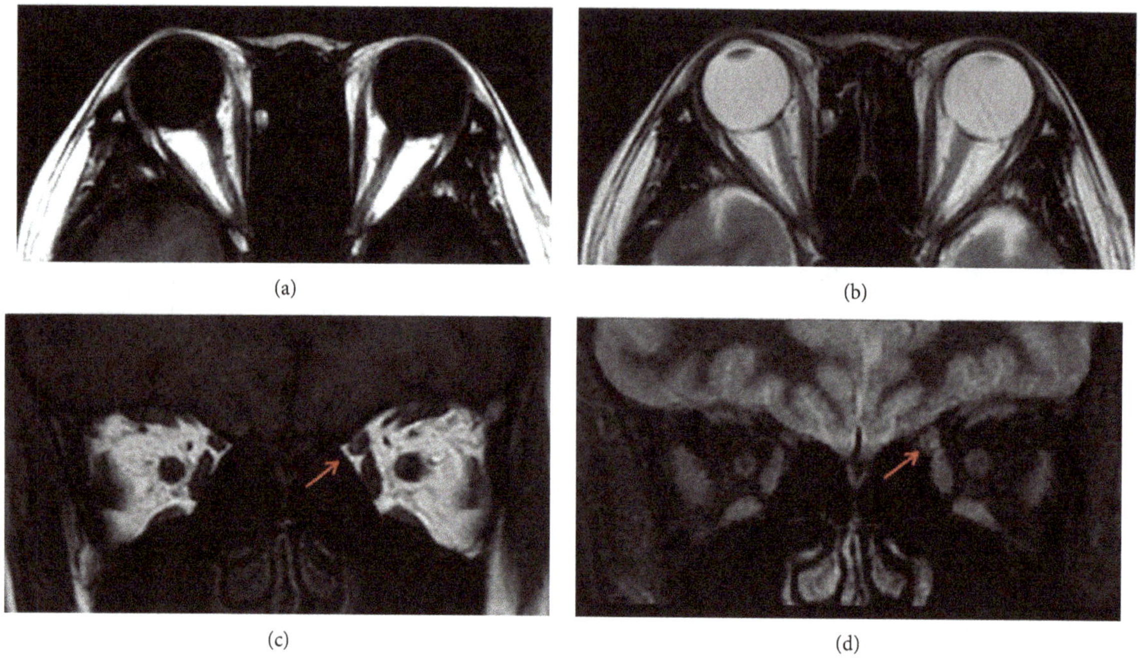

Figure 2: Magnetic resonance imaging (MRI) scans of the patient. The images showed a slight enlargement of the superior oblique muscle of the left eye (red arrow); however, neither enlargement nor abnormal signals were seen in the other four extraocular rectus muscles in either eye: (a) axial T1-weighted image, (b) axial T2-weighted image, (c) coronal T1-weighted image, and (d) coronal Short Tau Inversion Recovery (STIR) image.

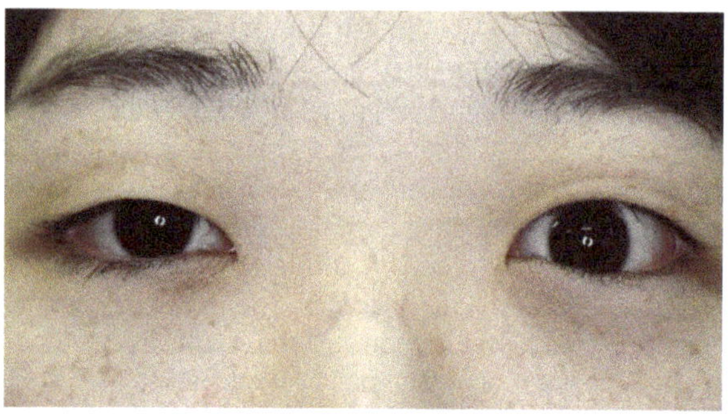

Figure 3: Clinical photograph of the patient at her last visit. Her eye position had improved.

Gerlach and Ferbert proposed that endocrine ophthalmology could be divided into two types: those that cause exophthalmos, due to inflammation of the orbital adipose tissues, and those that cause diplopia and extraocular muscle paralysis due to inflammation of the extraocular muscles—the latter type is quite infrequent [6]. This case is also considered to be of the latter type, but such a pathological condition is rare, and caution should be taken in the diagnosis.

The other difficulty in this case was how to differentiate the cause of the hypertrophy of the isolated superior oblique muscle. Extraocular muscle enlargement and increased orbital fat are important findings of TAO, and such MRI findings are useful for diagnosis. Usually, multiple extraocular muscles are enlarged in one or both eyes, and various ocular misalignments are often seen in TAO. According to previous reports, the extraocular muscle that is most commonly involved in TAO is the inferior rectus muscle, followed by the medial rectus muscle, the superior rectus muscle, and the lateral rectus muscle, in that order [7]. There was a relatively rare case of TAO, with enlargement of the isolated lateral rectus muscle, reported [8], but reports regarding the superior oblique muscle are quite rare. There seems to have been only one article, in French, that showed hypertrophy of the isolated superior oblique muscle associated with Graves' disease on computed tomography [9], but this case is the first report to be demonstrated by MRI.

In this case, extraocular myositis and acquired Brown syndrome [10] also had to be considered differential diseases. Regarding myositis, this patient was considered negative because she did not complain of pain in the orbit, there was no eye injection due to inflammation, and movement of her left eye was not restricted. Brown syndrome was also considered negative because she had no history of head trauma or surgery, and MRI revealed swelling of the muscle belly rather than the trochlear or superior oblique tendon.

In conclusion, isolated superior oblique muscle involvement may be a presenting symptom of Graves' disease. It should be taken into consideration that, in the early stages of TAO in adults, only the superior oblique muscle may be enlarged.

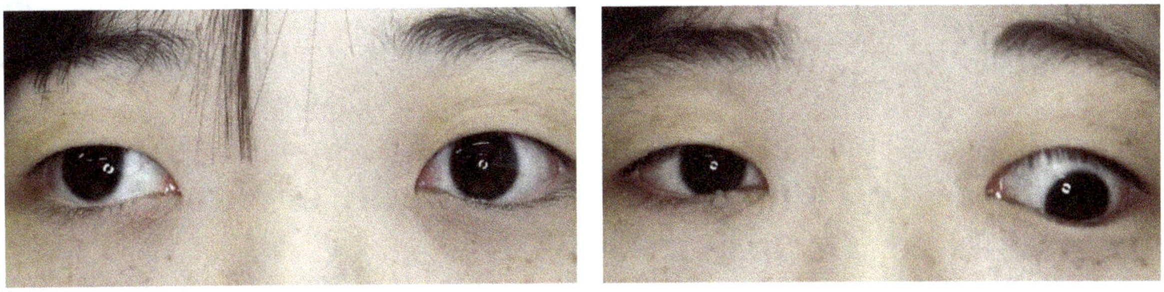

(a) (b)

FIGURE 4: Clinical photographs of the patient. Eye positions are shown for (a) left-eye fixed and (b) right-eye fixed conditions. The original abnormality of the eye position was confirmed as shown in (b).

Consent

Informed consent was obtained from the patient to use her medical records.

Authors' Contributions

Keiichi Aomatsu wrote and edited the manuscript as a major contributor. All authors read and approved the final manuscript.

Acknowledgments

We would like to express our deep gratitude to Yuzo Nakao, an emeritus professor of the Department of Ophthalmology, Kindai University Faculty of Medicine, for his appropriate advice in the treatment of this case. We thank Claire Barnes, PhD, from Edanz Group (https://en-author-services.edanzgroup.com/) for editing the draft of this manuscript.

References

[1] M. L. Moster, T. M. Bosley, M. L. Slavin, and S. E. Rubin, "Thyroid ophthalmopathy presenting as superior oblique paresis," *Journal of Clinical Neuro-Ophthalmology*, vol. 12, no. 2, pp. 94–97, 1992.

[2] V. M. Chen and L. R. Dagi, "Ocular misalignment in Graves disease may mimic that of superior oblique palsy," *Journal of Neuro-Ophthalmology*, vol. 28, no. 4, pp. 302–304, 2008.

[3] H.-J. Wu and R.-K. Tsai, "Thyroid-associated orbitopathy with superior oblique muscle involvement: a case report," *The Kaohsiung Journal of Medical Sciences*, vol. 20, no. 2, pp. 86–88, 2004.

[4] N. M. Thacker, F. G. Velez, J. L. Demer, and A. L. Rosenbaum, "Superior oblique muscle involvement in thyroid ophthalmopathy," *Journal of AAPOS*, vol. 9, no. 2, pp. 174–178, 2005.

[5] B. J. Kushner, "Errors in the three-step test in the diagnosis of vertical strabismus," *Ophthalmology*, vol. 96, no. 1, pp. 127–132, 1989.

[6] M. Gerlach and A. Ferbert, "Pure eye muscle involvement in endocrine orbitopathy," *European Neurology*, vol. 60, no. 2, pp. 67–72, 2008.

[7] Y. Nishida, S. Tian, B. Isberg, L. Tallstedt, and G. Lennerstrand, "MRI measurements of orbital tissues in dysthyroid ophthalmopathy," *Graefe's Archive for Clinical and Experimental Ophthalmology*, vol. 239, no. 11, pp. 824–831, 2001.

[8] M. Erdurmus, S. Celebi, S. Ozmen, and Y. Y. Bucak, "Isolated lateral rectus muscle involvement as a presenting sign of euthyroid Graves disease," *Journal of American Association for Pediatric Ophthalmology and Strabismus*, vol. 15, no. 4, pp. 395–397, 2011.

[9] M. C. Charif, A. Bernoussi, Z. Hajji et al., "Isolated hypertrophy of the superior oblique muscle in Basedow disease," *Bulletin de la Societe belge d'ophtalmologie*, vol. 295, pp. 11–15, 2005.

[10] D. S. Hughes, L. Beck, R. Hill, and J. Plenty, "Dysthyroid eye disease presenting as Brown's syndrome," *Acta Ophthalmologica*, vol. 71, no. 2, pp. 262–265, 1993.

32

Optical Coherence Tomography Angiography of Nonarteritic Cilioretinal Artery Occlusion Alone

Toyo Ikebukuro,[1] **Tsutomu Igarashi,**[1] **Shuhei Kameya,**[2] **Takeshi Arima,**[1] **Tomoyuki Kunishige,**[1] **and Hiroshi Takahashi**[1]

[1]*Department of Ophthalmology, Nippon Medical School, 1-1-5 Sendagi, Bunkyo-ku, Tokyo, Japan*
[2]*Department of Ophthalmology, Nippon Medical School Chiba Hokusoh Hospital, 1715 Kamagari, Inzai, Chiba, Japan*

Correspondence should be addressed to Toyo Ikebukuro; t-ikebukuro@nms.ac.jp

Academic Editor: Alexander A. Bialasiewicz

Cilioretinal artery occlusion (CLRAO) is a rare disease. Here, we report the case of a 70-year-old man with nonarteritic cilioretinal artery occlusion alone. The patient was allergic to fluorescein. Therefore, we followed the retinal circulation with optical coherence tomography angiography (OCTA). OCTA at 40 days postonset showed partial improvement in the retinal circulation.

1. Introduction

The retinal artery is a terminal artery responsible for blood flow in the inner retinal layer. Retinal artery occlusion (RAO) causes pallor and edematous changes in the retina and thickening of the inner retinal layer in the ischemic area. Basically, the central retinal artery plays a major role in retinal circulation, but this circulation is diverse. Cilioretinal arteries, which belong to the posterior ciliary artery system, usually arise from the peripapillary choroid or directly from one of the short posterior ciliary arteries. In a previous study, the incidence of cilioretinal arteries in 2,000 eyes of 1,000 people was evaluated by fundus photographs and fluorescein angiography. Among them, 959 people were patients of the department of ophthalmology, Baylor College of Medicine. Forty-one people were healthy young adult volunteers with no history of ophthalmic disease. Cilioretinal arteries were reported to be present in 49.5% of these people (34.9% in one eye only and 14.6% in both eyes) [1]. Cilioretinal artery occlusion (CLRAO) is a rare disease, occurring in only about 5% of RAO cases [2]. To date, fluorescein angiography (FA) has been a standard method for the diagnosis of RAO. However, recently, noninvasive microcirculation evaluation by optical coherence tomography angiography (OCTA) has become possible [3]. Here, we report a case of CLRAO that was followed up with OCTA because of an allergic reaction to fluorescein.

2. Case Presentation

We report a case of CLRAO in a 70-year-old male. He became aware of loss of vision in his left eye upon waking at 07:00 on November 14, 2018. He had no subjective symptoms when he went to bed at 23:00 the night before. After visiting a nearby eye clinic, he was referred to our hospital because of suspected left RAO. He arrived at our hospital at 15:00; thus, it was estimated that 8–16 hours had elapsed since the onset of RAO.

The patient had no history of risk factors for RAO, such as hypertension, hypercholesterolemia, or diabetes mellitus, and no family history of ophthalmologic disease, but had a history of smoking about 20 cigarettes a day. His visual acuity at the initial visit was 20/16 in the right eye and 20/40 in the left eye. On slit-lamp examination, no abnormalities were found in the anterior segment of the eye. Intraocular pressure was 17.0 mmHg in the right eye and 16.5 mmHg in the left eye.

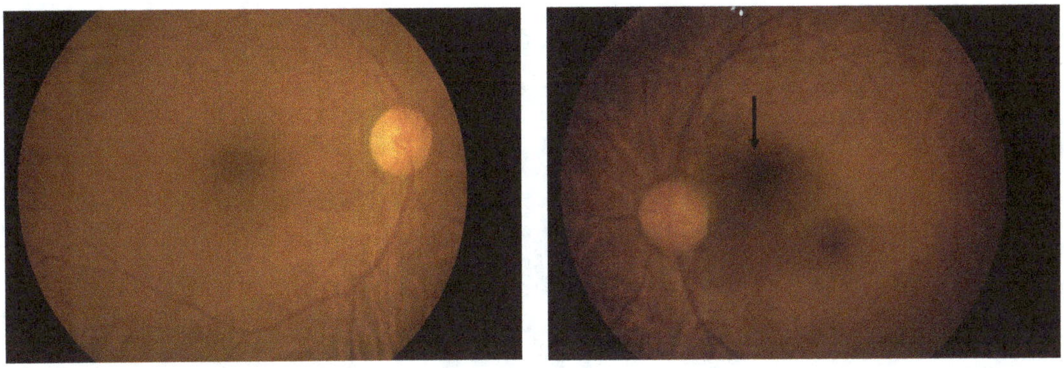

(a) (b)

Figure 1: Color fundus photographs of the (a) right eye and (b) left eye. (a) In the right eye, no obvious fundus abnormalities are apparent. (b) In the left eye, the cilioretinal artery extends from the upper temporal side of the optic nerve papillae to the temporal side. White change is seen in the retina along the cilioretinal artery.

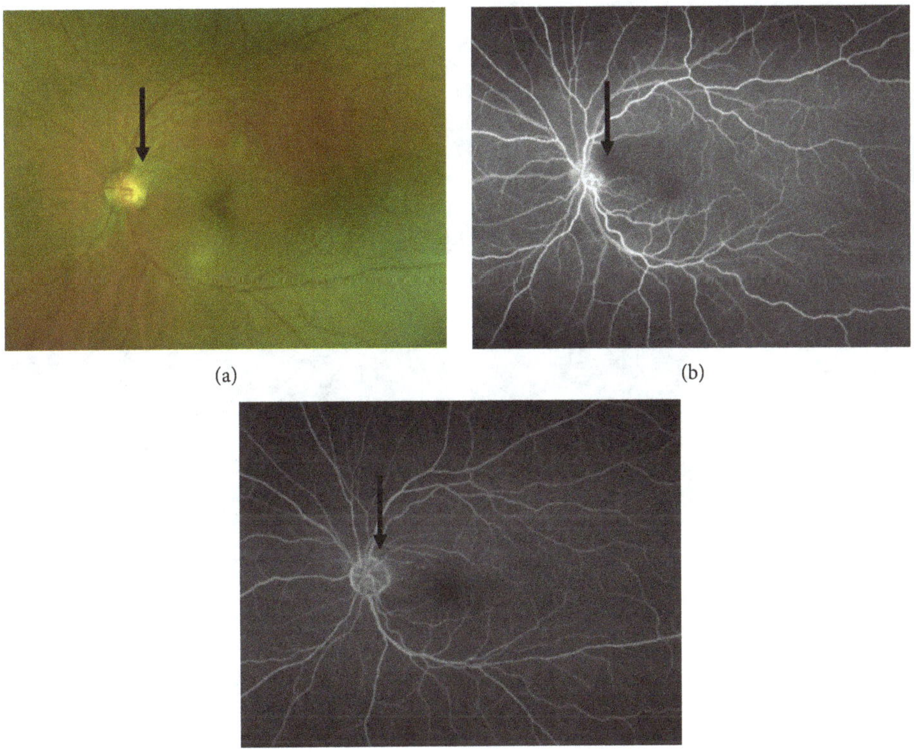

(a) (b) (c)

Figure 2: Fluorescein angiography (FA). (a) The left ocular fundus photograph. As in the fundus examination, the image shows a cilioretinal artery originating from the optic nerve papillae. White changes (arrow) are seen in the retina around the cilioretinal artery. (b) The image 20 s after the start of FA. Fluorescein staining of the cilioretinal artery was delayed (arrow). Subsequently, the cilioretinal artery was gradually refluxed from the distal side. (c) The image at 2 min and 39 s after the start of FA. The area around the cilioretinal artery was stained.

Fundus examination showed no abnormalities in the color tone of the optic nerve papillae, and the cup-to-disc ratio was 0.5 in both eyes. No abnormal findings were observed in the retina of the right eye, while a band-like white change was found in the superior macular area and in the superior temporal area in the left eye. The cilioretinal artery extended from the superior temporal side of the optic nerve papillae. The area of white change was consistent with the area of the cilioretinal artery, and therefore, CLRAO was suspected (Figure 1).

Then, FA and optical coherence tomography (OCT) and OCTA (RS-3000 Advance 2; NIDEK Co., Ltd., Aichi, Japan) were performed. After confirming that there were no problems with the blood test, the patient underwent FA using ultrawide-field retinal imaging device (OPTOS California; Nikon Healthcare Japan Inc., Tokyo, Japan). The results

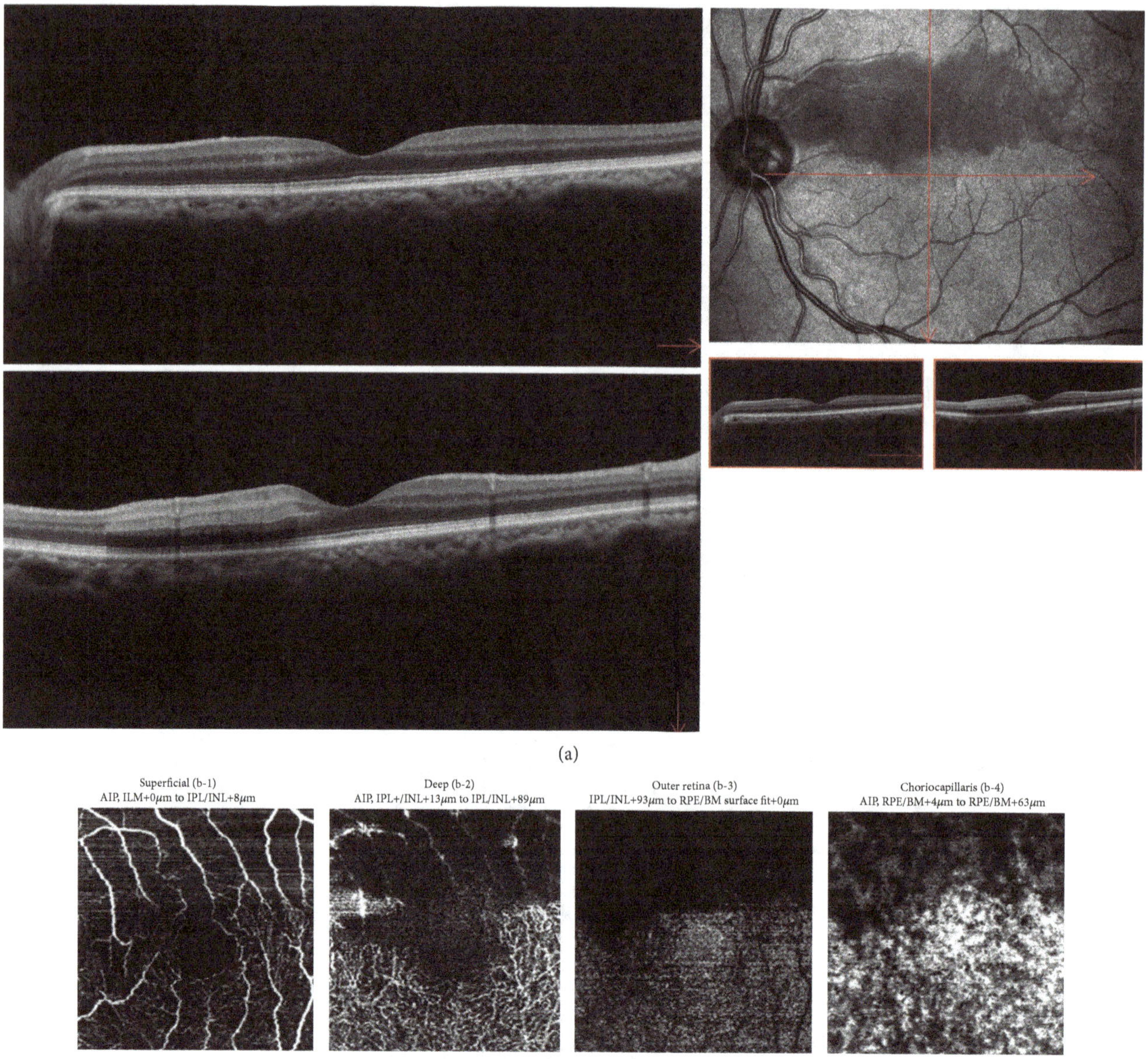

FIGURE 3: (a) Optical coherence tomography (OCT) and (b) optical coherence tomography angiography (OCTA) (onset): (b-1) superficial layer, (b-2) deep layer, (b-3) outer retina layer, and (b-4) choriocapillaris layer of OCTA. (a) OCT shows a thickening of the inner retinal layer consistent with the white change on the fundus photograph. On infrared reflectance images, the area of white change in the fundus photograph is depicted with low luminance, and the area of ischemia can be seen more clearly. (b) In OCTA, the flow sign is decreased in all layers.

showed delayed reflux in the cilioretinal artery of the left eye (Figure 2). After FA, although no abnormal vital signs were seen, a rash was found in the patient's chest, suggesting an allergic reaction to fluorescein. Therefore, OCTA was used to follow up his clinical course thereafter. OCT showed a thickening of the inner retinal layer consistent with the area of white change (Figure 3(a)). In infrared reflectance (IR) images, the area of white change in the fundus photograph was depicted with low luminance, and the area of ischemia could be seen more clearly. In OCTA, the flow sign in the superior macular white change area was reduced in the superficial retinal layer (Figure 3(b)). Due to edema of the inner layer of the retina, the flow signs of the deep, outer retina and choriocapillaris were unclear.

The patient was admitted to our hospital on the same day. After confirming no intracranial abnormalities by computed tomography, 240,000 units of urokinase-type plasminogen activator were administered per day for 3 days. The patient was also scheduled to receive alprostadil (prostaglandin E1) for 3 days; however, it caused vascular pain on the first day and was therefore stopped. Hyperbaric oxygen therapy could not be performed because of a history of spontaneous pneumothorax. Stellate ganglion block was performed five times by an anesthesiologist from the fourth day after onset.

Magnetic resonance angiography and ultrasonography of the carotid artery were performed to investigate cerebrovascular and carotid artery lesions, but no disease causing CLRAO was found. On day 5, oral kallidinogenase was

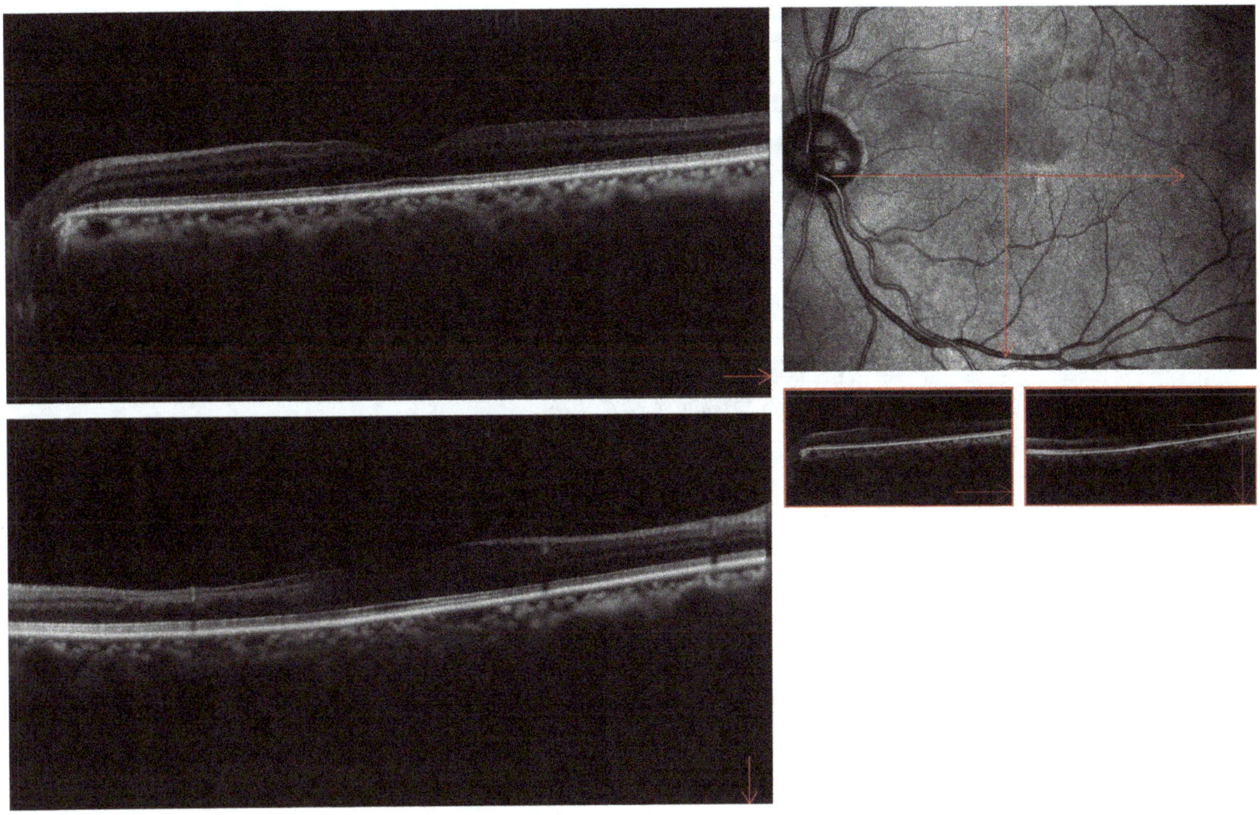

(a)

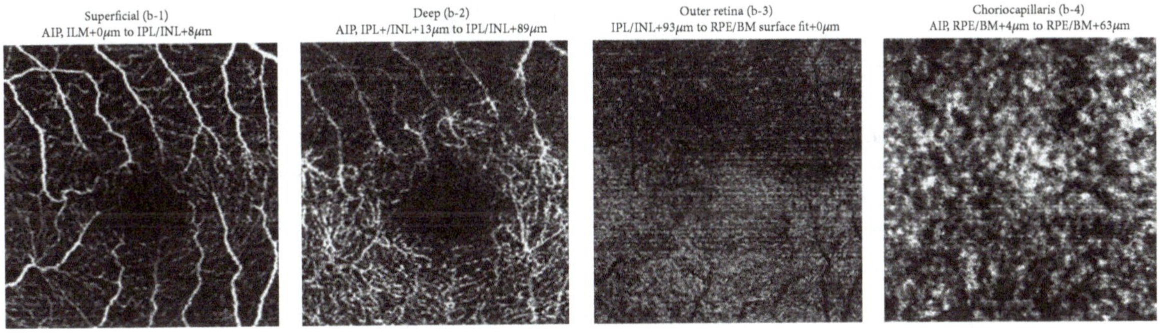

(b)

FIGURE 4: (a) OCT and (b) OCTA at 40 days from disease onset: (b-1) superficial layer, (b-2) deep layer, (b-3) outer retina layer, and (b-4) choriocapillaris layer of OCTA. (a) OCT shows thinning of the inner retinal layer consistent with the white change on the fundus photograph. (b) OCTA shows a decrease in the flow sign. Compared with at disease onset, the flow sign is improved in all layers, but the improvement is mainly in the superficial layer.

started, and his visual acuity gradually improved. On day 40, his left visual acuity eye was restored to 20/25, and OCT showed thinning of the lesion that had the white change. In OCTA, the flow sign was improved in all layers compared to that on day 1 (Figure 4). On day 56, visual field test showed a paracentral scotoma (Figure 5).

3. Discussion

In a previous study evaluating 2,000 eyes in 1,000 people using color fundus photography and FA, a cilioretinal artery was found in 49.5% of all patients and 32.1% of all eyes [1]. In the present case, a cilioretinal artery related to macular circulation was found in the left eye only. RAO is a rare disease, with an incidence of 1–10 per 100,000 population. Symptomatic CLRAO is even rarer, reported in 5.3–7.1% of all RAO cases [2].

CLRAO can be classified clinically into three categories: (1) nonarteritic CLRAO alone, (2) arteritic CLRAO associated with giant cell arteritis, and (3) CLRAO associated with central retinal vein occlusion [4]. The present case corresponds to nonarteritic CLRAO alone.

In the present case, visual acuity was 20/25 at 40 days after disease onset. The cilioretinal artery was occluded,

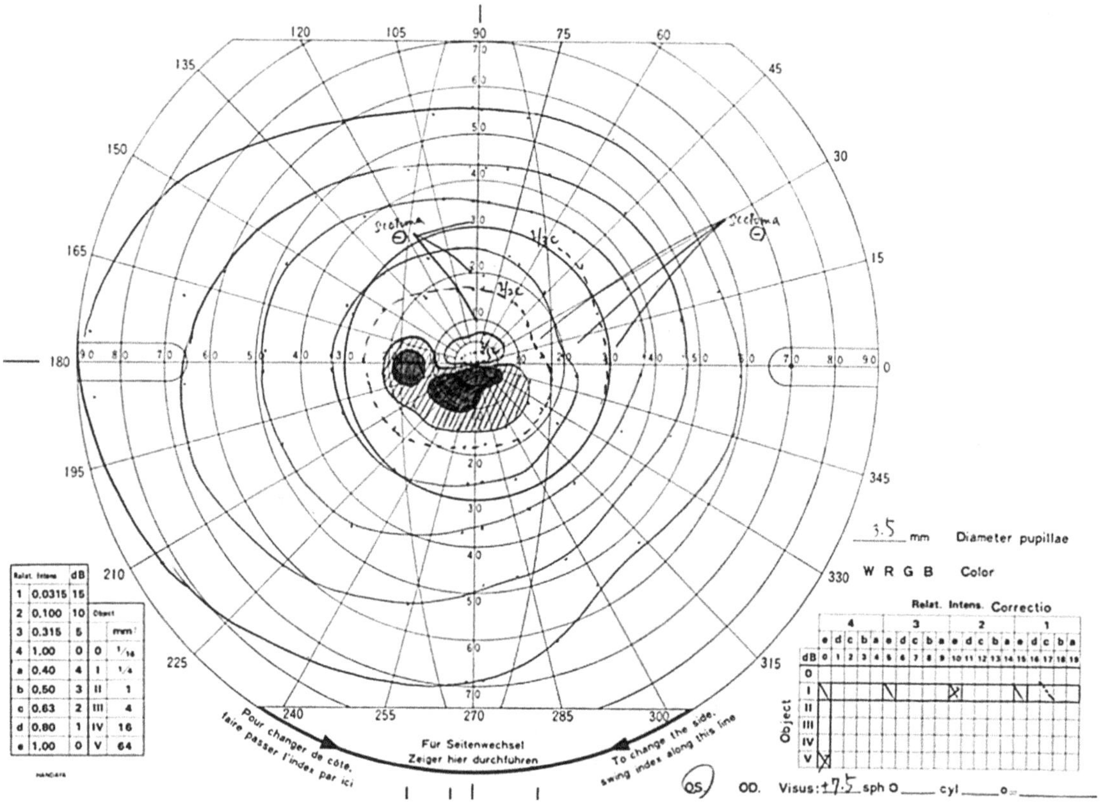

Figure 5: Visual field test by Goldmann perimetry at 56 days from disease onset. A scotoma is seen from slightly below center to the ear side. The location of this paracentral scotoma coincides with the location of cilioretinal artery occlusion.

resulting in ischemic changes in only the upper macula (the reflux area). Since this was partial ischemia of the macula, vision loss was considered to be mild. Important causes of RAO include hypertension, diabetes mellitus, vascular lesions, and a history of smoking. The risk factor in this patient was a history of smoking. Regarding treatment, hyperbaric oxygen therapy was not possible, but urokinase drip and stellate ganglion block could be administered. However, an allergic reaction to fluorescein made it impossible to follow up using FA. Therefore, OCTA was used to assess blood flow. On day 1, a decrease in the flow sign in all layers was observed in the ischemic area. On day 40, the flow sign had considerably improved in the superficial layer, the outer retina, and the choriocapillaris layers, while in the deep layer, although some improvement of blood flow was observed in areas close to the macula, no significant improvement in the flow sign was seen.

Abdellah reported that OCTA results in 11 cases of CRAO showed decreased flow in both the superficial and deep layers, but the superficial layer was more injured [5]. In the present case, there was more damage in the deep layer, which may suggest that CLRAO may be more damaging to the capillary network in the deep layer than in the superficial layer. However, this is only a case report and more cases are needed.

One disadvantage of OCTA is the effect of artifacts. The outer retina and choriocapillaris layers are nourished by choroidal vessels. Therefore, it is unlikely that retinal artery occlusion would cause circulatory failure in these layers. Decreased flow sign in the outer retina and choriocapillaris layers may be due to artifacts caused by edematous changes in the inner retinal layer.

Infrared reflectance (IR) images showed a hyporeflectant area clearly suggestive of ischemia that was consistent with the white change seen on the fundus examination and FA. Findings on IR images may therefore assist in the evaluation of ischemic areas in the acute phase of RAO.

Although susceptible to artifacts, OCTA is superior to FA in imaging in a patient with fluorescein allergy in cilioretinal artery occlusion.

References

[1] J. Justice, "Cilioretinal arteries. A study based on review of stereo fundus photographs and fluorescein angiographic findings," *Archives of Ophthalmology*, vol. 94, no. 8, pp. 1355–1358, 1976.

[2] S. Aktas, O. M. Uyar, E. Ozer, H. Aktas, and K. Eltutar, "Idiopathic isolated cilioretinal artery occlusion treated with hyperbaric oxygen therapy," *Türk Oftalmoloji Dergisi*, vol. 46, no. 5, pp. 244–247, 2016.

[3] T. E. de Carlo, A. Romano, N. K. Waheed, and J. S. Duker, "A review of optical coherence tomography angiography (OCTA)," *International Journal of Retina and Vitreous*, vol. 1, no. 1, p. 5, 2015.

[4] S. S. Hayreh, "Acute retinal arterial occlusive disorders," *Progress in Retinal and Eye Research*, vol. 30, no. 5, pp. 359–394, 2011.

[5] M. M. Abdellah, "Multimodal imaging of acute central retinal artery occlusion," *Medical Hypothesis Discovery & Innovation Ophthalmology Journal*, vol. 8, no. 4, pp. 283–290, 2019.

33

Macular Changes in a Mucopolysaccharidosis Type I Patient with Earlier Systemic Therapies

Augusto Magalhães,[1] Ana Maria Cunha,[1] Rodrigo Vilares-Morgado,[1] Elisa Leão-Teles,[2] Esmeralda Rodrigues,[2] Manuel Falcão,[1,3] Ângela Carneiro,[1,3] Jorge Breda,[1] and Fernando Falcão-Reis[1,3]

[1]*Department of Ophthalmology, Centro Hospitalar Universitário de São João, Porto, Portugal*
[2]*Pediatric Department, Reference Centre of Inherited Metabolic Diseases, Centro Hospitalar Universitário de São João, Porto, Portugal*
[3]*Department of Surgery and Physiology, Faculty of Medicine of University of Porto, Porto, Portugal*

Correspondence should be addressed to Ana Maria Cunha; ana.cunha.18@gmail.com

Academic Editor: Huban Atilla

Purpose. To describe retinal findings in a patient with mucopolysaccharidosis type I (MPS I) that underwent an early treatment with hematopoietic stem cell transplantation (HSCT) and enzyme replacement therapy (ERT). *Case Report.* We describe a case of a 12-year-old female with a biochemical and genetic diagnosis of MPS I. She underwent HSCT and ERT on the first year of life. The visual acuity was 5/10 in both eyes and she had bilateral grade 2 corneal haze. Spectral domain optical coherence tomography (SD-OCT) revealed thickening of the external limiting membrane (ELM) at the fovea. In the parafoveal and perifoveal regions, SD-OCT displayed a loss of the interdigitation, ellipsoid, and myoid zones and of the ELM accompanied by progressive thinning of the outer nuclear layer. Fundus infrared imaging revealed a hyperreflective ring centred on the fovea and hyporeflective areas in temporal parafoveal regions in both eyes. *En face* OCT imaging revealed two hyperreflective rings on the outer retinal level. *Conclusion.* This patient developed macular changes with foveal deposition of hyperreflective material and parafoveal thinning, despite early systemic treatment. Systemic therapies can provide an increase in life expectancy and stabilize visual acuity and corneal clouding, although their effect on retinal degeneration is unknown.

1. Introduction

Mucopolysaccharidosis (MPS) are a group of lysosomal storage disorders caused by inborn errors of glycosaminoglycan (GAG) metabolism [1]. MPS type I (MPS I) is an autosomal recessive disease due to deficiency of lysosomal hydrolase α-L-iduronidase [2], codified by the IDUA gene at locus 4p16.3 [3]. This enzyme is required to break down heparan and dermatan sulfate. As a result, these metabolites build up in several tissues [1].

The phenotypic spectrum of α-L-iduronidase deficiencies includes the mildest form, Scheie syndrome; the intermediate form, Hurler-Scheie syndrome; and the most severe form, Hurler syndrome [2]. Significant multisystemic involvement includes dysostosis multiplex, restrictive and obstructive pulmonary and respiratory disease, valvular disease, ocular and hearing disease, organomegaly, and central and peripheral neurological disease. Progressive neurodegeneration in early childhood characteristically complicates the Hurler phenotype, as opposed to the normal neurological development seen in the Scheie phenotype [1, 4].

Current treatments such as allogeneic hematopoietic stem cell transplantation (HSCT) and enzyme replacement therapy (ERT) have increased the life span of these patients and created the need to improve management of ocular disease [1].

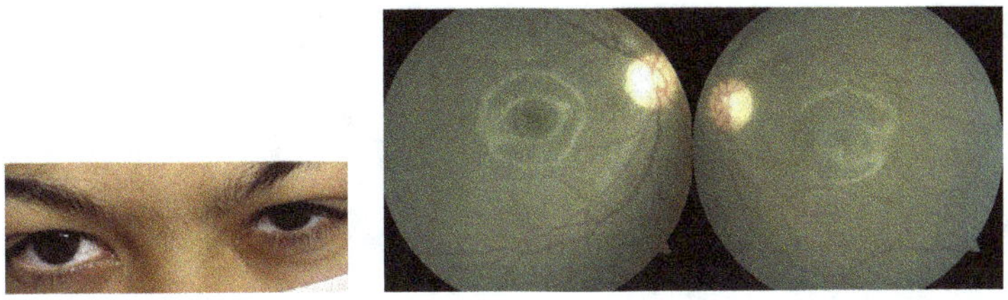

(a) (b)

Figure 1: Anterior segment photographs demonstrated mild grade corneal haze bilaterally (a). Fundus photography of the right and left eyes (b).

Ocular features of MPS I include corneal clouding, glaucoma, pigmentary retinopathy, optic nerve abnormalities (papilledema and atrophy), ocular motility disorders, and refractive errors [4].

We describe the spectral domain optical coherence tomography (SD-OCT) and infrared and *en face* OCT retinal findings in a 12-year-old patient with MPS I (Hurler's syndrome) who underwent treatment with HSCT and ERT during her first year of life.

2. Case Report

A 12-year-old Caucasian female child with the diagnosis of MPS I (Hurler's syndrome), with a severe genotype (homozygous status for the mutation c.1293G>A; p.W402X, exon 9, in the *IDUA* gene) began ERT at 5 months of age and was submitted to HSCT at 12 months. She started a severe graft versus host disease one month later, with important skin and pulmonary and gastrointestinal involvement. She was maintained on ERT for three years after HSCT, with no evidence of antibody development.

The patient presented typical dysmorphic features, short stature, slight cognitive impairment, and also interstitial respiratory disease. Her last analytics revealed a normal alpha-iduronidase leucocyte level (91 nmol/h/mg protein to the normal range: 53–105) and normal urinary GAGs (12 mg/mmol creatinine to the normal range: 4–11), although with an MPS I electrophoretic pattern.

Ophthalmologically, the best corrected visual acuity (BCVA) was 5/10 in both eyes (hyperopia of 1.5 dioptres). The anterior segment examination demonstrated bilateral grade 2 corneal haze (Figure 1). The corneal pachymetry was 544 μm in the right eye and 562 μm in the left eye, and the anterior chamber depth was 2.70 mm and 2.58 mm, respectively (Pentacam, Oculus, USA).

Fundus examination was clinically normal (Figure 1). However, the SD-OCT assessment revealed in the foveal area, in both eyes, increased thickness of the hyperreflective band of the external limiting membrane (ELM). The other outer retinal bands (the myoid, ellipsoid, and interdigitation zones, the retinal pigment epithelium (RPE), and Bruch's membrane) were within normal limits (Figure 2).

In the parafoveal and perifoveal regions, SD-OCT displayed a loss of the interdigitation, ellipsoid, and myoid zones, loss of the ELM, and thinning and eventual loss of the outer nuclear layer (ONL) (Figure 2). The scans, close to the fovea, also revealed small cysts in the ONL, inner nuclear layer (INL), and ganglion cell layer (GCL) (Figure 2).

Fundus infrared imaging revealed a bilateral hyperreflective ring centred on the fovea that was more evident in the left eye. It also revealed hyporeflective areas in the temporal extrafoveal regions in both eyes (Figure 3).

En face OCT images at the level of the outer retina revealed two hyperreflective rings. The inner ring corresponded to the limits of the disruption of the ellipsoid zone, and the external ring limits the disruption of the ELM on SD-OCT (Figure 3).

Electroretinography (ERG) was performed according to the International Society for Clinical Electrophysiology of Vision (ISCEV) standards. The ERG findings showed an absence of the dark-adapted (DA) 0.01 ERG response and a DA 10.0 with a diminished a-wave and b-wave. The light-adapted (LA) 3.0 ERG had a diminished b-wave and absence of the LA flicker 30 Hz ERG response (Figure 4).

3. Discussion

The main ocular manifestations of MPS I include corneal clouding, glaucoma, retinal pigmentary degeneration, and optic nerve abnormalities [1]. Earlier and more effective treatments have led to an increase in life expectancy of MPS I patients, and so it is currently possible to identify later manifestations of ocular diseases. Moreover, with the advent of new diagnostic technologies, namely, OCT, it is possible to identify retinal structural changes, even in the presence of a clinically normal fundus.

Our SD-OCT findings revealed, in both eyes, an increased thickness of the ELM in the foveal area; a loss of the interdigitation, ellipsoid, and myoid zones, of the ELM; and a thinning of the ONL in parafoveal and perifoveal regions. We also observed small cysts in the ONL, the INL, and the GCL.

Previous studies with SD-OCT in MPS I patients are scarce and include a limited number of patients. The thickening of the ELM at the fovea has been previously described [4–7]. However, in these previous studies, the patients were only treated with ERT, unlike our clinical case that received both HSCT and ERT. At the parafoveal and perifoveal regions, the photoreceptor inner and outer segment thinning has also been reported [5], but not the complete loss of the ellipsoid and myoid zones and the ELM. The thinning of the ONL, as described in our case, is a novel finding. Retinal cysts have been reported, usually at the ONL [4, 5]. Other possible OCT

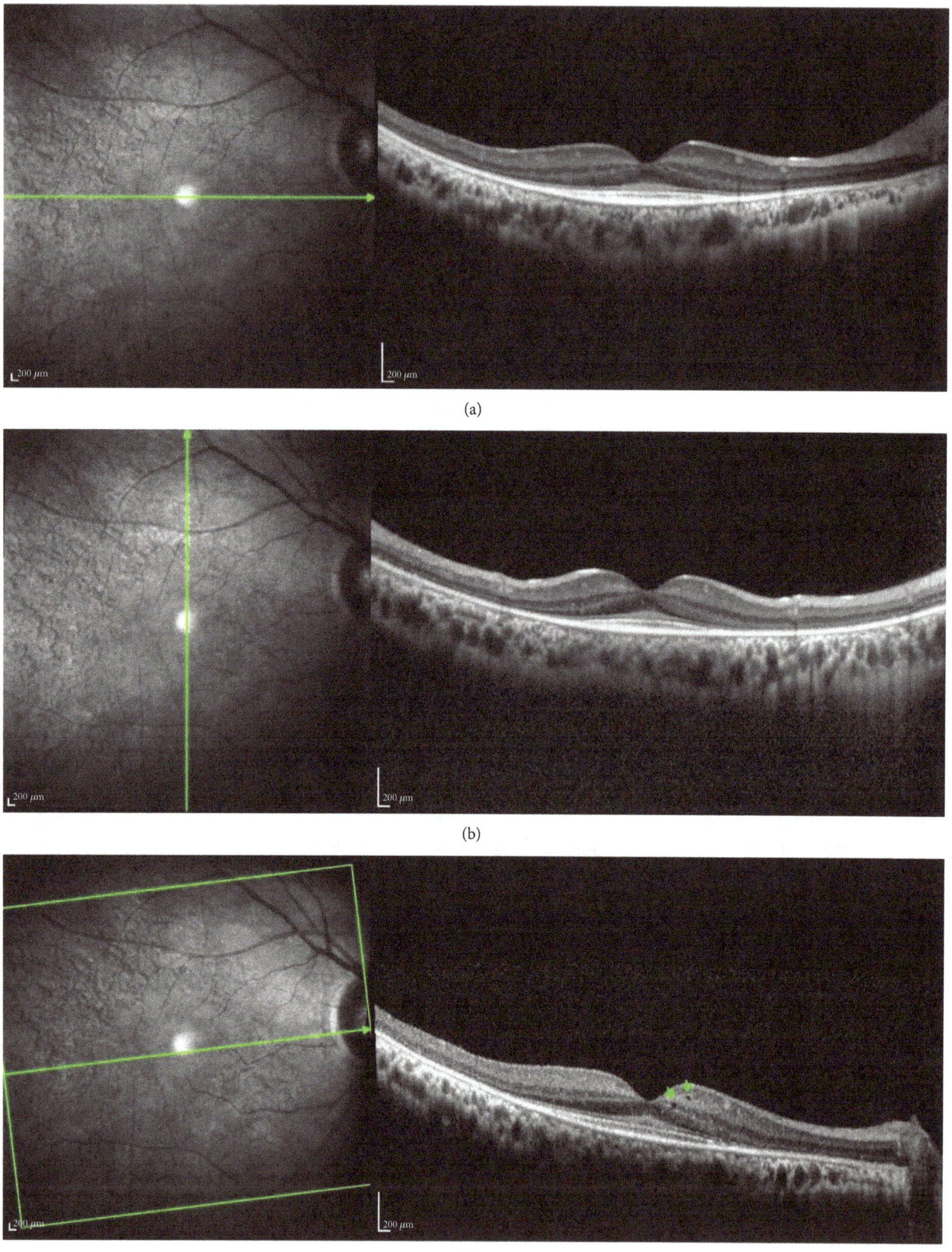

Figure 2: SD-OCT horizontal and vertical scans of fovea in the right eye (a, b). It demonstrates foveal increased thickness of hyperreflective band signal at the ELM, with intact myoid, ellipsoid, and interdigitation zones, RPE, and Bruch's membrane. In the parafoveal and perifoveal region, it demonstrated a progressive loss of interdigitation and ellipsoid zones, myoid zone, and ELM and thinning of the outer nuclear layer. SD-OCT horizontal scan, close to the fovea (c), demonstrated a small cyst in ONL, INL, and GCL (arrows). SD-OCT: spectral domain optical coherence tomography; ELM: external limiting membrane; RPE: retinal pigment epithelium; ONL: outer nuclear layer; INL: inner nuclear layer; GCL: ganglion cell layer.

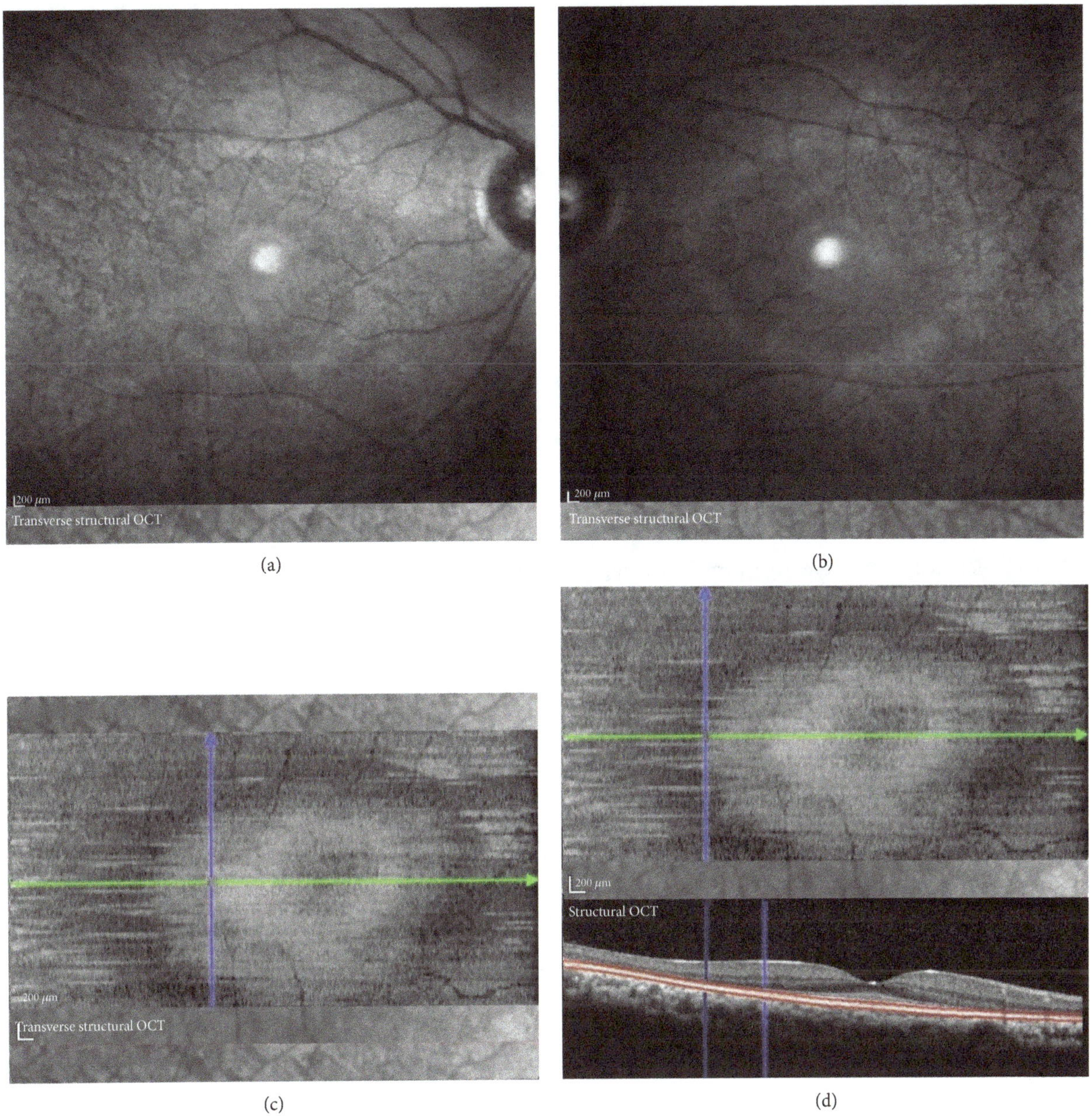

FIGURE 3: Continued.

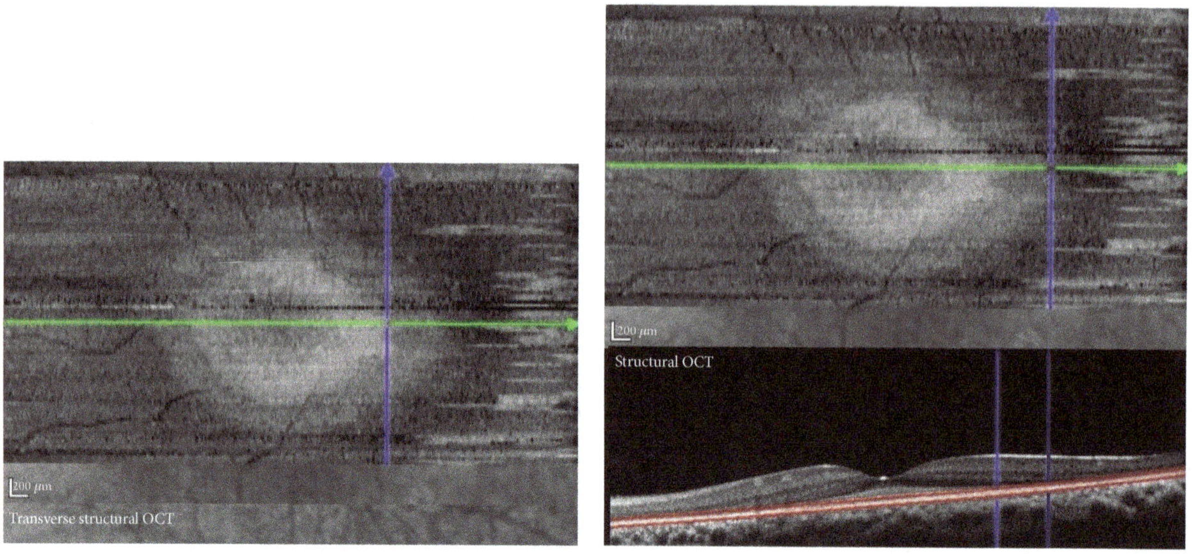

(e) (f)

Figure 3: Fundus infrared imaging revealed hyperreflective ring centred in the fovea and hyporeflective areas in temporal parafoveal regions in both eyes (a, b). *En face* SD-OCT images at the level of the outer retina revealed two hyperreflective rings corresponding to the disruption of the ellipsoid zone (c, e) and ELM (d, f). SD-OCT: spectral domain optical coherence tomography; ELM: external limiting membrane.

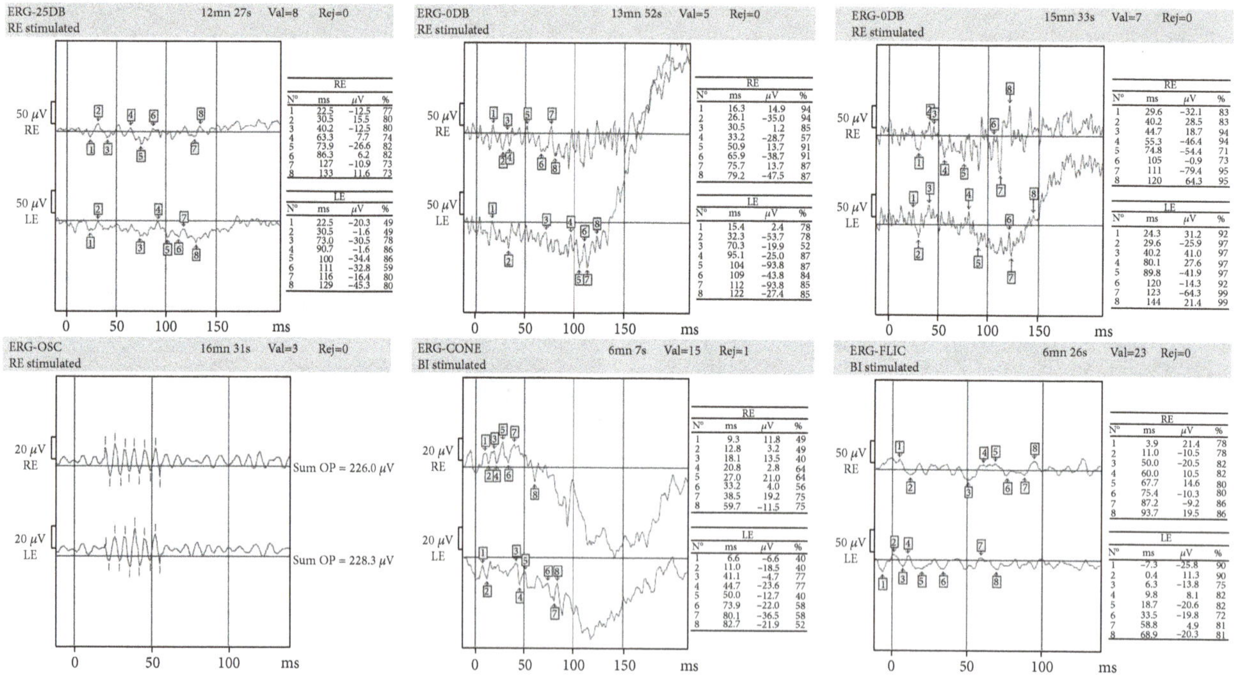

Figure 4: ERG findings. Absence of DA 0.01 ERG response and a DA 10.0 with a diminished a-wave and b-wave. LA 3.0 ERG with a diminished b-wave and absence of LA flicker 30 Hz ERG response. ERG: electroretinography; DA: dark-adapted; LA: light-adapted.

findings, not present in our case, include macular epiretinal membrane and macular edema-like changes [8].

The infrared and *en face* OCT findings correlate and have not been previously described. The fundus infrared image revealed a hyperreflective ring that is evident in the *en face* OCT images at the level of the outer retina, with two hyperreflective rings. These findings correspond to the area of the thickened ELM, and its limits correspond to the ellipsoid zone and ELM disruptions seen on SD-OCT B-scans. The hyperreflective ring has been reported in macular abnormalities such as retinitis pigmentosa [9], but it has not been previously described in MPS patients.

Retinopathy in MPS I occurs due to accumulation of GAG within the RPE cells and the interphotoreceptor matrix, followed by phagocytosis by Muller cells or retinal pigment epithelial cells, leading to progressive loss of photoreceptors

[4, 10]. Lazarus et al. suggested that the absence of lysosomal enzymes in the RPE induces RPE hypertrophy and can generate an altered GAG distribution of the interphotoreceptor matrix, which can subsequently affect the photoreceptor's cell-supportive function, leading to photoreceptor degeneration [11].

The cause for the increased hyperreflectance in the region of the ELM observed in our clinical case is not known. It may represent GAG accumulation in Müller cells, undigested abnormal photoreceptor outer segments (although unlikely given that it is internal to the ellipsoid line zone), or abnormal collagen deposition. We propose that our patient has attenuated enzyme action in Müller cells, allowing clearing of degraded GAG. However, at the fovea, the increased number of photoreceptors results in a higher load of GAG overwhelming local enzyme capacity leading to a consequent thickening of the ELM as seen on SD-OCT.

Electrophysiological tests are important for the evaluation of the functional integrity of the retina. In our clinical case, we identified a progressive rod-cone retinal degeneration with an attenuated ERG amplitude, which is the most commonly described pattern [12–14].

As previously reported, HSCT increases life expectancy and provides partial symptomatic improvement and is most effective when initiated early (during the first 2 years of life). Normal bone marrow cells from a matched donor appear to stabilize or improve visual acuity, corneal clouding, and optic nerve swelling in MPS I patients [1, 15]. The ERT replaces the enzyme deficiency via intravenous administration, and when treatment is started early in the patient's life, it is associated with stabilization of corneal clouding. Nevertheless, ERT does not cross the blood-brain barrier and presumably does not cross the blood-retina barrier either [4, 12]. For this reason, there are no reports of improved retinal function. This hypothesis is confirmed by the findings observed in our case report. The patient had a mild corneal clouding but retinal degeneration, despite having undergone early HSCT and being maintained for a long period of time with ERT with normal levels of lysosomal enzyme α-L-iduronidase (IDUA).

In conclusion, our patient presented macular changes with foveal deposition of a hyperreflective material at the level of the ELM and parafoveal thinning despite the early systemic treatment with HSCT and ERT and normal alpha-iduronidase levels. Systemic therapies provide an increase in life expectancy and stabilize visual acuity and corneal clouding, despite the fact that they do not seem to modify retinal degeneration. Further studies are required to determine the nature of the material and to truly evaluate the effect and incidence of the current therapies in MPS I retinal changes. With the increase in survival and improved technology, our comprehension of the disease evolution and the effect of available treatment can increase over time.

Disclosure

The study was conducted in the Department of Ophthalmology of São João Hospital, Porto, Portugal. Augusto Magalhães and Ana Maria should be considered as co-first authors.

Authors' Contributions

Augusto Magalhães and Ana Maria Cunha contributed equally to this work.

Acknowledgments

Several authors of this publication are members of the European Reference Network for Rare Hereditary Metabolic Disorders (MetabERN)—Project ID No. 739543.

References

[1] C. Fenzl, K. Teramoto, and M. Moshirfar, "Ocular manifestations and management recommendations of lysosomal storage disorders I: mucopolysaccharidoses," *Clinical Ophthalmology*, vol. 9, pp. 1633–1644, 2015.

[2] C. Meaney, G. Greenland, V. Adams et al., "Mutational analysis of 85 mucopolysaccharidosis type I families: frequency of known mutations, identification of 17 novel mutations and in vitro expression of missense mutations," *Human Genetics*, vol. 109, no. 5, pp. 503–511, 2001.

[3] A. Ganesh, Z. Bruwer, and K. Al-Thihli, "An update on ocular involvement in mucopolysaccharidoses," *Current Opinion in Ophthalmology*, vol. 24, no. 5, pp. 379–388, 2013.

[4] H. G. Mack, R. C. A. Symons, and G. de Jong, "Bull's eye maculopathy and subfoveal deposition in two mucopolysaccharidosis type I patients on long-term enzyme replacement therapy," *American Journal of Ophthalmology Case Reports*, vol. 9, pp. 1-6, 2018.

[5] S. Seok, I. J. Lyu, K. A. Park, and S. Y. Oh, "Spectral domain optical coherence tomography imaging of mucopolysaccharidoses I, II, and VI A," *Graefe's Archive for Clinical and Experimental Ophthalmology*, vol. 253, no. 12, pp. 2111–2119, 2015.

[6] C. T. Huang, S. Y. Chu, and Y. C. Lee, "Optical coherence tomography of chorioretinopathy caused by mucopolysaccharidoses," *Ophthalmology*, vol. 122, no. 7, pp. 1535–1537, 2015.

[7] S. Pitz, O. Ogun, M. Bajbouj, L. Arash, G. Schulze-Frenking, and M. Beck, "Ocular changes in patients with mucopolysaccharidosis I receiving enzyme replacement therapy a 4-year experience," *Archives of Ophthalmology*, vol. 125, no. 10, pp. 1353–1356, 2007.

[8] T. Usui, M. Shirakashi, M. Takagi, H. Abe, and K. Iwata, "Macular edema-like change and pseudopapilledema in a case of Scheie syndrome," *Journal of Clinical Neuro-Ophthalmology*, vol. 11, no. 3, pp. 183–185, 1991.

[9] Y. Makiyama, S. Ooto, M. Hangai et al., "Macular cone abnormalities in retinitis pigmentosa with preserved central vision using adaptive optics scanning laser ophthalmoscopy," *PLoS One*, vol. 8, no. 11, article e79447, 2013.

[10] J. L. Ashworth, S. Biswas, E. Wraith, and I. C. Lloyd, "The ocular features of the mucopolysaccharidoses," *Eye*, vol. 20, no. 5, pp. 553–563, 2006.

[11] H. S. Lazarus, W. S. Sly, J. W. Kyle, and G. S. Hageman, "Photoreceptor degeneration and altered distribution of interphotoreceptor matrix proteoglycans in the mucopolysaccharidosis VII mouse," *Experimental Eye Research*, vol. 56, no. 5, pp. 531–541, 1993.

[12] S. Laraway, J. Mercer, E. Jameson, J. Ashworth, P. Hensman, and S. A. Jones, "Outcomes of long-term treatment with laro-

nidase in patients with mucopolysaccharidosis type I," *The Journal of Pediatrics*, vol. 178, pp. 219–226.e1, 2016.

[13] J. P. Gills, R. Hobson, W. B. Hanley, and V. A. McKusick, "Electroretinography and fundus oculi findings in Hurler's disease and allied mucopolysaccharidoses," *Archives of Ophthalmology*, vol. 74, no. 5, pp. 596–603, 1965.

[14] R. C. Caruso, M. I. Kaiser-Kupfer, J. Muenzer, I. H. Ludwig, M. A. Zasloff, and P. A. Mercer, "Electroretinographic findings in the mucopolysaccharidoses," *Ophthalmology*, vol. 93, no. 12, pp. 1612–1616, 1986.

[15] V. Naik, U. Usgaonkar, and H. Albal, "Retinal changes in mucopolysaccharidosis I-A case report," *IP International Journal of Ocular Oncology and Oculoplasty*, vol. 4, no. 1, pp. 67–72, 2020.

A Solitary Choroidal Mass with Spontaneous Resolution

Fariba Ghassemi, Nazanin Ebrahimiadib, Hamid Riazi-Esfahani, Hassan Khojasteh, Zahra Mahdizad, and Elias Khalili Pour

Translational Ophthalmology Research Center, Farabi Eye Hospital, Tehran University of Medical Sciences, Tehran, Iran

Correspondence should be addressed to Elias Khalili Pour; ekhalilipour@gmail.com

Academic Editor: Stephen G. Schwartz

Background. To report an atypical case of a transient choroidal mass lesion with spontaneous resolution. *Case Presentation.* A solitary choroidal mass with an overlying neurosensory retinal detachment was seen in an otherwise healthy 31-year-old female. General physical examinations and serum chemistry were unremarkable. The patient had spontaneous resolution two weeks after initial examination without treatment. *Conclusions.* Inflammatory choroidal masses may be self-limited, but complete diagnostic measures must always be performed in these patients to distinguish between important causes such as tuberculosis, sarcoidosis, and tumors.

1. Background

Choroidal masses have wide differential diagnoses, such as tuberculosis, sarcoidosis, inflammatory diseases, and tumors, and timely diagnosis and treatment of each of these diseases are very important. We report an atypical case of a transient choroidal mass lesion that is spontaneously resolved without any treatment.

2. Case Presentation

A 31-year-old woman was referred to the retina ward of Farabi eye hospital with a history of sudden decreased vision and metamorphopsia in OD for 3 days. On clinical examination, the best-corrected visual acuity was 20/40 and 20/20 in OD and OS, respectively; with +3.00 diopters of hyperopic refraction in OD and Plano refraction in OS. Funduscopy of the OS was normal and the OD was remarkable for a serous retinal detachment (SRD) and a 4 to 5-disc diameter submacular elevated mass with extension beyond the inferior arcade (Figure 1(a)). Anterior segment examination was normal in both eyes without inflammatory findings. No cells or flare in the vitreous cavity, signs of retinitis, or vasculitis were observed.

Spectral-domain optical coherence tomography (SD-OCT) confirmed a dome-shaped elevated choroidal mass with associated SRD (Figure 1(b)) OD. Enhanced depth OCT (EDI-OCT) of the OD demonstrated a homogenous hyporeflective elevated choroidal lesion, with compression of the choroidal vascular structures (Figure 1(c)). Ultrasonography confirmed a hyperechoic choroidal mass (Figure 1(d)). Early-phase fluorescein angiography (FA) showed pooling consistent with SRD and multiple hyperfluorescent dots over the mass with the persistence of these dots through late phases without disc leakage (Figure 1(e)). Indocyanine green angiography (ICGA) revealed diffuse and multiple foci of small, round, hypocyanescent dots in both early and late phases (Figure 1(f)).

A complete metastatic workup for detecting malignancy including genitourinary system evaluation (Pap smear, ultrasonography, and urine analysis), gastrointestinal system analysis (upper and lower endoscopy, liver function tests, and abdominopelvic computed tomography with contrast), breast examination, and consult with an internist was done, and all were negative for any malignancy. Other evaluations

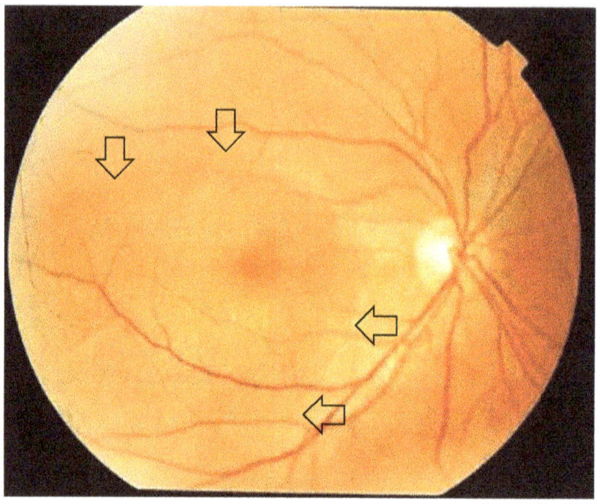

(a)

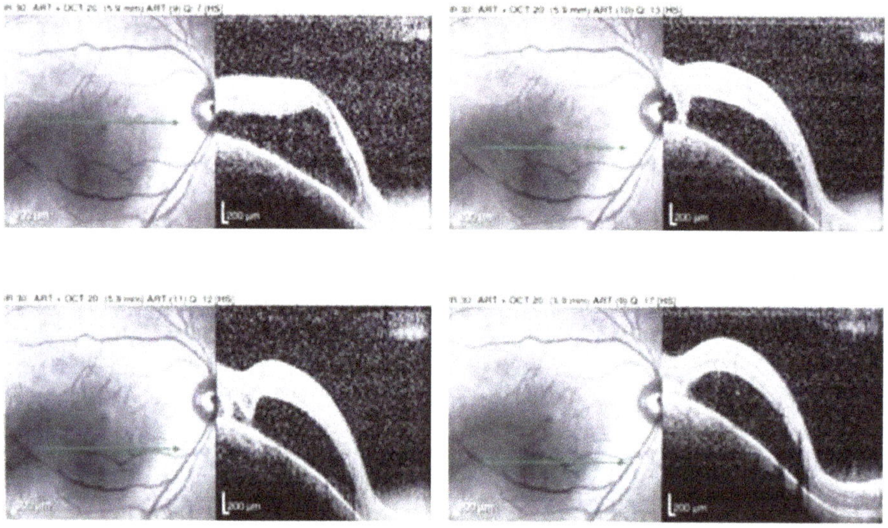

(b)

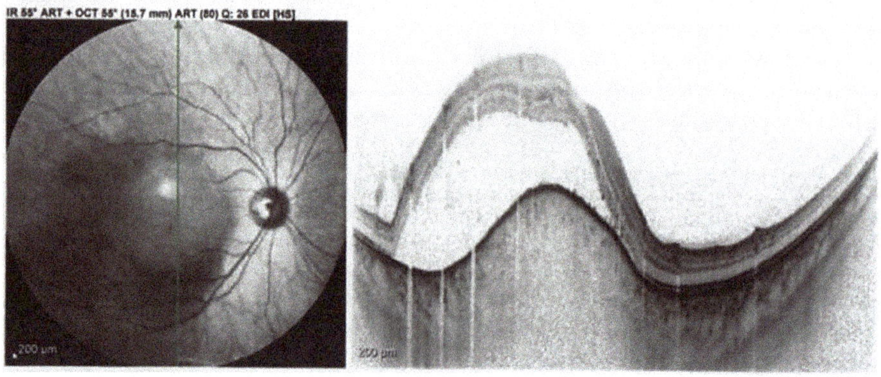

(c)

FIGURE 1: Continued.

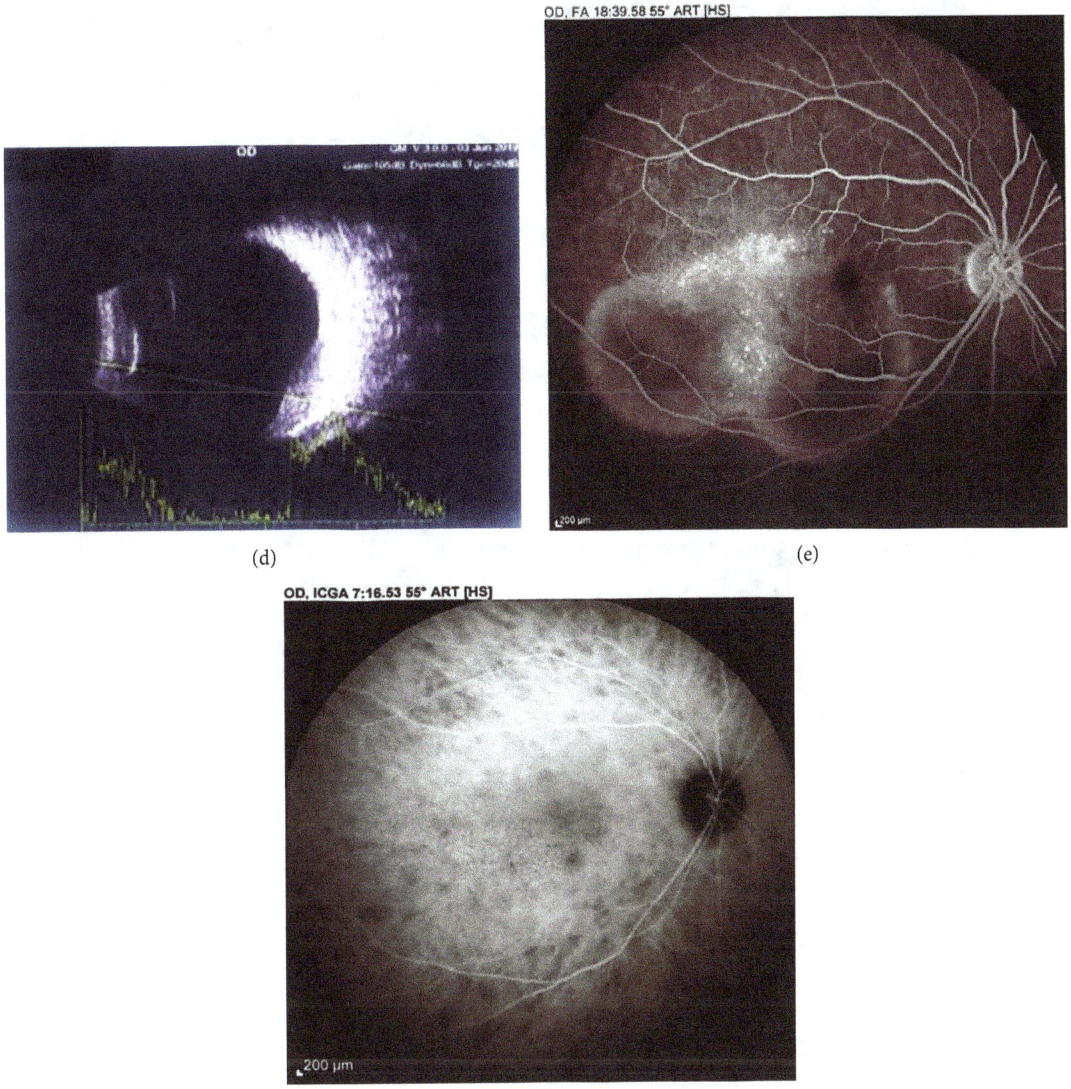

(d) (e) (f)

FIGURE 1: Initial examination of the right eye. Color fundus photo shows subretinal fluid (arrows) and elevated subretinal mass extending beyond the inferior arcade (a). Horizontal scans of optical coherence tomography (OCT) from the fovea to inferior vascular arcade shows subretinal fluid with a dome-shaped elevated choroidal mass in the macular area (b). Vertical scan of enhanced depth imaging optical coherence tomography shows a homogenous hyporeflective elevated lesion in the choroid (c). Ultrasonography shows a hyperechoic choroidal mass with medium to low internal reflectivity (d). Fluorescein angiography in the late phase shows the pooling of dye in the subretinal area and multiple hyperfluorescent dots over the lesion (e). Midphase indocyanine green angiography reveals multiple small, round, hypocyanescent dots in the posterior and midperipheral fundus (f).

including sarcoidosis (serum angiotensin-converting enzyme and calcium), tuberculosis (chest X-ray, QuantiFERON Gold, and purified protein derivative (PPD) skin test), syphilis (The Venereal Disease Research Laboratory test (VDRL) and rapid plasma reagin (RPR)), and lupus (Anti-nuclear antibodies (ANA), anti-double-stranded DNA antibody (anti-dsDNA)) were negative. Inflammatory markers (erythrocyte sedimentation rate and C-reactive protein) were within normal limits, and the chest X-ray showed no abnormalities. Two weeks after initial evaluation the patient showed spontaneous resolution with improvement in central vision (BCVA: 20/25) and metamorphopsia. Reevaluation was consistent with decreased SRD and choroidal mass volume. Interestingly, there was disruption of the ellipsoid zone (EZ) and multifocal accumulation of hyperreflective material not previously seen on initial OCT (Figures 2(a) and 2(b)). Ultrasonography confirmed the decrease in the size of choroidal mass (Figure 2(c)).

One month after initial presentation visual acuity returned to 20/20 without any refractive error or symptoms. OCT and ultrasonography showed nearly complete resolution choroidal mass effect, SRD, and EZ disruption (Figure 2(d)).

3. Discussion and Conclusion

The differential diagnosis of a solitary choroidal mass is broad, including inflammatory, neoplastic, and infectious

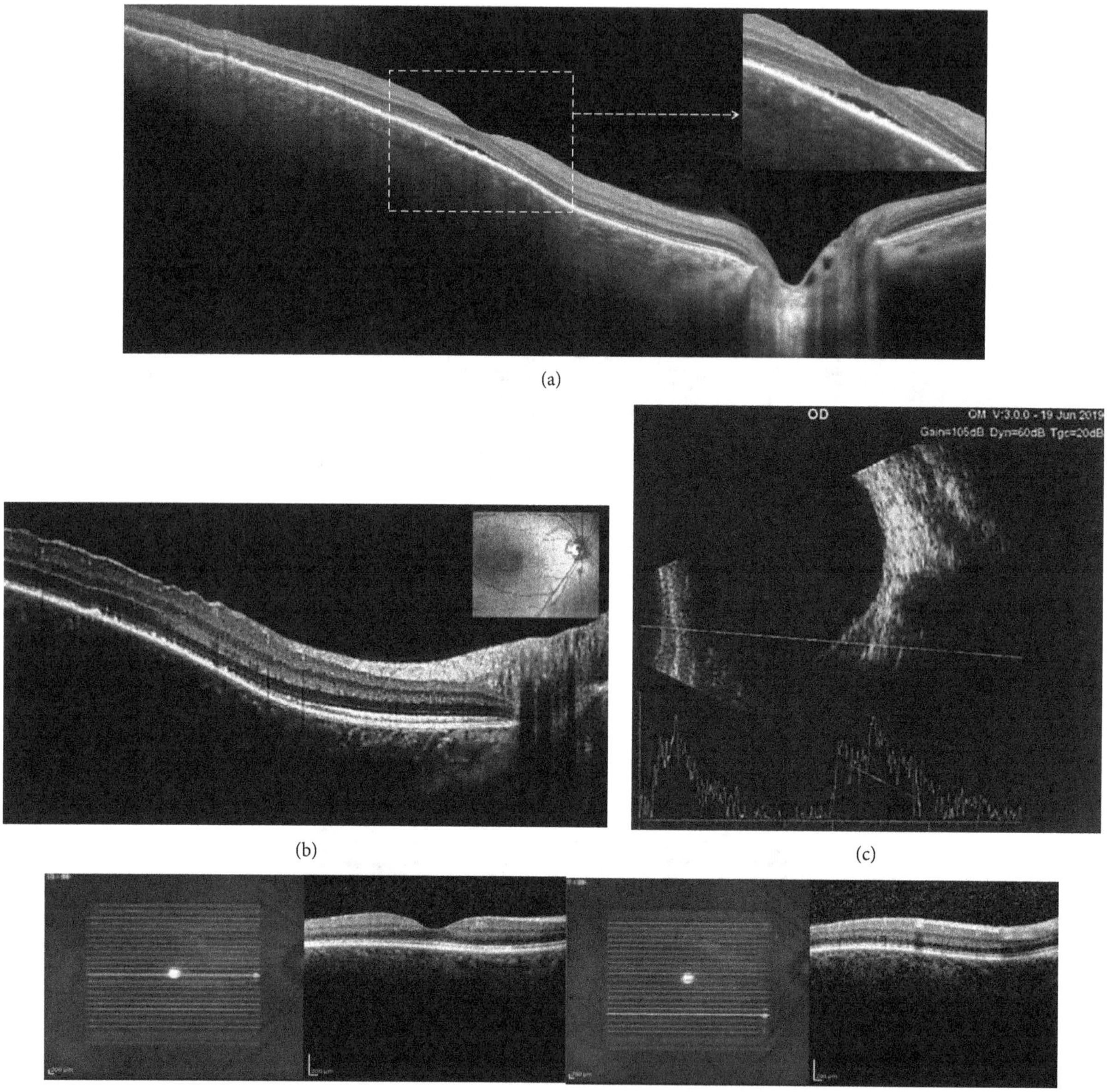

FIGURE 2: Follow-up examinations. Optical coherence tomography two weeks after initial presentation showed improvement of subretinal fluid, decreasing the size of the choroidal mass, disruption of the ellipsoid zone, and accumulations of hyperreflective material of variable size and shape under the fovea (a) and the corresponding retina over the choroidal mass (b). Ultrasonography two weeks after the initial presentation revealed decreasing the size of choroidal mass (c). OCT one month after initial presentation showed near-complete resolution of choroidal mass and SRF, EZ restoration, and disappearance of hyperreflective materials over RPE and outer retina.

diseases [1]. Multiple hypofluorescent spots on mid- and late-phase ICGA are indicative of an inflammatory process involving the choroid, such as Vogt-Koyanagi-Harada disease, acute multifocal posterior placoid pigment epitheliopathy (APMPPE), multifocal choroiditis, posterior scleritis, lupus choroidopathy, syphilis, tuberculosis, and sarcoidosis.

Sarcoidosis can affect the eyes in up to 79% of patients with systemic disease, but ocular involvement as a presenting symptom occurs in less than 30% of cases [2]. Although granulomatous or nongranulomatous uveitis is the most common finding, choroidal involvement is a rare manifestation in the absence of anterior uveitis (approximately 5% of patients), and a unifocal lesion is very rare [2, 3].

Kawasaki et al. reported a case presented with a mass resembling ocular metastases in association with Bartonella Hensle that despite treatment ended up with low visual acuity [4]. Our patient had a full recovery and did not show macular star or disc swelling and did not have any history of cat exposure, so that is so unlikely to have Bartonella.

History and laboratory workup, as well as the course of the disease, were not compatible with another diagnosis such as tuberculosis, syphilis, lupus, APMPPE, and multifocal choroiditis.

Even rare, nodular posterior scleritis has been reported [5] and can be considered as another possible diagnosis. Although sudden onset, loss of vision, SRD [5], and findings in FA (a localized starry sky appearance) and ICGA (hypofluorescent dark dots present up to the intermediate phase of angiography) [6] are compatible with the diagnosis but contrary to our case, majority of posterior scleritis patients present with ocular pain (78%) and edema in Tenon space ("T" sign in ultrasonography), and only 13% of patients exhibit subretinal localized granuloma [7–9]. To our knowledge, there is no report of spontaneous resolution of nodular posterior scleritis without any treatment.

MEWDS was first described in 1984 as a transient chorioretinal disease of obscure etiology and regularly influences healthy young ladies. The most prominent feature of the disease is the presence of numerous, tiny yellow-white spots that resolve spontaneously within a few weeks [10, 11].

Full recovery of BCVA and transient course in our case excluded malignancy and narrowed the differential to infectious diseases such as tuberculosis and bartonellosis and inflammatory etiologies such as sarcoidosis, posterior scleritis, and atypical forms of multiple evanescent white dot syndrome (MEWDS). Our patient's fundus examination in the initial presentation did not show the classic white dots of MEWDS. Presumably, the presence of a large amount of SRD could obscure this perception [12–14]. Considering hypofluorescent spots in ICGA, the disruption of the EZ and the accumulation of hyperreflective material in the outer retina may characterize an atypical subtype of MEWDS not previously described.

Shields et al. have previously described 60 patients with an idiopathic inflammatory condition characterized by a solitary choroidal mass without a specific cause and named this condition solitary idiopathic choroiditis (SIC). They made the diagnosis clinically and described the course of disease in two stages: active and inactive. Fifty percent of subjects showed late-phase hypocyanescence over the choroidal lesion. Our case was similar to a typical active SIC, but the case did not show the complete inactive stage characteristics, including discrete, nummular, yellow-white lesion without SRD [15].

In conclusion, inflammatory choroidal masses may undergo spontaneous resolution. A complete diagnostic workup should be performed in these patients to differentiate them from other etiologies.

Acknowledgments

This study is funded by the Translational Ophthalmology Research Center, Farabi eye hospital, Tehran University of Medical Sciences (TUMS). This submission has not been published anywhere previously and that it is not simultaneously being considered for any other publication.

References

[1] N. Arej, A. Fadlallah, and E. Chelala, "Choroidal tuberculoma as a presenting sign of tuberculosis," *International Medical Case Reports Journal*, vol. Volume 9, pp. 365–368, 2016.

[2] J. E. Thorne and A. J. Brucker, "Choroidal white lesions as an early manifestation of sarcoidosis," *Retina*, vol. 20, no. 1, pp. 8–14, 2000.

[3] E. B. Turkoglu, S. E. Lally, and C. L. Shields, "CHOROIDAL SARCOID granuloma simulating prostate carcinoma metastasis," *Retinal Cases & Brief Reports*, vol. 11, pp. S226–S228, 2017.

[4] A. Kawasaki and D. L. Wilson, "Mass lesions of the posterior segment associated with Bartonella henselae," *British Journal of Ophthalmology*, vol. 87, no. 2, pp. 248-249, 2003.

[5] P. J. McCluskey, P. G. Watson, S. Lightman, J. Haybittle, M. Restori, and M. Branley, "Posterior scleritis," *Ophthalmology*, vol. 106, no. 12, pp. 2380–2386, 1999.

[6] C. Auer and C. P. Herbort, "Indocyanine green angiographic features in posterior scleritis," *American Journal of Ophthalmology*, vol. 126, no. 3, pp. 471–476, 1998.

[7] C. M. Calthorpe, P. G. Watson, and A. C. E. McCartney, "Posterior scleritis: a clinical and histological survey," *Eye*, vol. 2, no. 3, pp. 267–277, 1988.

[8] Z. Z. Dong, Y. F. Gan, Y. N. Zhang, Y. Zhang, J. Li, and H. H. Zheng, "The clinical features of posterior scleritis with serous retinal detachment: a retrospective clinical analysis," *International Journal of Ophthalmology*, vol. 12, no. 7, pp. 1151–1157, 2019.

[9] R. Agrawal, A. Lavric, M. Restori, C. Pavesio, and M. S. Sagoo, "Nodular posterior scleritis," *Retina*, vol. 36, no. 2, pp. 392–401, 2016.

[10] L. M. Jampol, P. A. Sieving, D. Pugh, G. A. Fishman, and H. Gilbert, "Multiple evanescent white dot syndrome: I Clinical Findings," *JAMA Ophthalmology*, vol. 102, no. 5, pp. 671–674, 1984.

[11] G. N. Papaliodis, "Multiple evanescent white dot syndrome," in *Uveitis: A Practical Guide to the Diagnosis and Treatment of Intraocular Inflammation*, G. N. Papaliodis, Ed., pp. 217-218, Springer International Publishing, Cham, 2017.

[12] H. N. Shelsta, R. R. Rao, H. K. Bhatt, and L. M. Jampol, "Atypical presentations of multiple evanescent white dot syndrome without white dots: a case series," *Retina*, vol. 31, no. 5, pp. 973–976, 2011.

[13] M. K. Shin, I. S. Byon, S. W. Park, and J. E. Lee, "Serous retinal detachment accompanied by MEWDS in a myopic patient with dome-shaped macula," *Ophthalmic Surgery, Lasers & Imaging Retina*, vol. 45, no. 3, pp. 253–255, 2014.

[14] D. L. Chao, M. Marsiglia, B. Ahmad et al., "Peripapillary serous detachment in multiple evanescent white dot syndrome," *Retina*, vol. 35, no. 3, pp. 521–524, 2015.

[15] J. A. Shields, C. L. Shields, H. Demirci, and S. Hanovar, "Solitary idiopathic Choroiditis," *Archives of Ophthalmology*, vol. 120, no. 3, pp. 311–319, 2002.

35

Peripapillary Pachychoroid Syndrome (PPS): Diagnosing and Treating a Rare Entity

Peggy Bouzika, Ilias Georgalas, Maria-Evanthia Sotirianakou, Aristotelis Karamaounas, Chrysanthos Symeonidis, Konstantinos Tyrlis, Stylianos Blounas, Ekaterini Mani, and Tryfon Rotsos

Retina Service, 1st Department of Ophthalmology, National and Kapodistrian University of Athens, General Hospital of Athens "G. Gennimatas", Athens, Greece

Correspondence should be addressed to Tryfon Rotsos; tryfonrotsos@hotmail.com

Academic Editor: Maurizio Battaglia Parodi

Two cases with peripapillary pachychoroid syndrome (PPS) along with the challenges concerning correct diagnosis and treatment are presented. In the first case, the patient presented with painless unilateral gradual visual loss. Fundoscopy and optical coherence tomography (OCT) revealed cystoid macular edema (CME) in the left eye (LE), extending from the temporal optic disc margin towards the fovea, with no additional findings. Enhanced-depth imaging- (EDI-) OCT provided additional information and increased choroidal thickness nasally to the macula and pachyvessels in the outer choroidal layer, findings supportive of PPS. Photodynamic therapy (PDT) was applied at the leakage sites. Two months later, CME and subretinal fluid (SRF) had resolved, and VA had significantly improved. In the second case, a patient presented with reduced vision and metamorphopsia bilaterally over the previous 5 days. Fundoscopy revealed CME in both eyes. OCT confirmed the presence of CME in the papillomacular area in the right eye; similarly, CME was recorded in the macula of the LE with SRF located subfoveally. EDI-OCT showed increased choroidal thickness in both eyes. Treatment was administered, originally with dorzolamide eye drops along with eplerenone tablets, and then dexamethasone eye drops that eventually led to significant anatomic and functional improvement. It is important for ophthalmologists to be able to recognize the unique clinical entity of PPS, as its resemblance to disorders with similar features may lead to misdiagnoses and unnecessary, or even incorrect, interventions.

1. Introduction

Peripapillary pachychoroid syndrome (PPS) is a relatively novel pathological entity within the pachychoroid disease spectrum (PDS). Although it shares common findings with central serous chorioretinopathy (CSC), it is considered a separate disease. It is characterized by pachychoroid features around the optic nerve head (ONH) and is associated with intraretinal and/or subretinal fluid in the nasal macula. Prominent choroidal pachyvessels, observed on indocyanine green angiography (ICGA), are accompanied by peripapillary retinal pigment epithelium (RPE) mottling and, occasionally, choroidal folds. ONH edema has also been observed in some patients [1].

The aim of this case series is to present 2 cases with PPS along with the challenges concerning correct diagnosis and treatment of this newly recognized disease.

2. Case 1

A 72-year-old white male presented with unilateral, painless, and gradual visual loss. Regarding his past ophthalmic history, the patient had been previously treated with intravitreal antivascular endothelial growth factor (anti-VEGF) injections for branch retinal vein occlusion. Specifically, he had received 5 aflibercept injections in his left eye. The patient saw no improvement in his vision, so he opted for another medical opinion.

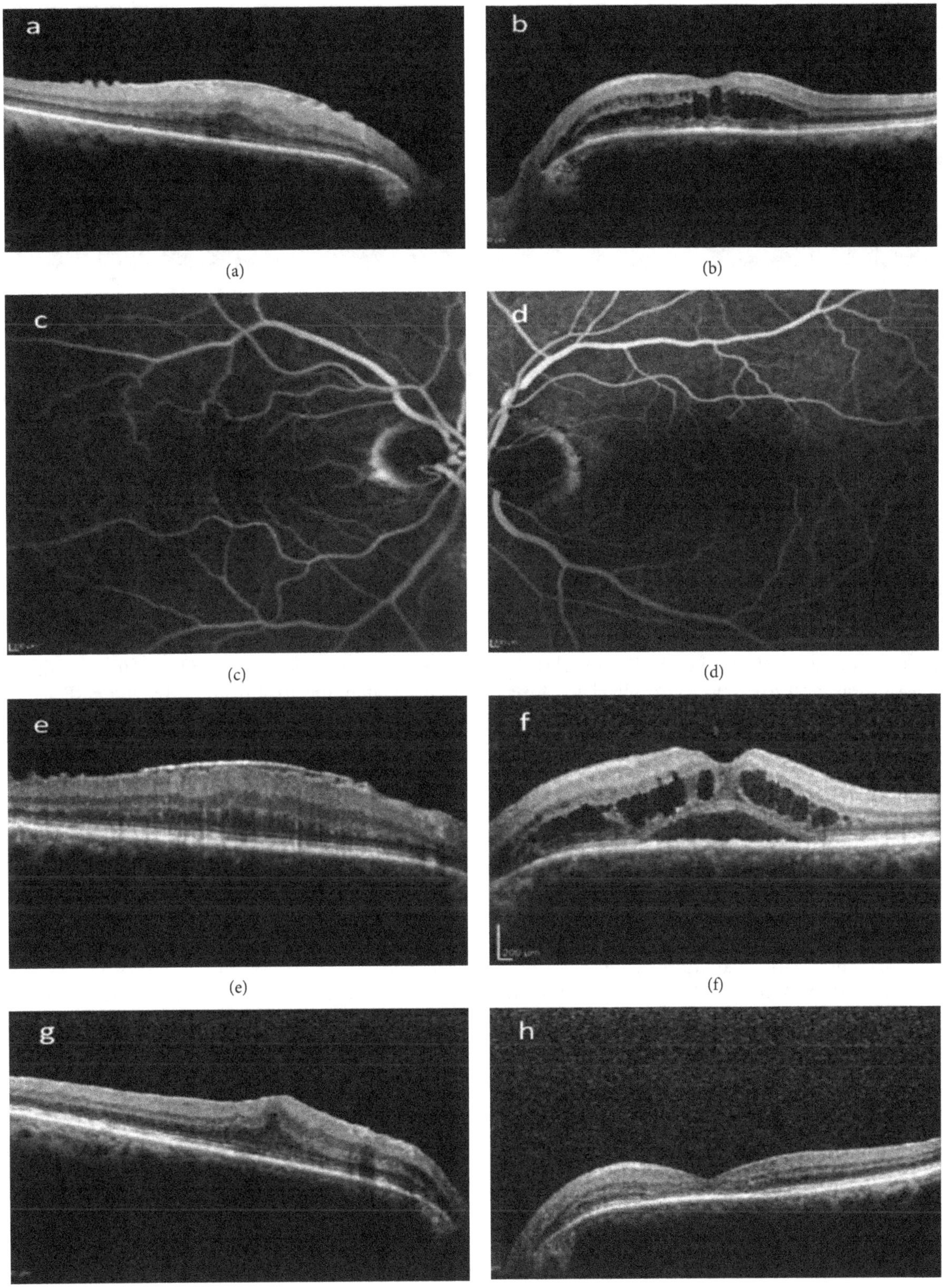

(a) (b) (c) (d) (e) (f) (g) (h)

FIGURE 1: Continued.

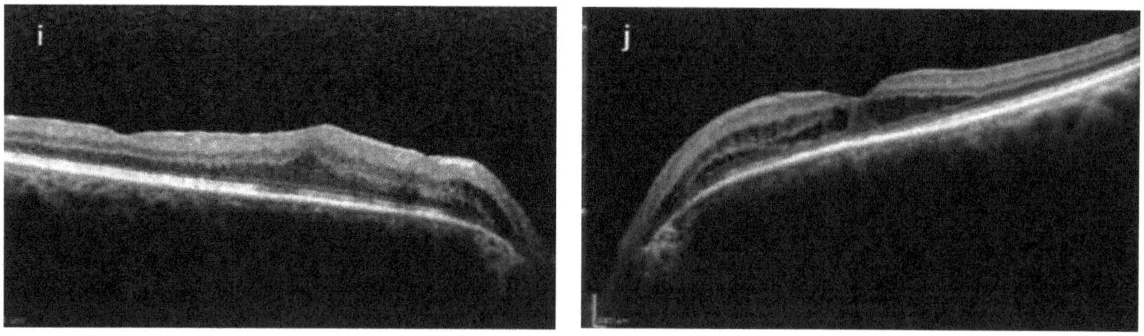

(i) (j)

Figure 1: OCT images at presentation showing ERM in the RE (a) and CME in the LE (b). FA of the RE (c) and LE (d) showed very mild hyperfluorescence in the fovea of the LE and mild late staining of the ONH, temporally, in both eyes. Three months later, the OCT of the RE remained unchanged (e), while in the LE there is additional SRF in the fovea (f). OCT images after ERM peeling in RE (g) and topical treatment with dexamethasone and nepafenac drops in the LE (h); the accumulations of SRF and IRF have almost completely resolved. OCTs six months later: the RE (i) is stable, while CME has reappeared in the LE (j).

At baseline, visual acuity (VA) was 20/50 in the right eye (RE) and 20/40 in the left eye (LE). Examination of the anterior segment showed mild cataract in the RE and was unremarkable in the LE. Fundoscopy and optical coherence tomography (OCT) of the macula (Heidelberg Spectralis HRA&OCT; Heidelberg Engineering, Heidelberg, Germany) revealed an epiretinal membrane (ERM) in the RE and cystoid macular edema (CME) in the LE (Figures 1(a) and 1(b)). The CME was localized between the ONH and fovea, extending from the temporal optic disc margin towards the fovea. Apart from a Salus-Gunn sign noted on the superior arcade close to the ONH, no additional findings, such as retinal hemorrhages, exudates, or cotton-wool spots, were observed in the LE. Fluorescein angiography (FA) was also performed; mild hyperfluorescence in the fovea of the LE during the late phase was observed (Figures 1(c) and 1(d)). The patient was placed on a course of dorzolamide eye drops bid in the LE.

Three months later, the CME in the LE still persisted, while subretinal fluid (SRF) had developed in the fovea (Figures 1(e) and 1(f)). A combination of dexamethasone qid and nepafenac 3 mg/ml bid eye drops was initiated in the LE. During the following months, the intraretinal and subretinal fluid started to gradually decrease leading to visual improvement. A small amount of intraretinal fluid (IRF) remained in the papillomacular area of the LE. The patient also underwent pars plana vitrectomy with ERM peeling in his RE with an aim to further improve his vision (Figures 1(g) and 1(h)).

After six months, the CME in the LE increased once again (Figures 1(i) and 1(j)). Systemic administration of acetazolamide tablets (250 mg qid) was added to the treatment. Two months later, SRF redeveloped in the fovea of the LE, leading to a severe VA decrease (counting fingers). Although FA did not reveal significant findings, ICGA showed increased hyperfluorescence due to choroidal hyperpermeability in 4 distinct foci in the posterior pole of the LE, located in the superior and inferior arcades close to the ONH (Figures 2(a)–2(d)). Enhanced-depth imaging- (EDI-) OCT provided additional information, i.e., increased choroidal thickness nasally to the macula and pachyvessels in the outer choroidal layer of the posterior pole, findings supportive of PPS (Figures 2(e) and 2(f)). Photodynamic therapy (PDT) was applied at the leakage sites; intravenous verteporfin (Visudyne, Novartis AG, Basel, Switzerland) was administered over a period of 10 minutes, and treatment was applied 15 minutes after the beginning of the infusion. The light energy used was 25 J/cm^2 for half-fluence. Two months after the treatment, CME and SRF had resolved (Figures 2(g) and 2(h)) and VA had significantly improved (20/32). Six months later, CME was once more observed in the LE (Figure 2(i)). Dexamethasone eye drops qid were initiated and resulted in almost complete IRF resorption (Figure 2(j)).

3. Case 2

A 70-year-old man presented with bilaterally reduced vision and metamorphopsia over the previous 5 days. The patient also suffered from systemic hypertension and coronary artery disease. He was under treatment with methylprednisolone per os, 32 mg per day over the previous 2 weeks, prescribed by his general practitioner for persistent cough.

VA was 20/63 in the RE and 20/40 in the LE. Ophthalmic examination showed normal intraocular pressure and mild cataract in both eyes. Fundoscopy revealed CME in the posterior pole of both eyes. OCT (Heidelberg Spectralis HRA&OCT; Heidelberg Engineering, Heidelberg, Germany) confirmed the presence of CME in the papillomacular area in the RE; similarly, CME was recorded in the macula of the LE with a small amount of SRF located subfoveally (Figures 3(a) and 3(b)). FA showed 3 small hyperfluorescent areas perifoveally in the RE, and 1 hyperfluorescent area adjacent to the ONH in the LE due to window defects (Figures 3(c)–3(f)). A diagnosis of CSC was hypothesized, and the patient was prescribed dorzolamide eye drops tid and acetazolamide tablets 250 mg bid.

On his follow-up examination 10 days later, there was anatomic deterioration observed in his RE with the appearance of SRF subfoveally; the LE showed a slight

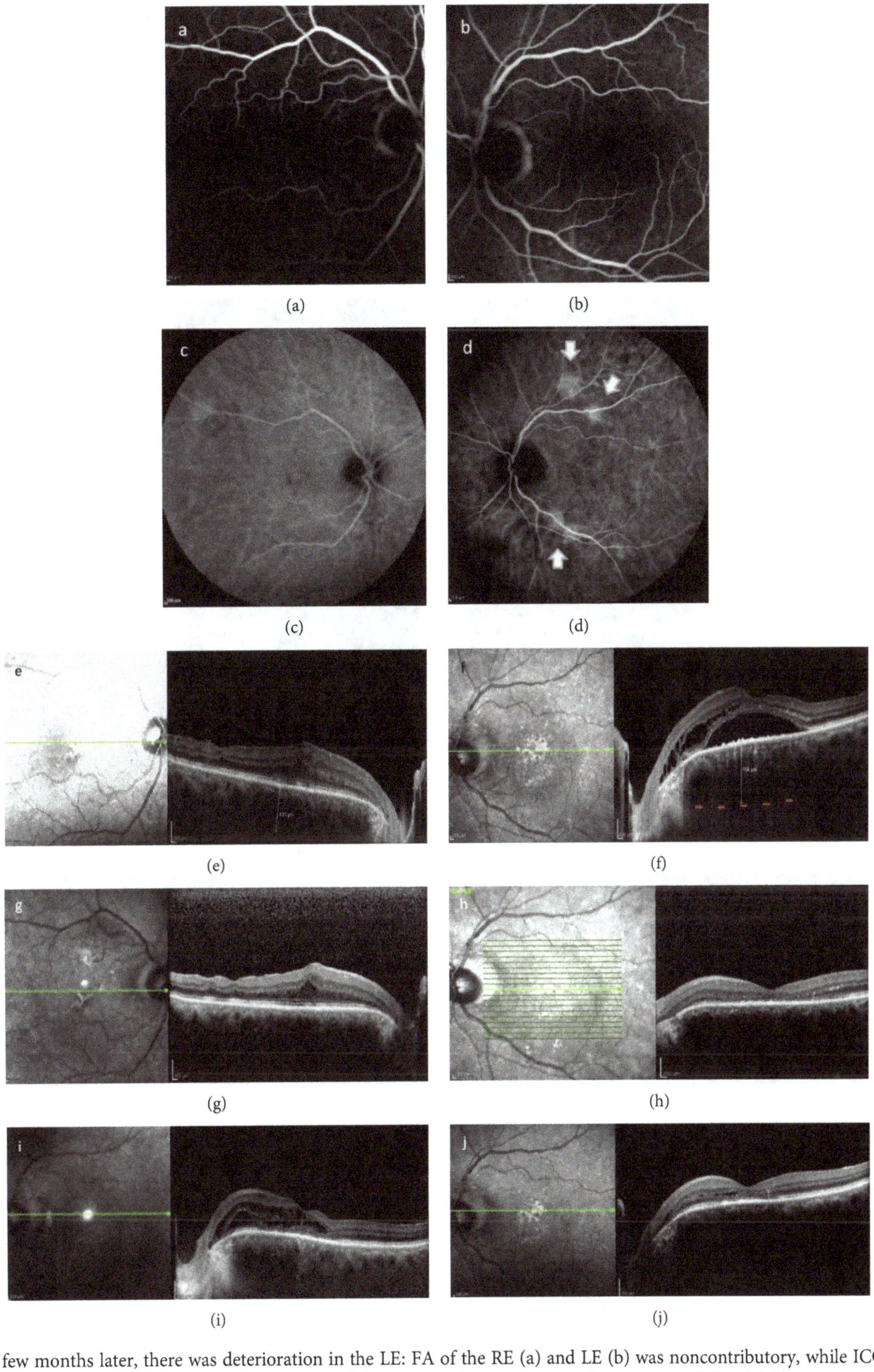

FIGURE 2: A few months later, there was deterioration in the LE: FA of the RE (a) and LE (b) was noncontributory, while ICGA (c and d) showed hyperfluorescence in 4 foci during the late phase of the exam in the LE corresponding to areas of choroidal hyperpermeability (white arrows, (d)). EDI-OCT revealed increased choroidal thickness [max thickness: 431 μm in the RE (e) and 554 μm in the LE (f)], with pachyvessels (LE > RE) located mostly nasally to the fovea and IRF/SRF accumulation in the fovea of the LE (f). OCT images of RE (g) and LE (h) after PDT treatment in LE, showing resolution of CME and SRF in LE. CME observed in the LE 6 months later (i), and fluid absorption after treatment with dexamethasone drops in the LE (j).

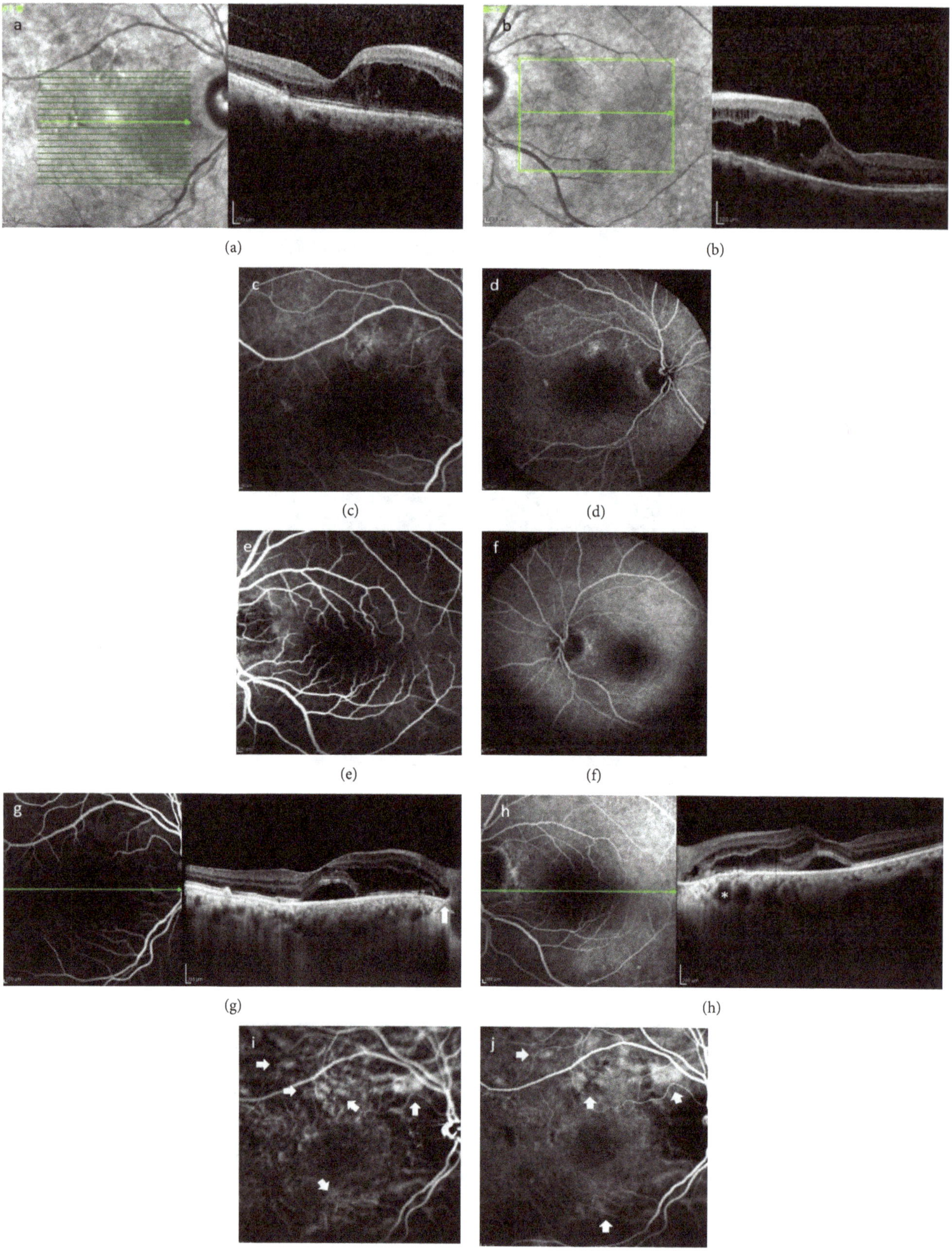

Figure 3: Continued.

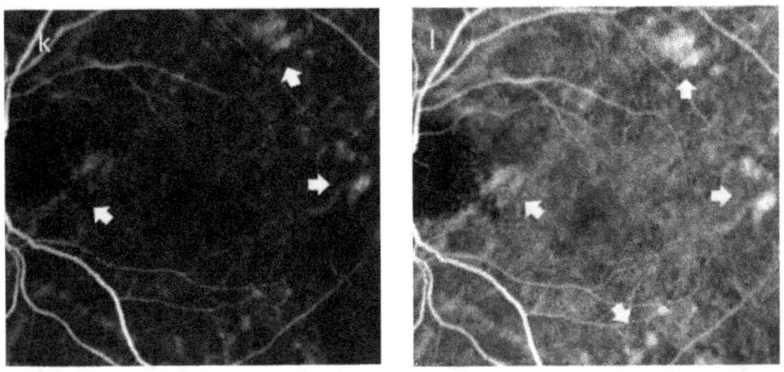

(k) (l)

Figure 3: OCT images of RE (a) and LE (b) with CME in the papillomacular area of both eyes and SRF in the LE. FA pictures of RE (c and d) and LE (e and f) showing several small window defects causing hyperfluorescence. Ten days later, the EDI-OCT performed (g and h) showed increased choroidal thickness and pachyvessels (asterisk, (h)) in both eyes (LE > RE) with additional SRF subfoveally in the RE (g); the IRF in the LE was slightly reduced, while SRF persisted (h). PFP was present temporally to the optic disc margin in the RE (white arrow, (g)). ICGA revealed pachyvessels (white arrows), especially superiorly to the ONH in the RE (i and j) and adjacent to the optic disc inferiorly in the LE (k and l), corresponding to hyperfluorescent areas of choroidal hyperpermeability noted during the mid-phase.

improvement, with a small reduction in the amount of IRF present. EDI-OCT showed increased choroidal thickness in both eyes; additionally, there were choroidal pachyvessels adjacent to the temporal edge of the ONH in the LE (Figures 3(g) and 3(h)). ICGA was also performed and demonstrated dilated choroidal vessels, with hyperfluorescent areas in the posterior pole of both eyes, indicative of choroidal hyperpermeability (Figures 3(i)–3(l)). These choroidal alterations led to a new diagnosis of PPS. Topical treatment (dorzolamide drops) remained unaltered with a switch of acetazolamide tablets to eplerenone tablets 25 mg bid.

During the following 3 months, VA improved significantly (20/25 bilaterally); the SRF had regressed in both eyes, and only a small amount of IRF remained temporally to the optic disc (Figures 4(a) and 4(b)). One month later, deterioration was observed with a limited quantity of SRF in the RE and an increased quantity of IRF temporally of the optic disc in the LE (Figures 4(c) and 4(d)). The patient was treated with dexamethasone eye drops qid. After a month, OCT scans showed complete fluid absorption in the RE and only a small amount of IRF in the LE (Figures 4(e) and 4(f)). During the following two months, dexamethasone drops were gradually tapered and VA remained stable at 20/25 bilaterally.

4. Discussion

This case series highlights the difficulties in diagnosing PPS as well as the variability in both the course of the disease and its response to different treatment modalities. PPS was first described by Phasukkijwatana et al. [2] in 2017 as a distinct pathology within the PDS. Currently, the PDS includes pathologies, such as CSC, polypoidal choroidal vasculopathy, and PPS, conditions which seem to overlap to some extent. The basic features of these choroidopathies are a focal or diffuse increase in choroidal thickness, the presence of choroidal pachyvessels, i.e., dilated choroidal vessels in Haller's layer which lead to attenuation of the inner choroid, and choroidal vascular hyperpermeability. It is important to note that it is not the mere augmentation in choroidal thickness that appears to contribute to the pathogenesis of PDS but rather the increased diameter of the larger choroidal vessels, which may account for the full extent of the choroidal thickness increase [3].

PPS can be differentiated from other disease entities within the PDS due to the presence of pachychoroid features notably in the peripapillary area. Studies in normal eyes have shown that there is a regional variation of choroidal thickness, with the thickest region beneath the fovea and the thinnest nasally [4]. In PPS, the thickest choroidal region is located nasally to the fovea. The IRF and/or SRF that subsequently develop also appear to be extending from the temporal edge of the optic disc towards the macular center. All these findings were present in both cases presented here. In a study by Xu at al [5], data from 35 patients with PPS was used in order to elucidate the peripapillary preference of IRF accumulation in PPS. Specifically, it was noted that, while increased choroidal hydrostatic pressure contributes to diseases, such as CSC, the absence of RPE around the ONH along with the unique peripapillary arteriolar anastomosis present in that area may facilitate the transmission of pressure directly to the inner retina in the peripapillary region, hence facilitating the peripapillary location of PPS.

PPS has also been shown to occur bilaterally and more frequently in hyperopic patients, with crowded optic discs [3]. None of our patients had the latter characteristics, though our second patient did present with PPS findings in both eyes. OCT of the RE revealed a small cystoid space immediately temporal to the optic disc margin, which appears to be a distinct accumulation from the diffuse IRF or SRF present. This "peripapillary fluid pocket" (PFP) has been previously described and is thought to represent a possible entry site of fluid from the choroid to the retina and a biomarker of PPS [5].

Other ocular pathologies causing SRF accumulation, with or without ONH edema, are occasionally considered in the differential diagnosis of PPS; uveal effusion syndrome is strongly associated with nanophthalmic eyes and scleral, rather than choroidal, thickening. Posterior scleritis is a painful entity which causes exudative retinal detachment and

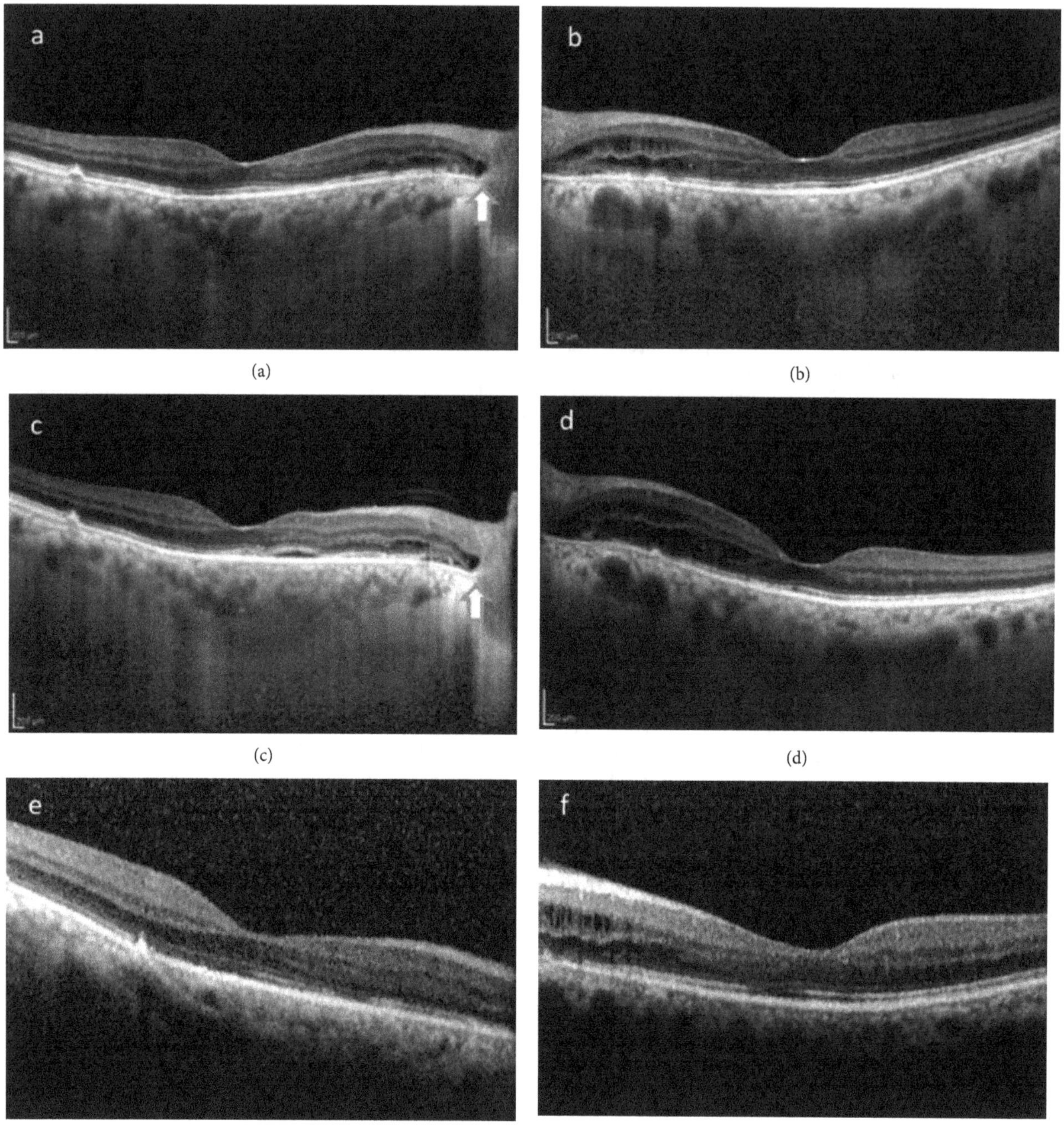

FIGURE 4: ECI-OCT 3 months after topical and systemic treatment with CAIs and diclofenac drops showed resorption of SRF in both eyes (a and b) with some IRF remaining temporally to the optic disc (LE > RE). A relapse was noted one month later: EDI-OCT showed a small amount of SRF in RE (c) and deterioration with the presence of IRF in the LE (d). OCT after treatment with dexamethasone eye drops: the RE is completely dry (e), and a small amount of IRF remains temporally to the ONH in the LE (f). The arrow denotes the PFP persisting in the RE.

choroidal folds, whereas optic disc pit maculopathy may lead to papillomacular detachment, even though the exact source of fluid is still debatable. Our patient had none of the characteristic features of the aforementioned clinical entities.

Currently, there is no established treatment for PPS. Several therapeutic modalities have been tested in the past, such as topical and/or systemic carbonic anhydrase inhibitors (CAIs), intravitreal anti-VEGF injections, and PDT, with variable outcomes [2, 5–7]. In some cases, there was no immediate response to treatment with most patients showing anatomical improvement with VA stabilization. A recent study by Iovino et al. [8] supports the use of PDT for PPS since in their cohort, best-corrected VA significantly improved from baseline to month 3. On the other hand, in a recent PPS case report, it is emphasized that CME in PPS may show significant fluctuations and sometimes observation should be the initial approach especially if vision is not considerably affected [9].

Vision was significantly affected in both our patients, hence rendering observation inadequate as a management option. The least invasive approach was selected with the administration of CAIs topically and systemically; these agents have long been used for the management of CME as they can increase fluid absorption across the RPE [10]. Similarly, eplerenone, a mineralocorticoid receptor antagonist, was used in the second patient, to suppress the effect of increased choroidal thickness and congestion caused by stimulation of such receptors in the choroid [11]. Results were not as favorable as expected, and PDT was employed in order to reduce choroidal hyperperfusion. After PDT, VA in our first patient improved considerably.

The beneficial effect of topical prednisolone on the peripapillary IRF in PPS was recently described by Pothof et al. [12]. In this paper, authors hypothesize that choroidal hyperpermeability resulting in PPS might be secondary to an underlying inflammatory process, hence the positive effect of steroids. Both patients presented here received topical dexamethasone, and both demonstrated a great improvement regarding IRF absorption. This topical treatment may need to be applied over extended periods of time or combined with other therapeutic modalities such as PDT in order to bring about long-lasting results and facilitate the prevention of relapses. In any case, topical steroids, either dexamethasone or prednisolone, may be a simple yet viable treatment for PPS, especially when other options, such as PDT, are unavailable.

5. Conclusions

It is important for ophthalmologists to be able to recognize PPS as it constitutes a challenging diagnosis and a unique clinical entity. Its resemblance to disorders with similar features may lead to misdiagnoses and unnecessary, or even incorrect, interventions. Further studies, with a greater number of patients and longer follow-up periods, are warranted for an effective management of PPS.

Consent

The patient in the study has given consent for the clinical study to be published.

Disclosure

This paper was presented as a virtual abstract in the 2021 Euretina Congress (https://www.karger.com/Article/Pdf/519205).

References

[1] V. Castro-Navarro, F. Behar-Cohen, W. Chang et al., "Pachychoroid: current concepts on clinical features and pathogenesis," *Graefe's Archive for Clinical and Experimental Ophthalmology*, vol. 259, no. 6, pp. 1385–1400, 2021.

[2] N. Phasukkijwatana, K. B. Freund, R. Dolz-Marco et al., "Peripapillary pachychoroid syndrome," *Retina*, vol. 38, no. 9, pp. 1652–1667, 2018.

[3] C. M. G. Cheung, W. K. Lee, H. Koizumi, K. Dansingani, T. Y. Y. Lai, and K. B. Freund, "Pachychoroid disease," *Eye*, vol. 33, no. 1, pp. 14–33, 2019.

[4] R. Margolis and R. F. Spaide, "A pilot study of enhanced depth imaging optical coherence tomography of the choroid in normal eyes," *American Journal of Ophthalmology*, vol. 147, no. 5, pp. 811–815, 2009.

[5] D. Xu, E. Garg, K. Lee et al., "Long-term visual and anatomic outcomes of patients with peripapillary pachychoroid syndrome," *British Journal of Ophthalmology*, vol. 106, no. 4, pp. 576–581, 2020.

[6] B. Alonso-Martín, B. de-Lucas-Viejo, M. Gimeno-Carrero, M. Ferro-Osuna, and J. Sambricio, "Diagnostico mediante imagen multimodal en sindrome paquicoroideo peripapilar: a proposito de un caso," *Archivos de la Sociedad Española de Oftalmología (English Edition)*, vol. 95, no. 5, pp. 248–253, 2020.

[7] P. Sen, J. Sreenivasan, and P. Maitra, "A case of peripapillary pachychoroid syndrome treated with anti-vascular endothelial growth factor injections," *Indian Journal of Ophthalmology - Case Reports*, vol. 1, no. 2, pp. 346–348, 2021.

[8] C. Iovino, E. Peiretti, F. Tatti et al., "Photodynamic therapy as a treatment option for peripapillary pachychoroid syndrome: a pilot study," *Eye*, vol. 36, no. 4, pp. 716–723, 2022.

[9] S. Hubschman, K. Hou, D. Sarraf, and I. Tsui, "An unusual presentation of peripapillary pachychoroid syndrome," *American Journal of Ophthalmology Case Reports*, vol. 25, article 101338, 2022.

[10] T. J. Wolfensberger, "The role of carbonic anhydrase inhibitors in the management of macular edema," *Documenta Ophthalmologica*, vol. 97, no. 3/4, pp. 387–397, 1999.

[11] M. Zhao, I. Célérier, E. Bousquet et al., "Mineralocorticoid receptor is involved in rat and human ocular chorioretinopathy," *The Journal of Clinical Investigation*, vol. 122, no. 7, pp. 2672–2679, 2012.

[12] A. B. Pothof, P. Fernández-Avellaneda, F. Behar-Cohen, J. P. Martinez Ciriano, and S. Yzer, "Potential treatment for peripapillary pachychoroid syndrome," *Retinal Cases and Brief Reports*, vol. Publish Ahead of Print, 2021.

36

A Case of Terson-Like Syndrome in a Patient with Viral Meningoencephalitis

Masumi G. Asahi,[1] Stephanie J. Weiss,[2,3] Krishi Peddada,[2] and Deepika Malik[2,4,5]

[1] *Western University of Health Sciences, 309 E 2nd St., Pomona, CA 91766, USA*
[2] *Drexel University College of Medicine, 219 N. Broad St., 3rd Floor, Philadelphia, PA 19107, USA*
[3] *Weill Cornell Medical College, 1305 York Ave., New York, NY 10021, USA*
[4] *Moore Eye Institute, 100 W Sproul Rd., Springfield, PA 19064, USA*
[5] *Philadelphia College of Osteopathic Medicine, 4170 City Ave., Philadelphia, PA 19131, USA*

Correspondence should be addressed to Deepika Malik; deepika_malik@yahoo.com

Academic Editor: Kevin J. Blinder

The proposed mechanism of Terson's syndrome is increased intracranial pressure that leads to dilation of the retrobulbar optic nerve and compression of the central retinal vein. Terson's syndrome has been associated with many conditions that increase intracranial pressure such as venous sinus thrombosis, Moyamoya disease, leukemia, direct head trauma, and intraocular hemorrhage related to shaken baby syndrome. We present a novel case of a patient with recent viral prodrome found to have papilledema and multilayered retinal hemorrhages consistent with Terson syndrome. Computed tomography and magnetic resonance venography of the brain did not reveal any subdural, subarachnoid, or intracranial hemorrhages. However, cerebrospinal fluid analyses were significant for increased opening pressure and elevated protein levels, which were suggestive of viral meningoencephalitis. We describe this case as a Terson-like syndrome because the etiology of intraocular hemorrhage is increased intracranial pressure. However, this case does not fit the traditional presentation of Terson's syndrome as the intracranial pressure is secondary to meningeal inflammation instead of subdural, subarachnoid, or intracranial hemorrhage. We strongly feel that it is important for physicians to be aware of the link between viral meningoencephalitis and retinal conditions such as Terson-like syndrome because it can facilitate rapid diagnosis and treatment.

1. Introduction

In 1881, German ophthalmologist Moritz Litten described vitreous bleeding occurring with subarachnoid hemorrhage, a condition that later became named Terson's syndrome. The cause was presumed to be subarachnoid blood being transmitted directly forward through the optic nerve sheath [1]. More recently, Terson's syndrome has been understood in the context of increased intracranial pressure resulting from any number of conditions that cause subdural, subarachnoid, or intracranial hemorrhage. Some of the conditions associated with Terson's syndrome include venous sinus thrombosis, Moyamoya disease, leukemia, direct head trauma, and intraocular hemorrhage related to shaken baby syndrome [2–6]. In Terson's syndrome, increased intracranial pressure causes rapid effusion of cerebrospinal fluid into the optic nerve sheath [1, 7], which in turn results in dilation of the retrobulbar optic nerve and subsequent compression of the central retinal veins [1, 7]. The venous obstruction causes venous stasis, venous hypertension, and distension, ultimately resulting in rupture of thin retinal vessels and subsequent hemorrhage [1, 2, 7].

Viruses can cause central nervous system (CNS) infections and contribute significantly to the disease burden in humans globally [8]. While most viral CNS infections are benign and self-limiting, some can cause severe inflammation and result in severe long-term neurologic dysfunction [8]. Viral meningoencephalitis is typically associated with fever, headache, photophobia, and neck stiffness whereas viral encephalitis is associated with fever, seizures, focal neurologic deficits, and decreased consciousness [9]. Thus far, the only reported ocular complications linked to viral meningoencephalitis include sixth nerve palsy, optic neuritis, and papilledema [10–12]. We describe a case of viral

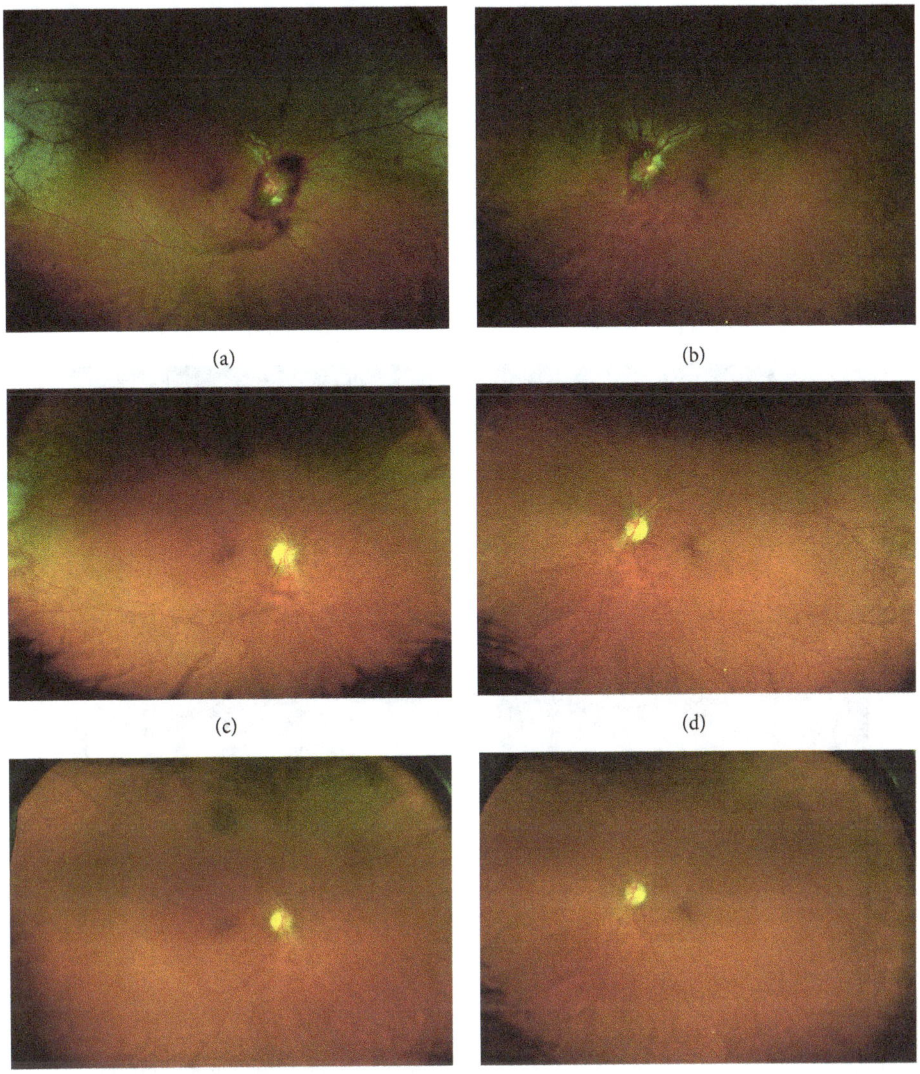

(a) (b) (c) (d) (e) (f)

FIGURE 1: Optos Fundus Photos showing (a) right eye and (b) left eye at presentation showing preretinal hemorrhages, flame hemorrhages, and intraretinal blot hemorrhages with optic disc edema consistent with Terson syndrome. (c, e) Right eye and (d, f) left eye showing disc pallor consistent with optic atrophy and resolving hemorrhages with persistent inferior preretinal hemorrhages inferior to the disc at (c, d) 3-month follow-up and at (e, f) 4-month follow-up.

meningoencephalitis with multilayered retinal hemorrhages suggestive of a Terson-like syndrome.

2. Case Presentation

A 50-year-old African American female presented with a three-week history of intractable headache, confusion, vertical binocular diplopia, photophobia, and difficulty with balance. Examination revealed best corrected visual acuities of 20/25 in the right eye (OD) and 20/20 in the left eye (OS) with intraocular pressures (IOP) of 14 mmHg in both eyes (OU). No afferent pupillary defect was noted, extraocular motility (EOM) was full OU, and confrontational visual fields were full OU. Anterior segment examination in both eyes was unremarkable. Funduscopic examination of both eyes revealed grade-four optic disc edema, blurring of optic disc margin, and obscuration of vasculature of the optic nerve. Preretinal and intraretinal hemorrhages were present in both eyes, largely concentrated in the peripapillary retina, but extending to the mid-peripheral retina (Figures 1(a) and 1(b)). Optic nerve swelling was confirmed on optical coherence tomography (OCT) of the retinal nerve fiber layer (Figures 2(a) and 2(b)). Fluorescein angiography revealed hyperfluorescence of the optic disc OU (Figures 3(a) and 3(b)).

Computed tomography of the head, magnetic resonance imaging of the brain, and magnetic resonance venography of the brain were unremarkable and had no evidence of intracranial mass, hemorrhage, or ischemia. Cerebrospinal fluid (CSF) analysis revealed an opening pressure of 30 cm H_2O, 77 white blood cells/mm^3 with 94% lymphocytes, 93 mg/dL protein, and 73 mg/dL glucose. Bacterial and fungal cultures of the CSF were negative. CSF studies for Lyme, syphilis, herpes simplex virus, and West Nile virus were unremarkable. A limited panel consisting of laboratory studies

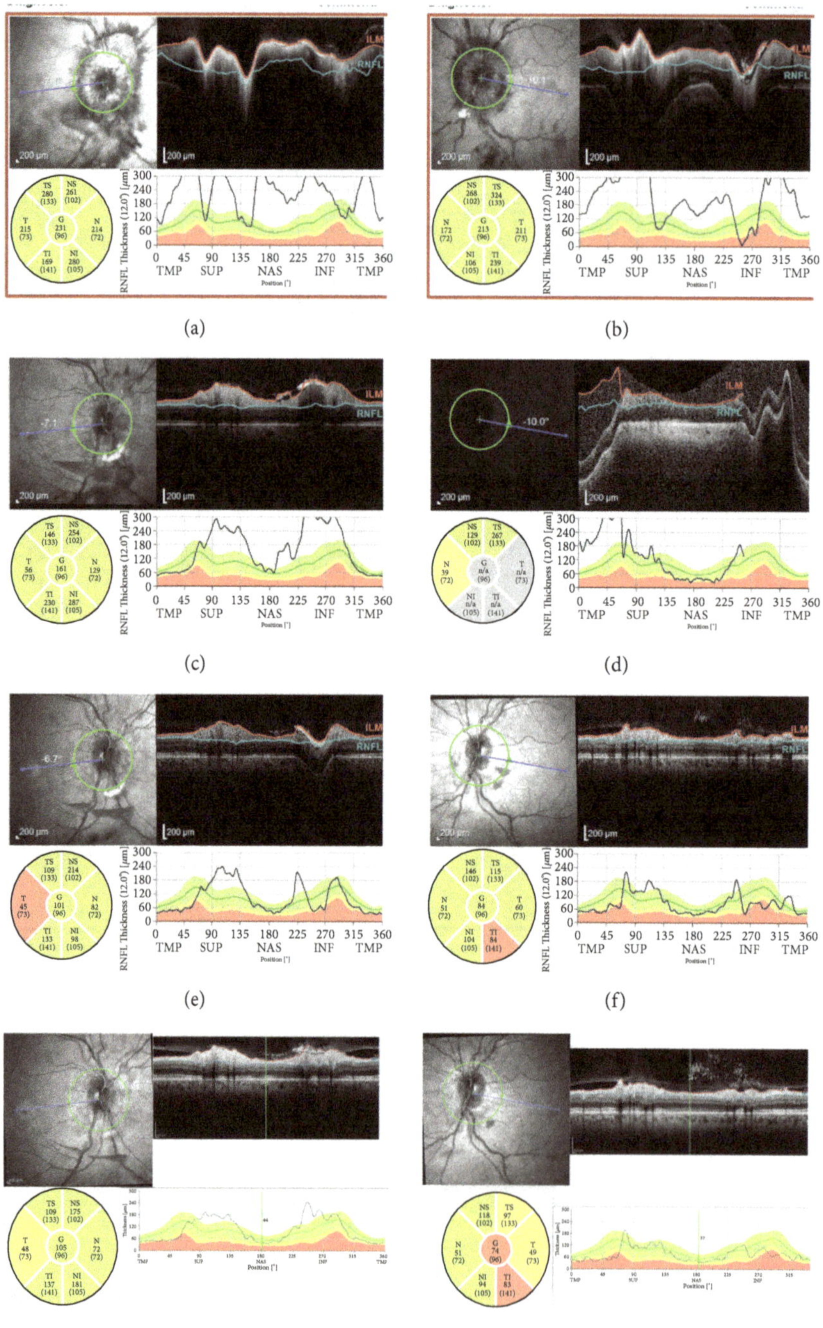

(a) (b) (c) (d) (e) (f) (g) (h)

Figure 2: Retina Nerve Fiber Layer (RNFL) Optical Coherence tomography (OCT) of the (a, c, e, g) right eye and (b, d, f, h) left eye showing (a, b) disc edema at presentation, (c, d) improving disc edema at six-week follow-up, and (e, f) near resolution of disc edema at twelve weeks and (g, h) sixteen weeks. Sectoral thickness measured in microns, and thickness of cross-section in temporal (TMP), superior (SUP), nasal (NAS), and inferior (INF) graphed against normative population data set.

for enterovirus, syphilis, ANA, and p-ANCA was negative. A respiratory viral panel for adenovirus, cytomegalovirus, influenza, parainfluenza, rhinovirus, and respiratory syncytial virus was negative on Polymerase Chain Reaction testing. Based on the patient's presentation and cerebrospinal fluid findings, she was diagnosed with viral meningoencephalitis. She was monitored as an inpatient with conservative management. During the hospital course, the patient noted improvement in her double vision and headaches. A repeated lumbar puncture 5 days later revealed opening pressure of 4 cm H_2O, 38 white blood cells/mm^3, 75 mg/dL protein, and 57 mg/dL glucose. The patient was subsequently discharged from the hospital.

Follow-up examinations with serial OCT of the optic nerve showed continued progressive improvement in disc edema (Figures 2(a)–2(h)) along with complete resolution

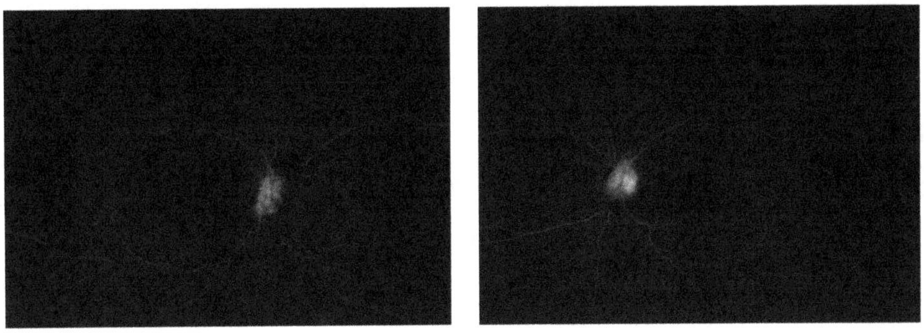

(a) (b)

FIGURE 3: Fluorescein angiography (FA) taken at six minutes of (a) right and (b) left eye showing disc hyperfluorescence without disc leakage and surrounding peripapillary hemorrhages.

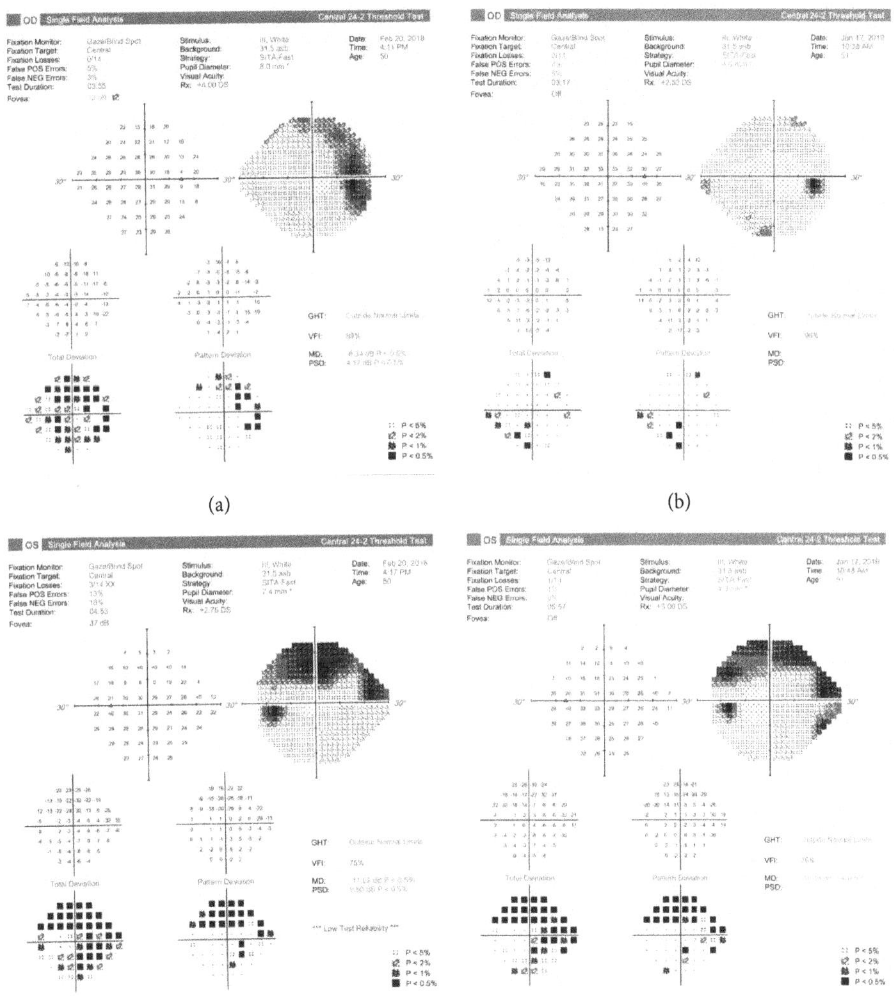

(a) (b) (c) (d)

FIGURE 4: Humphrey visual field of the patient of the right eye shows scattered deficits both upon presentation (a) and almost one year later (b). A dense superior arcuate defect seen in the left eye on presentation (c) is consistent and has not progressed almost one year later (d). This superior arcuate defect corresponds to inferotemporal thinning of the retinal nerve fiber layer on OCT of the left eye.

of papilledema and peripapillary hemorrhages (Figures 1(a)–1(f)). Mild residual pallor of both optic nerves was observed at the end of one year. OCT revealed borderline temporal thinning of the right optic nerve. The left optic nerve had borderline temporal thinning, borderline superotemporal thinning, and inferotemporal thinning. The findings of persistent disc pallor and inferotemporal nerve fiber layer thinning on OCT were consistent with the persistent visual field deficit documented on Humphrey visual fields (Figures 4(a)–4(d)).

3. Discussion

This case report presents a patient in whom increased intracranial pressure was associated with hemorrhage from the peripapillary retinal vessels [13]. Based on the papilledema and peripapillary hemorrhages, we hypothesize that a Terson-like mechanism of increased intracranial pressure led to dilation of the central retinal veins and subsequent retinal hemorrhaging. The mechanism of increased intracranial pressure was presumed to be due to inflammation from viral meningoencephalitis. In encephalitis, inflammation is a key part of the pathway as cytokines increase permeability of blood vessels and leak plasma proteins into the CSF [13]. The subarachnoid exudates of proteinaceous material and leukocytes can diminish the resorptive capacity of arachnoid granulations and obstruct CSF flow, leading to hydrocephalus and interstitial edema [13]. The combination of vasogenic and cytotoxic edema can result in elevated intracranial pressure in patients with viral meningoencephalitis. This case is an important addition to the literature because it provides an etiology for some of the approximately 5.3% of patients with meningitis or meningoencephalitis with retinal hemorrhages [14]. Such hemorrhages have been described in a wide range of CNS infections ranging from West Nile Virus to Rickettsia [15, 16].

Our patient was managed conservatively, as intraretinal hemorrhages tend to resolve spontaneously in most cases [17]. Vision typically improves with resolution of the intraretinal hemorrhages, but permanent vision impairment can occur. In patients with persistent vitreous hemorrhage or premacular hemorrhage, pars plana vitrectomy has been shown to be effective treatment [18]. One must carry a high degree of suspicion for Terson's syndrome, and we recommend early fundoscopic screening in cases of visual disturbances with unknown etiology. Although this case was not a classic presentation of Terson's syndrome, it may be possible that Terson's syndrome itself may be associated with a wider spectrum of neurological disease entities and is more common than previously thought.

References

[1] P. Czorlich, C. Skevas, V. Knospe et al., "Terson syndrome in subarachnoid hemorrhage, intracerebral hemorrhage, and traumatic brain injury," *Neurosurgical Review*, vol. 38, no. 1, pp. 129–136, 2015.

[2] H. S. Kim, S. W. Lee, S. K. Sung, and E. K. Seo, "Terson syndrome caused by intraventricular hemorrhage associated with moyamoya disease," *Journal of Korean Neurosurgical Society*, vol. 51, no. 6, pp. 367–369, 2012.

[3] A. Takkar, P. Kesav, V. Lal, and A. Gupta, "Teaching NeuroImages: Terson syndrome in cortical venous sinus thrombosis," *Neurology*, vol. 81, no. 6, pp. e40–e41, 2013.

[4] E. W. Hoving, M. Rahmani, L. I. Los, and V. W. Renardel De Lavalette, "Bilateral retinal hemorrhage after endoscopic third ventriculostomy: iatrogenic terson syndrome," *Journal of Neurosurgery*, vol. 110, no. 5, pp. 858–860, 2009.

[5] E. Buschini, U. Lorenzi, A. Fea, F. Machetta, and F. Grignolo, "Terson syndrome and leukemia: a case report," *Clinical Ophthalmology*, vol. 3, no. 8, pp. 681–683, 2014.

[6] Y. M. Wang, E. Nudleman, D. Vinocur, and D. J. Kuo, "Terson syndrome before induction chemotherapy for acute lymphoblastic leukemia," *Journal of Pediatric Hematology/Oncology*, vol. 40, no. 2, pp. 141-142, 2018.

[7] Z. Michalewska, J. Michalewski, and J. Nawrocki, "Possible methods of blood entrance in Terson syndrome," *Ophthalmic Surgery, Lasers & Imaging*, vol. 41, pp. S42–S49, 2010.

[8] N. Deigendesch and W. Stenzel, "Acute and chronic viral infections," in *Handbook of Clinical Neurology*, vol. 145 of *Handbook of Clinical Neurology*, pp. 227–243, Elsevier, 2018.

[9] D. E. Bronstein, W. D. Shields, and C. A. Glaser, "Encephalitis and meningoencephalitis," in *Feigin and Cherry's Textbook of Pediatric Infectious Diseases*, J. D. Cherry, G. J. Harrison, S. L. Kaplan et al., Eds., p. 492, Elsevier Saunders, Philadelphia, Penn, USA, 7th edition, 2014.

[10] S. Hasan, H. B. Basri, L. P. Hin, and J. Stanslas, "Encephalitis followed by optic neuritis: a case report and review of literature," *Pakistan Journal of Medical Sciences*, vol. 29, no. 3, pp. 859–862, 2013.

[11] K. Hellgren, Å. Fowler, A. Rydberg, and R. Wickström, "Ophthalmological findings in children with encephalitis," *Acta Ophthalmologica*, vol. 95, no. 1, pp. 66–73, 2017.

[12] D. Dubey, M. Toledano, and A. McKeon, "Clinical presentation of autoimmune and viral encephalitides," *Current Opinion in Critical Care*, vol. 24, no. 2, pp. 80–90, 2018.

[13] F. Kuhn, R. Morris, C. D. Witherspoon, and V. Mester, "Terson syndrome: results of vitrectomy and the significance of vitreous hemorrhage in patients with subarachnoid hemorrhage," *Ophthalmology*, vol. 105, no. 3, pp. 472–477, 1998.

[14] D. S. Pachapure, D. M. B S, and D. M. T Achar, "Occurrence of ocular fundal changes in cases of infective meningitis and meningoencephalitis in our hospital," *IOSR Journal of Dental and Medical Sciences*, vol. 13, no. 1, pp. 54–59, 2014.

[15] C. K. Chan, S. A. Limstrom, D. G. Tarasewicz, and S. G. Lin, "Ocular features of west nile virus infection in north america. a study of 14 eyes," *Ophthalmology*, vol. 113, no. 9, pp. 1539–1546, 2006.

[16] M. Khairallah, A. Ladjimi, M. Chakroun et al., "Posterior segment manifestations of Rickettsia conorii infection," *Ophthalmology*, vol. 111, no. 3, pp. 529–534, 2004.

[17] G. Kumar, J. Kalita, and U. K. Misra, "Raised intracranial pressure in acute viral encephalitis," *Clinical Neurology and Neurosurgery*, vol. 111, no. 5, pp. 399–406, 2009.

[18] R. Narayanan, S. C. Taylor, A. Nayaka et al., "Visual outcomes after vitrectomy for terson syndrome secondary to traumatic brain injury," *Ophthalmology*, vol. 124, no. 1, pp. 118–122, 2017.

37

Hyperbaric Oxygen Therapy in Retinal Arterial Occlusion: Epidemiology, Clinical Approach and Visual Outcomes

Ana Sofia Lopes,[1] **Rita Basto**,[1] **Susana Henriques**,[1] **Luísa Colaço**,[1] **Filomena Costa e Silva**,[1] **Isabel Prieto**,[1] **and Francisco Guerreiro**[2]

[1]*Department of Ophthalmology of Professor Doutor Fernando Fonseca E.P.E. Hospital (Amadora-Sintra), Lisbon, Portugal*
[2]*Underwater and Hyperbaric Medicine Center, Armed Forces Hospital—Lisbon Pole, Lisbon, Portugal*

Correspondence should be addressed to Ana Sofia Lopes; anasofialopes16@gmail.com

Academic Editor: Cristiano Giusti

Purpose. To evaluate the efficacy and safety of hyperbaric oxygen therapy (HBOT) in patients with acute retinal artery occlusion (RAO). Secondarily, to analyse the epidemiology and the clinical approach. *Methods.* Retrospective study of 13 patients submitted to HBOT between 2013 and 2018. The analysed parameters consisted of: systemic history, time between symptoms onset and treatment, initial approach, number of HBOT sessions, complications of HBOT and best corrected visual acuity—BCVA (of the total sample, central RAO—CRAO—group, and branch RAO—BRAO group). *Results.* Arterial hypertension was the most prevalent systemic risk factor (53.8%). Initial therapies were 100% normobaric oxygen administration, topical and oral hypotensive medication, eye massage and aspirin. CRAO was observed in 69.2% and BRAO in 30.8% of the cases, with clinically significant visual improvement (a decrease in logMAR of 0.3) in 55.5% and 75%, respectively. Time between symptoms onset and treatment had a median of 9 hours. The median number of HBOT sessions was 7, without complications. *Conclusions.* HBOT provide BCVA improvement in patients with RAO, when it is performed in an early time after the symptom onset. It seems to be an effective and safe therapeutic option for a pathology that still remains without approved treatment.

1. Introduction

Retinal artery occlusion (RAO) is a rare ophthalmological emergency, with embolism being the most common aetiology [1–4]. It is manifested by acute painless monocular vision loss and a meaningful visual improvement (three lines in Snellen chart) is expected only in 10% of the cases [1–7]. The time of ischemia is classically the critical prognosis factor for the visual outcome, considering that the retina is the tissue of the human body with the highest oxygen consumption, being therefore very sensitive to variations in oxygen [1, 4, 8, 9]. Animal models of central RAO (CRAO) have demonstrated that an ischemic insult to the retinal tissue greater than 90 minutes (min) will lead to some degree of inner retina damage and it will be irreversible if greater than 240 min [10]. As opposed to animal models, in humans there is no clear timeline until irreversible anoxic retinal damage occurs (some authors suggest elapsed time of around 6–6.5 hours, h) [11]. RAO remains without approved treatment and traditional options are not effective enough, having globally a nonsignificant visual outcome improvement [4, 6].

Hyperbaric oxygen therapy (HBOT) delivers 100% oxygen by a pressure greater than 1 atmosphere (atm), increasing plasma oxygen transportation and diffusion, with positive effects in vascular perfusion and neuroprotection, in the presence of an adequate vascular supply. Its pathophysiological mechanisms are based on the retinal double vascular supply, in which the choroidal capillary vessels that supply the outer retina will bypass the occlusion and oxygenate inner ischemic retina until spontaneous reperfusion occurs [1, 2, 4, 8]. Normally, under normobaric conditions the choroidal circulation supplies 60% of the oxygen needed by the retina, which increases to 100% under hyperbaric conditions [4]. HBOT also decrease edema and preserve compromised tissue adjacent to ischaemic area [1, 2, 8]. Karaman et al. demonstrated, in mice models of CRAO, that the apoptotic index of retinal inner cells was lower in the group submitted to HBOT in the reperfusion phase than in control group [12]. Also in an animal experiment in a CRAO mice model, Gaydar et al. showed that HBOT diminished cell loss from 58% to 30%, which was related to increased survival of cells in the retinal inner layer [13]. According to the Tenth European Consensus Conference on Hyperbaric Medicine (2016), the European Committee of Hyperbaric Medicine (ECHM) indicate that CRAO cases have Type 2 recommendation (where HBOT is suggested, as it is supported by acceptable levels of evidence) and level C evidence (when the conditions do not allow for proper randomised controlled trials—RCTs—but there is ample and international expert consensus) [14]. The class of recommendation of HBOT by American College of Cardiology/American Heart Association (ACC/AHA) clinical practice guidelines is IIb (where it is not unreasonable to perform procedure/administer treatment) [15]. Also, Undersea and Hyperbaric Medicine Society (UHMS) refer that patients presenting CRAO within 24 h of symptom onset should be considered for HBOT [4].

The main purpose of this study was to evaluate the efficacy and the safety of HBOT in patients with RAO. *The secondary purpose* was to analyse the epidemiology and the clinical approach. The efficacy was evaluated by the: analyses of the best corrected visual acuity (BCVA) improvement, number of HBOT sessions and time between symptoms onset and HBOT. The safety was evaluated by the analyses of frequency and severity of complications.

2. Case Presentation

2.1. Methods. Retrospective study of 13 patients (13 eyes) with RAO from the Professor Doutor Fernando Fonseca E.P.E. Hospital (HFF, Lisbon, Portugal) were submitted to HBOT at the Underwater and Hyperbaric Medicine Center of the Armed Forces Hospital—Lisbon Pole, between September 2013 and June 2018. Inclusion criteria consisted of: RAO documented by fluorescein angiography; absence of patent cilioretinal artery; time between symptoms onset and treatment no longer than 24 h; absence of previous ophthalmic pathology with relevant impact on BCVA; regular follow-up with documented BCVA; and tolerance to HBOT. All consecutive patients meeting the criteria during the period considered were included in the study and this was performed according to the principles of the Helsinki Declaration (2013).

Data was collected for the study through consultation of patients' clinical records. The parameters studied were: demographic (patients' age and sex) and epidemiological factors (personal systemic history, as dyslipidemia, arterial hypertension, diabetes, smoking habits, cerebrovascular or coronary disease, arrhythmia or other relevant factor for arterial occlusion; and type of retinal occlusion between CRAO and branch RAO—BRAO); time between symptoms onset and treatment; the initial approach in the Emergency Room; number of HBOT sessions; complications of HBOT (frequency and severity); and BCVA (total sample, CRAO group and BRAO group). BCVA was analysed before and after each session of HBOT, quantified initially in the Snellen chart in decimal scale and then converted to the logarithm of the minimal angle of resolution (logMAR) scale to perform the statistical analysis. In case of very low vision (<0.05 in Snellen chart), BCVA was assessed by semiquantitative scale, the capability to count-fingers (CF), to see hand movement (HM) or light perception (LP) at a distance of 30 cm. Decimal value attributed to CF, HM and LP was 0.014, 0.005 and 0.0001, respectively, as described in some previous studies [2, 16]. A clinically significant visual improvement was defined as a decrease in logMAR of 0.3 [1, 2, 5].

The HBOT protocol applied had two phases: patients were initially submitted to two daily sessions of 100% oxygen at 2.5 atm during 90 min during the first three consecutive days; then, patients were submitted to additional sessions (1 per day) if BCVA improvement occurred and until it stabilized, or the treatment was interrupted if no subjective BCVA gain occurred after the first three consecutive sessions. This method followed the treatment algorithm of UHMS [4].

A statistical analysis was performed with the SPSS program (Statistical Package for Social Sciences, version 22.0). Continuous variables were presented as median with minimum and maximum values. Wilcoxon signed-rank test was applied to analyse the BCVA variation before and after HBOT. A p-value <0.05 was considered to be statistically significant.

2.2. Results

(a) Demographic factors: the study included 13 eyes from 13 patients, 8 males and 5 females, with a median age of 70 years (min. 41; max. 83);
(b) Epidemiological factors:
   (i) Personal systemic history: arterial hypertension was the most prevalent (53.8%, number of patients—$n = 7$), followed by cerebrovascular disease (30.8%, $n = 4$), dyslipidemia (23.1%, $n = 3$), coronary disease (7.7%, $n = 1$), arrhythmia (7.7%, $n = 1$) and smoking habits (7.7%, $n = 1$);
   (ii) Type of retinal occlusion: CRAO was observed in 69.2% ($n = 9$) of the cases and BRAO in 30.8% ($n = 4$);
(c) Time between symptoms onset and treatment: median of 9 h (min. 2; max. 20), with 77% of cases up to 12 h;
(d) The initial approach in the Emergency Room consisted of: administration of normobaric oxygen in 69.2% ($n = 9$), topical hypotensive application and oral acetazolamide in 53.8% each ($n = 7$), and eye massage and oral administration of aspirin in 46.1% each ($n = 6$);
(e) Number of HBOT sessions: median of 7 (min. 3; max. 18), which corresponds to a total of 10.5 h of treatment;
(f) Complications of HBOT: no complications were observed;
(g) BCVA:
   (i) Difference between pre and post-HBOT BCVA: there was a statistically significant improvement in BCVA of the total sample, the CRAO group and the BRAO

TABLE 1: BCVA pre and post-HBOT (decimal and logaritmic scales; values in median with range—minimum and maximum values).

		Total	CRAO	BRAO
BCVA pre-HBOT	Decimal scale	0.005 (min. 0.0001; max. 0.2)	0.005 (min. 0.0001; max. 0.014)	0.15 (min. 0.1; max. 0.2)
	Logaritmic scale	2.3 (min. 4; max. 0.7)	2.3 (min. 4; max. 1.85)	0.82 (min.1; max. 0.7)
BCVA post-HBOT	Decimal scale	0.2 (min. 0.005; max. 1)	0.05 (min. 0.005; max. 1)	0.9 (min. 0.6; max. 1)
	Logaritmic scale	0.7 (min. 2.3; max. 0)	1.3 (min. 2.3; max. 0)	0.045 (min. 0.22; max. 0)
p-value (*<0.05)		0.007*	0.03*	0.005*

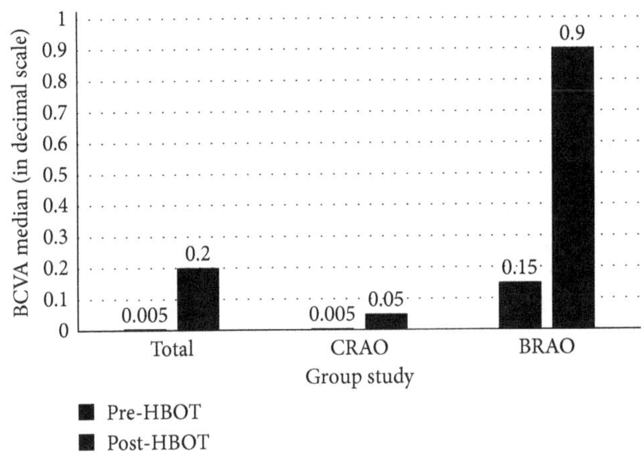

FIGURE 1: BCVA pre and post-HBOT (in decimal scale).

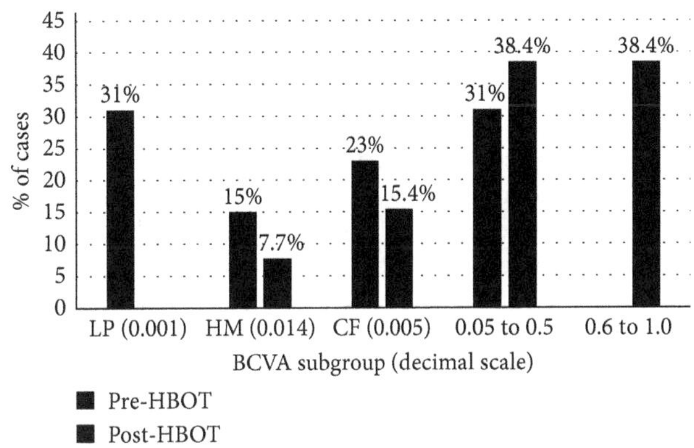

FIGURE 2: Prevalence of BCVA subgroups (in decimal scale) for the total sample.

group, with this one having a better outcome, as detailed in Table 1 and Figure 1;

(ii) Clinically significant improvement of BCVA: it was observed in 61.5% ($n = 8$) of cases in the total sample ($n = 13$). In the group of patients who improved ($n = 8$), 62.5% ($n = 5$) were patients with CRAO and 37.5% ($n = 3$) were patients with BRAO. These results correspond also to an improvement in 55.5% ($n = 5$) of cases in the CRAO group ($n = 9$) and in 75% ($n = 3$) of cases in the BRAO group ($n = 4$). Best results were observed when HBOT was performed within 9 h of symptom onset. The detailed prevalence of BCVA subgroups (in decimal scale) for the total sample is shown in Figure 2.

3. Discussion

According to our study, HBOT seems to be an effective and safe option in the treatment of patients with RAO, in case of an early administration. It may be an option to consider also because there is no approved treatment yet for RAO, the current alternative therapies do not have similar outcomes and without treatment there is little chance of visual improvement by the natural history [1, 2, 4].

The results of our study are in agreement with the literature and other studies, as patients responded well to HBOT, showing a clinically significant BCVA improvement in 61.5% ($n = 8$) of cases in the total sample, of which 62.5% ($n = 5$) belongs to the CRAO group and 37.5% ($n = 3$) belongs to the BRAO group [1, 2, 11, 17]. Coelho et al. observed a clinical significant BCVA improvement in 71.4% of the patients following HBOT and Hadanny et al. a BCVA improvement in 67.2% [2, 11]. Hadanny et al. also demonstrated a significant mean improvement in BCVA (logMar) of 0.526 ± 0.688, from 2.14 ± 0.50 to 1.61 ± 0.78 ($p < 0.01$), with 67% of the patients achieving a BCVA gain >0.3 logMar [11]. Also, an improvement from HM to CF has been described to be clinically relevant, and corresponds to an interval of 4 lines (in 0.1 log-unit steps) [2, 16]. Our results are in accordance with these. We observed an evolution of 31% of cases with LP to 0% after treatment, 15% of cases with HM to 7.7% and 23% to 15.4% of cases with CF.

The median number of HBOT sessions is also a parameter that contributes to the analysis of the efficacy of this therapeutic option. The median number of our study, which corresponds to a total of 10.5 h of treatment, is in line with what Wu et al. reported in his recent meta-analysis of seven randomized controlled trials (251 eyes, with the most effective treatment length over 9 hours) [6]. It is also noteworthy that, according to UHMS, the optimum number of HBOT sessions depends on the severity and duration of the patients' symptoms and the degree of response to them. Most patients stabilize within 1 week of symptom onset [4].

Our good results may be related to the early timing between symptoms and treatment (median of 9 h and 77% of cases within 12 h of symptom onset) and, the absence of other ophthalmic pathology. It is well known that the period of time until the treatment is considered the critical factor for the visual prognosis, between the several factors that may influence it. This is based on the main pathophysiological mechanism of an early HBOT, in case of RAO, of the hyperbaric oxygen supply to the inner and outer retinal layers through the choroid [1, 2, 4, 17–19]. However, the best time to perform treatment is controversial. Ideally, the shorter the time delay until treatment, the better the likelihood of recovering ischemic retina that is threatened but viable (penumbra) [4]. Coelho et al., Beiran et al. and Hertzog et al. described that HBOT is most useful up to 8 h of visual loss and Butler et al. documented that the best evidence is a delay up to 12 h of visual loss [2, 5, 9, 20]. The UHMS refer that HBOT should be started in the first 24 h after the onset of the symptoms, and some ophthalmology literature includes strongest evidence for symptomatic improvement in cases with less than 12 hours' delay [4, 9, 21, 22]. Despite this traditional critical prognostic factor, Hadanny et al. recently reported that having cherry-red spot (CRS) macula in the fundoscopy at presentation is associated with a prominent VA improvement and a higher success of the treatment, than the patients without CRS at presentation. It was observed a clinically significant visual improvement in 86.0% of patients with CRS compared with 49.4% of patients without CRS at presentation ($p = 0.0001$). In this context, the authors documented that CRS can be used as a marker for irreversible anoxic retinal damage for patients candidates for HBOT. They even highlight that it, rather than the time delay from symptoms onset, should be used as the most important marker for treatment success [11].

The safety of HBOT is another factor that supports this therapeutic option. It is essential to preclude any contraindication to treatment in advance, as well as to perform a regular patient follow-up. In our study, no patient had complications. According to the literature and some similar studies, the most prevalent complication of HBOT is ear barotrauma, which usually have a full spontaneous resolution in few days [2, 4].

We also highlight the type of occlusion as essential factor for visual prognosis, influencing treatment response: BRAO have a better prognosis, as our study showed in the comparison between the CRAO and BRAO groups. Most studies include only cases of CRAO. Wu et al.'s recent meta-analysis included both CRAO and BRAO cases, with good visual outcome in both groups, concluding that oxygen therapy is considered an effective method of treatment for RAO diseases. It reported a global improvement in BCVA between 58.8% and 90%. This study also stands out for including the comparison between a group under HBOT, a group under normobaric oxygen and a group not submitted to oxygen therapy, as well as the result of traditional therapies. Oxygen therapy groups were more likely to have visual improvement (5.61x more); the group under HBOT presented better final visual outcome and with statistical significance; there was no statistical significance between HBOT alone and combined treatment with traditional therapies, nor between the CRAO and BRAO groups (despite both groups presented favorable visual outcomes) [6].

Considering that RAO is the ocular equivalent of an acute cerebral ischemic event by the AHA and American Stroke Association (ASA), having the same risk factors and aetiology, management of RAO should also include secondary prevention of further vascular events, such as cerebral ischemia, myocardial infarction, and cardiovascular death. In this context, RAO may be a "warning sign" for the concomitant evolution of systemic vascular pathologies, thus implying a timely medical articulation with Internal Medicine, Cardiology and/or Neurology. The prevalence of vascular risk factors in our study is consistent with other studies, highlighting the arterial hypertension, dyslipidemia, and brain and cardiovascular diseases [3, 23, 24].

There are still few studies regarding this issue. Many of them have relatively small study samples and some of them differ not only in the definition of the ideal "time window" to perform HBOT but also on the HBOT protocol, regarding that there is no consensus for treatment or guideline-based therapy [1, 2]. Thus, the discussion of this issue may contribute to an improvement of the clinical practice.

The main limitations of our study were the retrospective profile and sample size (however, this is a rare pathology and not all patients are indicated for HBOT). *Aspects to highlight* are: the inclusion of CRAO and BRAO cases, considering that most studies include only CRAO cases; and the great impact on clinical practice of this issue, whereas HBOT appears to be a promising therapeutic option in a pathology without an approved effective treatment and with a bad visual prognosis according to its natural history.

To conclude, HBOT may improve the BCVA in patients with RAO when it is provided in the first 24 h after the onset of symptoms. Further studies with more patients are necessary to better analyze the value and safety of HBOT in the treatment of RAO, as well as the exact "time window" to perform it.

References

[1] A. Soares, N. L. Gomes, L. Mendonça, and C. Ferreira, "The efficacy of hyperbaric oxygen therapy in the treatment of central retinal artery occlusion," *BMJ Case Reports*, vol. 2017, pp. 1–3, 2017.

[2] P. Coelho, A. P. Ferreira, R. Gonçalves et al., "Hyperbaric oxygen therapy following central retinal artery occlusion—a retrospective case series analysis," *Oftalmologia*, vol. 42, no. 2, 2018.

[3] M. Dattilo, N. J. Newman, and V. Biousse, "Acute retinal arterial ischemia," *Annals of Eye Science*, vol. 3, no. 6, pp. 1–13, 2018.

[4] H. Murphy-Lavoie, F. Butler, and C. Hagan, "Central retinal artery occlusion treated with oxygen: a literature review and treatment algorithm," *Undersea & Hyperbaric Medicine*, vol. 39, no. 5, pp. 943–953, 2012.

[5] I. Beiran, I. Goldenberg, Y. Adir, A. Tamir, A. Shupak, and B. Miller, "Early hyperbaric oxygen therapy for retinal artery occlusion," *European Journal of Ophthalmology*, vol. 11, no. 4, pp. 345–350, 2001.

[6] X. Wu, S. Chen, S. Li et al., "Oxygen therapy in patients with retinal artery occlusion: a meta-analysis," *PLoS One*, vol. 13, no. 8, pp. 1–11, 2018.

[7] S. S. Hayreh and M. B. Zimmerman, "Central retinal artery occlusion: visual outcome," *American Journal of Ophthalmology*, vol. 140, no. 3, pp. 376.e1–376.e, 2005.

[8] C. V. Pereira, S. Pina, A. R. Azevedo et al., "Oclusão arteriolar retiniana e a oxigenoterapia hiperbárica," *Oftalmologia*, vol. 38, no. 1, pp. 43–47, 2014.

[9] L. M. Hertzog, G. W. Meyer, S. Carson, M. B. Strauss, and G. B. Hart, "Central retinal artery occlusion treated with hyperbaric

oxygen," *Journal of Hyperbaric Medicine*, vol. 7, no. 1, pp. 33–42, 1992.

[10] S. S. Hayreh, M. B. Zimmerman, A. Kimura, and A. Sanon, "Central retinal artery occlusion, retinal survival time," *Experimental Eye Research*, vol. 78, no. 3, pp. 723–736, 2004.

[11] A. Hadanny, A. Maliar, G. Fishlev et al., "Reversibility of retinal ischemia due to central retinal artery occlusion by hyperbaric oxygen," *Clinical Ophthalmology*, vol. 11, pp. 115–125, 2017.

[12] S. Karaman, B. Ozkan, Y. Yazir et al., "Comparison of hyperbaric oxygen versus iloprost treatment in an experimental rat central retinal artery occlusion model," *Graefe's Archive for Clinical and Experimental Ophthalmology*, vol. 254, no. 11, pp. 2209–2215, 2016.

[13] V. Gaydar, D. Ezrachi, O. Dratviman-Storobinsky, S. Hofstetter, B. C. Avraham-Lubin, and N. Goldenberg-Cohen, "Reduction of apoptosis in ischemic retinas of two mouse models using hyperbaric oxygen treatment," *Investigative Ophthalmology & Visual Science*, vol. 52, no. 10, pp. 7514–7522, 2011.

[14] D. Mathieu, A. Marroni, and J. Kot, "Tenth European consensus conference on hyperbaric medicine: recommendations for accepted and nonaccepted clinical indications and practice of hyperbaric oxygen treatment," *Diving and Hyperbaric Medicine*, vol. 47, no. 1, pp. 24–32, 2017.

[15] R. J. Gibbons, S. Smith, and E. Antman, "American college of cardiology; American heart association: American college of cardiology/American heart association clinical practice guidelines: Part I. Where do they come from?" *Circulation*, vol. 107, no. 23, pp. 2979–2986, 2003.

[16] K. Schulze-Bonsel, N. Feltgen, H. Burau, L. Hansen, and M. Bach, "Visual acuities "hand motion" and "counting fingers" can be quantified with the Freiburg visual acuity test," *Investigative Opthalmology & Visual Science*, vol. 47, no. 3, pp. 1236–1240, 2006.

[17] A. Cope, J. Eggert, and E. O'Brien, "Retinal artery occlusion: visual outcome after treatment with hyperbaric oxygen," *Diving and Hyperbaric Medicine*, vol. 41, no. 3, pp. 135–139, 2011.

[18] D. D. Varma, S. Cugati, A. W. Lee, and C. S. Chen, "A review of central retinal artery occlusion: clinical presentation and management," *Eye*, vol. 27, no. 6, pp. 688–697, 2013.

[19] J. N. Weiss, "Hyperbaric oxygen treatment of nonacute central retinal artery occlusion," *Undersea & Hyperbaric Medicine*, vol. 36, no. 6, pp. 401–405, 2009.

[20] F. K. Butler, C. Hagan, and H. Murphy-Lavoie, "Hyperbaric oxygen therapy and the eye," *Undersea & Hyperbaric Medicine*, vol. 35, no. 5, pp. 333–387, 2008.

[21] H. K. Li, B. J. Dejean, and R. A. Tang, "Reversal of visual loss with hyperbaric oxygen treatment in a patient with Susac syndrome," *Ophthalmology*, vol. 103, no. 12, pp. 2091–2098, 1996.

[22] J. Yotsukura and E. Adachi-Usami, "Correlation of electroretinographic changes with visual prognosis in central retinal artery occlusion," *Ophthalmologica*, vol. 207, no. 1, pp. 13–18, 1993.

[23] M. Dattilo, V. Biousse, and N. J. Newman, "Update on the management of central retinal artery occlusion," *Neurologic Clinics*, vol. 35, no. 1, pp. 83–100, 2017.

[24] R. L. Sacco, S. E. Kasner, J. P. Broderick et al., "An updated definition of stroke for the 21st century: a statement for healthcare professionals from the American Heart Association/American Stroke Association," *Stroke*, vol. 44, no. 7, pp. 2064–2089, 2013.

38

Failure of XEN Gel Stent Implantation as a Stand-Alone Procedure in Congenital Glaucoma: Case Report of Secondary Congenital Glaucoma in Neurofibromatosis Type 1

Hannah Schellhase, Matthias Fuest, David Kuerten, Peter Walter, and Niklas Plange

Department of Ophthalmology, Universitätsklinikum Aachen, Pauwelsstr. 30, 52057 Aachen, Germany

Correspondence should be addressed to Hannah Schellhase; hschellhase@ukaachen.de

Academic Editor: Pradeep Venkatesh

A XEN gel stent implant procedure was performed in a one-year-old child with severe unilateral congenital glaucoma. At the age of 6 weeks, an uncomplicated 360° trabeculotomy had been performed, which resulted in intraocular pressure (IOP) control for only 4 months. The gel stent implantation was performed ab interno without complications. However, 1 month later, the stent was repelled into the anterior chamber due to the elasticity of Tenon's layer. A first revision surgery was performed, with excision of Tenon's layer and implantation of a new gel stent under sight. At the age of 18 months, a second revision surgery was performed because of an encapsulated Tenon cyst with insufficient IOP control, again with the implantation of a new stent. At that time, a progressive upper eyelid swelling was apparent. Eyelid biopsy led to the diagnosis of neurofibromatosis type 1, presenting with an orbital plexiform neurofibroma. Further insufficient IOP control resulted in a cyclodestructive procedure and loss of light perception during follow-up. XEN gel stent implantation in congenital glaucoma in infants is more challenging than that in adult patients. Gel stent implantation ab interno may be difficult due to the thickness and elasticity of Tenon's layer. Gel stent dislocation may occur, even months after surgery. Trabeculectomy might be a better approach after failed trabeculotomy in congenital glaucoma. An underlying systemic disease might become apparent late during follow-up.

1. Introduction

Congenital glaucoma is a rare disease but still an important cause of childhood ocular morbidities. Typical clinical signs are corneal clouding, megalocornea, epiphora, and buphthalmos. Paediatric glaucoma surgery is the first treatment of choice. However, it is challenging due to the differences in anatomy and tissue behaviour, compared with adult eyes. Angle surgery, such as trabeculotomy, is the preferred initial surgical option for congenital glaucoma; it has high success rates and a good safety profile [1, 2]. However, in case of failure of the initial intervention, further surgical treatment becomes more challenging. Then, trabeculectomy and tube shunt implantation may be necessary, with challenging bleb-related postoperative care. Ciliodestructive procedures are considered to be options of last resort [3, 4].

The XEN gel stent (Allergan, Dublin, Ireland) is a tubular implant designed to affect IOP control with a filtering bleb, as an alternative to conventional trabeculectomy. The implantation is performed ab interno using a minimally invasive approach, avoiding surgical manipulation of the conjunctiva. However, bleb encapsulation often occurs and bleb revision may be necessary in 28% of pseudophakic and up to 50% of phakic adult patients [5].

We report the failure of XEN gel stent implantation in a child with unilateral secondary congenital glaucoma in neurofibromatosis type 1 (NF1). We discuss the implications for possible use of the XEN gel stent in children.

2. Case Presentation

A 6-week-old female was referred for glaucoma evaluation after the mother had identified left eye enlargement and tearing. The newborn's medical history was uneventful, with full-term delivery. No family history of congenital glaucoma or other inherited diseases was evident. On examination, the child was unable to fixate with the left eye (OS) and strongly resisted occlusion of the right eye (OD). A buphthalmos OS was apparent, with a large corneal diameter and cloudy corneal stroma (Figure 1). Examination under anaesthesia (EUA) was performed, revealing suspected unilateral congenital glaucoma OS. After the induction of anaesthesia, IOP was measured as 11 mmHg OD and 40 mmHg OS using iCare rebound tonometry (iCare® PRO, Icare, Vanda, Finland). All IOP measurements during further examinations were performed using this rebound tonometer. Corneal diameters were 10 mm horizontally OD and 12 mm horizontally OS. Handheld slit lamp examination revealed a clear cornea OD and corneal oedema and extensive Haab's striae OS. Corneal thickness, measured using ultrasound pachymetry, was 550 μm OD; OS could not be measured due to extensive corneal oedema. The iris did not show any structural abnormalities, and no ectropium uveae was apparent. Gonioscopic evaluation of the OS was not possible due to the corneal oedema. Dilated fundus examination showed a healthy optic nerve with a cup-to-disc ratio of 0.4 OD and, due to limited visibility, a presumed terminal excavation OS. Axial lengths, measured using A-scan ultrasound, were 16.5 mm OD and 20.5 mm OS.

The patient was diagnosed with congenital unilateral glaucoma and buphthalmos OS. She underwent 360° trabeculotomy using an illuminated microcatheter (iTrack™250, Ellex, Minneapolis, MN, USA). A paediatric examination at 6 weeks of age did not reveal any systemic disease or other ocular or nonocular malformations. Over the next 4 months, IOP ranged from 14 to 20 mmHg OS. The corneal oedema declined significantly. Amblyopia treatment with occlusion was not tolerated because of severe amblyopia and advanced glaucomatous optic disc damage.

Five months posttrabeculotomy, IOP was found to be elevated in OS up to 30 mmHg. Travoprost and dorzolamide-timolol in fixed combination twice daily were prescribed to lower IOP. The patient underwent a second EUA. The angle OS was closed, with anterior synechia on gonioscopy. We assumed that anterior synechiae had developed after the 360° trabeculotomy, although no gonioscopic evaluation was possible at the initial examination due to the corneal oedema. Therefore, a 360° synechiolysis of the anterior synechia was performed using a standard surgical spatula with a gonioscopic lens with two paracenteses. This intervention produced satisfying IOP (up to 21 mmHg) for 3 months. This surgical intervention had to be repeated 3 months later, after IOP had again increased and angle OS was closed on gonioscopy.

After another rise in IOP (39 mmHg OS at age 1 year), we decided to perform a filtering surgery using the XEN gel stent via a conventional ab interno approach, along with subconjunctival injection of 0.1 mL mitomycin C (MMC) 0.2 mg/mL. We assumed that XEN implantation might incur less surgical trauma than a standard trabeculectomy, especially considering postsurgical complications. The XEN gel stent procedure is a minimally invasive glaucoma surgery that affects a defined externalisation of the aqueous humour to a subconjunctival filtering zone. The XEN gel stent is designed as an advancement of the trabeculectomy, with less risk of severe complications. Over the next month, IOP ranged from 8 to 15 mmHg OS without use of medication, and the patient showed a diffuse functional filtering bleb. No adverse events were present, such as flattening of the anterior chamber or choroidal detachment.

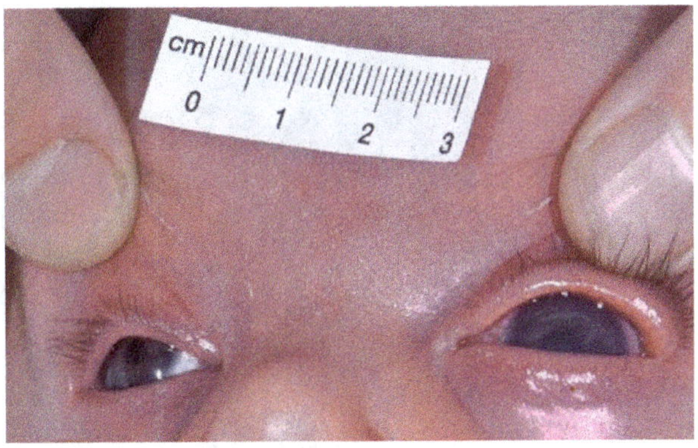

FIGURE 1: Photograph of the patient at age 6 weeks. The left eye shows buphthalmos and corneal oedema.

However, 1 month later, increased IOP was again apparent. EUA revealed the XEN implant to be dislocated too far into the anterior chamber. About 50% of the XEN implant was visible in the anterior chamber; the implant was still in contact with the inner part of the scleral tunnel. During this first XEN revision surgery, the implant could not be repositioned without opening the conjunctiva because of the strong Tenon's layer. The stent was removed, and a new XEN gel stent was implanted under sight ab interno after tenonectomy had been performed. The new XEN implant was positioned in the same quadrant, as the conjunctiva was already surgically opened. After surgery, IOP remained under control for 5 months.

At the age of 18 months, IOP increased again to a level in the high 30s, despite the use of medication (travoprost and dorzolamide-timolol in fixed combination twice daily). A further EUA showed an encapsulated Tenon cyst, with correct position of the implant. As Tenon revision surgeries regularly need to be performed in adults, we decided to perform a second XEN revision surgery. However, while removing the scarring Tenon's layer, the implant was dislocated completely into the anterior chamber. Six months after implantation, the stent was still highly mobile inside the child's sclera. A new XEN gel stent (the third XEN gel stent) was implanted ab interno, as filtration and IOP control had been achieved in the previous months.

At that time, a progressive eyelid swelling became noticeable. A histopathological biopsy of the eyelid was taken, which revealed a spindle cell tumour and 5% KI 67 fraction positivity, indicating a perineural tumour. A further paediatric examination led to the suspected diagnosis of neurofibromatosis. A magnetic resonance imaging (MRI) scan revealed a retroocular tumour (suspected plexiform neurofibroma) OS with extraorbital portions in the eyelid and left temple (Figure 2). In addition, optic nerve gliomas on both optic

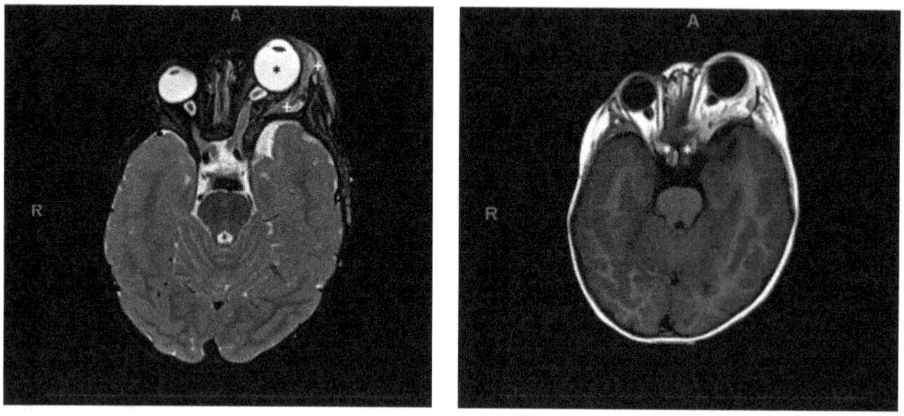

(a) (b)

Figure 2: Magnetic resonance imaging. (a) Axial T2-weighted magnetic resonance image shows buphthalmos and exophthalmos of the left eye (asterisks denote the left eye). Also seen are neurofibromas in the left orbit, eyelid, and temple (plus signs denote the tumour). (b) Axial T1-weighted magnetic resonance image shows glioma of both optic nerves with diffuse enlargement (asterisks denote the tumours).

nerves were found (Figure 2). The diagnosis of neurofibromatosis type 1 (NF1) was confirmed. Chemotherapy with carboplatin and vincristine along with mitogen-activated protein kinase (MEK) inhibitor therapy (trametinib) was initiated. MRI examinations and visual function tests were performed at 3-month intervals. Eye status and IOP were measured at least on a monthly basis.

IOP was under control for another 6 months with medication use but was then found again to be elevated to 32 mmHg. To reduce the burden of another surgical approach (e.g., shunt surgery) and because of the limited visual prognosis (only light projection), a laser ciliodestructive procedure was performed. Over the next 2 years, IOP ranged from 17 to 28 mmHg OS. Loss of light perception was documented during chemotherapy. Through until the last follow-up (at age 3 years), IOP was 28 mmHg OS under medication (travoprost and dorzolamide-timolol in fixed combination twice daily). No IOP-derived pain perception was apparent. A functional filtering bleb could not be seen.

3. Discussion

The management of congenital glaucoma is complex. Surgical intervention is considered the treatment of choice. Angle surgeries, including goniotomy and trabeculotomy (including 360° trabeculotomy using a microcatheter), are considered first-line procedures and may reach success rates of about 80% [1, 2, 6]. Filtering surgeries, such as trabeculectomy and glaucoma shunt surgery (i.e., Ahmed valve or Baerveldt implant), have been performed in the past and follow first-line treatment [3, 4, 7]. In children, success rates of trabeculectomy with MMC may reach 60% in the first years after surgery, but long-term complications, such as blebitis and endophthalmitis, may occur [3, 4]. Glaucoma drainage devices in paediatric patients can show a success ratio of about 50% after 10 years, with sight-threatening complications in 10% of cases [7].

The XEN gel stent may be an alternative surgical approach to other filtering procedures in challenging cases of congenital glaucoma, avoiding early complications due to overfiltration and with limited surgical trauma to the conjunctiva when using the ab interno approach. A case series of three children with congenital glaucoma has recently reported good outcomes of the XEN gel stent in 2 years of follow-up [8]. Case 1 showed successful IOP values after 2 years. In case 2, a combination of XEN gel stent and Kahook Dual Blade goniotomy was performed; a revision surgery with implantation of a second XEN gel stent was necessary because the stent was located within Tenon's layer. This new stent was implanted using a transconjunctival ab externo approach. Case 3 was a 10-year-old girl with complex secondary glaucoma and retinopathy of prematurity. During XEN stent implantation, a cataract surgery with iridectomy was performed simultaneously. IOP was well controlled, without any revision surgery after 2 years. Thus, no standard XEN implantation was performed in any of the cases.

In contrast, we failed to achieve long-term IOP control in our young patient after XEN gel stent implantation. In our perception, there is one major lesson to learn from our case. The elasticity and thickness of a child's Tenon's layer result in more difficult placement of the XEN gel implant. The implant may be repelled, even months after surgery, into the anterior chamber. Placement of the XEN implant above Tenon's layer, just under the conjunctiva, or a surgical incision of the conjunctiva with excision of Tenon's layer might be necessary for improved results.

No postoperative complications, such as cataract, ocular hypotony, choroidal detachment, or expulsive bleeding, were seen in our case. A larger case series would be necessary to evaluate the risks and benefits of the XEN gel implantation as a stand-alone procedure in congenital glaucoma in comparison with other filtering surgical procedures, such as trabeculectomy, after failed angle surgery. The main burden of filtering surgery in children (i.e., the high risk of conjunctival scarring) also remains a significant issue in XEN gel stent surgery.

The treatment of congenital glaucoma is even more complex when associated with systemic diseases such as NF1 [9–12]. Neurofibromatosis is a rare phakomatosis that mainly affects the skin and peripheral nervous system. There are two types: neurofibromatosis type 1 (NF1 or von Recklinghausen syndrome) and type 2, which is characterised by acoustic and/or central neurofibromatosis. Around 85% of patients suffer from NF1, as did our patient. Typical features of the disease are multiple neural tumours (neurofibromas), pigmented skin lesions (cafe au lait spots), and pigmented iris hamartomas (Lisch nodules). In addition, approximately 15%–20% of children with NF1 develop an optic pathway tumour, as did our patient [11, 12]. In our patient, increasing swelling of the eyelid began approximately 12 months after birth and was first considered to be secondary because of the initial exophthalmos. Eyelid biopsy at the age of 18 months and later MRI examination revealed the diagnosis NF1. Paediatric full body examination did not identify any pathology until that date. Unfortunately, vision-threatening optic nerve gliomas were found on both sides, posing a high risk of blindness.

To summarise, XEN gel stent surgery might be an alternative approach to conventional filtering techniques in congenital glaucoma after failed angle surgery. However, XEN placement and revision surgeries may be more challenging in infants than in adults. Further studies are needed to establish whether the XEN gel stent might offer any advantages over filtration surgeries. Until then, trabeculectomy should be considered a standard procedure after failed trabeculotomy. Moreover, little is known about the long-term survival of the XEN gel stent itself [13].

References

[1] O. Barkan, "Goniotomy for the relief of congenital glaucoma," *British Journal of Ophthalmology*, vol. 32, no. 9, pp. 701–728, 1948.

[2] I. Chang, J. Caprioli, and Y. Ou, "Surgical management of Pediatric glaucoma," *Developments in Ophthalmology*, vol. 59, pp. 165–178, 2017.

[3] S. A. Tanimoto and J. D. Brandt, "Options in pediatric glaucoma after angle surgery has failed," *Current Opinion in Ophthalmology*, vol. 17, no. 2, pp. 132–137, 2006.

[4] H. Jayaram, R. Scawn, F. Pooley et al., "Long-term outcomes of trabeculectomy augmented with mitomycin C undertaken within the first 2 years of life," *Ophthalmology*, vol. 122, no. 11, pp. 2216–2222, 2015.

[5] R. A. Widder, T. S. Dietlein, S. Dinslage, P. Kühnrich, C. Rennings, and G. Rössler, "The XEN45 Gel Stent as a minimally invasive procedure in glaucoma surgery: success rates, risk profile, and rates of re-surgery after 261 surgeries," *Graefe's Archive for Clinical and Experimental Ophthalmology*, vol. 256, no. 4, pp. 765–771, 2018.

[6] Y. M. El Sayed and G. I. Gawdat, "Microcatheter-assisted trabeculotomy versus 2-site trabeculotomy with the rigid probe trabeculotome in primary congenital glaucoma," *Journal of Glaucoma*, vol. 27, no. 4, pp. 371–376, 2018.

[7] E. O'Malley Schotthoefer, T. L. Yanovitch, and S. F. Freedman, "Aqueous drainage device surgery in refractory pediatric glaucomas: I. Long-term outcomes," *Journal of American Association for Pediatric Ophthalmology and Strabismus*, vol. 12, pp. 33–39, 2008.

[8] O. U. Smith, D. S. Grover, M. E. Emanuel, D. G. Godfrey, and R. L. Fellman, "XEN gel stent in pediatric glaucoma," *Journal of Glaucoma*, vol. 29, no. 4, pp. e19–e22, 2020.

[9] T. Colás-Tomás, E. Gutiérrez-Díaz, P. Tejada-Palacios, A. Barceló-Mendiguchía, and E. Mencía-Gutiérrez, "Management of congenital glaucoma in neurofibromatosis type 1: a report of two cases," *International Ophthalmology*, vol. 30, no. 2, pp. 211–214, 2010.

[10] M. S. Payne, J. M. Nadell, Y. Lacassie, and A. H. Tilton, "Congenital glaucoma and neurofibromatosis in a monozygotic twin: case report and review of the literature," *Journal of Child Neurology*, vol. 18, no. 7, pp. 504–508, 2003.

[11] R. A. Lewis, L. P. Gerson, K. A. Axelson, V. M. Riccardi, and R. P. Whitford, "von Recklinghausen Neurofibromatosis: II. Incidence of Optic Gliomata," *Ophthalmology*, vol. 91, no. 8, pp. 929–935, 1984.

[12] R. Listernick, J. Charrow, M. Greenwald, and M. Mets, "Natural history of optic pathway tumors in children with neurofibromatosis type 1: a longitudinal study," *The Journal of Pediatrics*, vol. 125, pp. 63–66, 1994.

[13] R. A. Widder, P. Kühnrich, M. Hild, C. Rennings, A. Szumniak, and G. F. Rössler, "Intraocular degradation of XEN45 gel stent 3 years after its implantation," *Journal of Glaucoma*, vol. 28, no. 12, pp. e171–e173, 2019.

Permissions

All chapters in this book were first published by Hindawi Publishing Corporation; hereby published with permission under the Creative Commons Attribution License or equivalent. Every chapter published in this book has been scrutinized by our experts. Their significance has been extensively debated. The topics covered herein carry significant findings which will fuel the growth of the discipline. They may even be implemented as practical applications or may be referred to as a beginning point for another development.

The contributors of this book come from diverse backgrounds, making this book a truly international effort. This book will bring forth new frontiers with its revolutionizing research information and detailed analysis of the nascent developments around the world.

We would like to thank all the contributing authors for lending their expertise to make the book truly unique. They have played a crucial role in the development of this book. Without their invaluable contributions this book wouldn't have been possible. They have made vital efforts to compile up to date information on the varied aspects of this subject to make this book a valuable addition to the collection of many professionals and students.

This book was conceptualized with the vision of imparting up-to-date information and advanced data in this field. To ensure the same, a matchless editorial board was set up. Every individual on the board went through rigorous rounds of assessment to prove their worth. After which they invested a large part of their time researching and compiling the most relevant data for our readers.

The editorial board has been involved in producing this book since its inception. They have spent rigorous hours researching and exploring the diverse topics which have resulted in the successful publishing of this book. They have passed on their knowledge of decades through this book. To expedite this challenging task, the publisher supported the team at every step. A small team of assistant editors was also appointed to further simplify the editing procedure and attain best results for the readers.

Apart from the editorial board, the designing team has also invested a significant amount of their time in understanding the subject and creating the most relevant covers. They scrutinized every image to scout for the most suitable representation of the subject and create an appropriate cover for the book.

The publishing team has been an ardent support to the editorial, designing and production team. Their endless efforts to recruit the best for this project, has resulted in the accomplishment of this book. They are a veteran in the field of academics and their pool of knowledge is as vast as their experience in printing. Their expertise and guidance has proved useful at every step. Their uncompromising quality standards have made this book an exceptional effort. Their encouragement from time to time has been an inspiration for everyone.

The publisher and the editorial board hope that this book will prove to be a valuable piece of knowledge for researchers, students, practitioners and scholars across the globe.

List of Contributors

Renato Pejic and Marija Simic Prskalo
University Clinical Hospital Mostar, Department of Ophthalmology, Bosnia and Herzegovina

Josip Simic
Faculty of Health Studies, University in Mostar, Bosnia and Herzegovina

Ruchi Goel and Shalin Shah
Ophthalmology, Maulana Azad Medical College, New Delhi, India

Ravindra Kumar Saran
Pathology, Govind Ballabh Pant Hospital, New Delhi, India

Somnath Chakraborty
Retina Institute of Bengal, Siliguri, India

Jay Umed Sheth
Surya Eye Institute and Research Center, Mumbai, India

Sahel Khazaei, Mehrdad Motamed Shariati, Naser Shoeibi and Seyedeh Maryam Hosseini
Eye Research Center, Mashhad University of Medical Sciences, Mashhad, Iran

Mohammad Arjmand
Sabzevar University of Medical Sciences, Heshmatie Hospital, Sabzevar, Iran

Jeanne M. Gunzinger, Katrin Fasler, Daniel Barthelmes, Christian Böni and Sandrine A. Zweifel
Department of Ophthalmology, University Hospital Zurich, Zurich 8091, Switzerland

Peter Maloca
Institute of Molecular and Clinical Ophthalmology Basel (IOB), Basel, Switzerland
Department of Ophthalmology, University Hospital Basel, Basel 4056, Switzerland
CTlab, Department of Ophthalmology, University Hospital Basel, Basel, Switzerland
Moorfields Eye Hospital, London, UK

Pascal W. Hasler
Institute of Molecular and Clinical Ophthalmology Basel (IOB), Basel, Switzerland
Department of Ophthalmology, University Hospital Basel, Basel 4056, Switzerland
OCTlab, Department of Ophthalmology, University Hospital Basel, Basel, Switzerland

Nicola McDowell
Institute of Education, Massey University, Albany Drive, Palmerston North 4474, New Zealand

Gordon N. Dutton
Department of Vision Sciences, Glasgow Caledonian University, Cowcaddens Road, Glasgow G4 0BA, UK

Ayman G. Elnahry, Ahmed A. Abdel-Kader, Karim A. Raafat and Khaled Elrakhawy
Department of Ophthalmology, Faculty of Medicine, Cairo University, Cairo, Egypt

Yuka Kasuya, Ichiya Sano, Shinji Makino and Hidetoshi Kawashima
Department of Ophthalmology, Jichi Medical University, Shimotsuke, Tochigi, Japan

Isha Agarwal, Mayuresh Naik and HarinderSingh Sethi
Department of Ophthalmology, V.M.M.C. & Safdarjung Hospital, Ring Road, Ansari Nagar, New Delhi 110029, India

Sepideh Ghods, Hooshang Faghihi and Bahman Inanloo
Retina Ward, Farabi Eye Hospital, Tehran University of Medical Sciences, Tehran, Iran

Elias Khalili Pour and Hamid Riazi-Esfahani
Eye Research Center, Farabi Eye Hospital, Tehran University of Medical Sciences, Tehran, Iran
Retina Ward, Farabi Eye Hospital, Tehran University of Medical Sciences, Tehran, Iran
Translational Ophthalmology Research Center, Farabi Eye Hospital, Tehran University of Medical Sciences, Tehran, Iran

Nazimul Hussain
Department of Ophthalmology, Mediclinic Parkview Hospital, Dubai, UAE
Department of Ophthalmology, Al Zahra Hospital, Sharjah, UAE

Massimo Lorusso, Eleni Nikolopoulou and Tommaso Micelli Ferrari
Department of Ophthalmology, Ente Ecclesiastico "F. Miulli" Hospital, Acquaviva delle Fonti, Bari, Italy

Luisa Micelli Ferrari
Department of Ophthalmology, "G. Moscati" Hospital, Taranto, Italy

Nazanin Ebrahimiadib and Mohammad Zarei
Eye Research Center, Farabi Eye Hospital, Tehran University of Medical Sciences, Tehran, Iran

Violet Zaker Esteghamati
Imam Khomeini General Hospital, School of Medicine, Tehran University of Medical Sciences, Tehran, Iran

Naoko Ishiguro, Yoshiko Yamawaki, Kei Mizobuchi and Tadashi Nakano
Department of Ophthalmology, The Jikei University School of Medicine, Tokyo, Japan

Takaaki Hayashi
Department of Ophthalmology, The Jikei University School of Medicine, Tokyo, Japan
Department of Ophthalmology, Katsushika Medical Center, The Jikei University School of Medicine, Tokyo, Japan

sutomu Yasukawa
Department of Ophthalmology and Visual Science, Nagoya City University Graduate School of Medical Sciences, Aichi, Japan

Shigeru Honda
Department of Ophthalmology and Visual Sciences, Osaka City University Graduate School of Medicine, Osaka, Japan

Annahita Amireskandari, Elena Nguyen, David Hinkle and Thomas Mauger
Department of Ophthalmology, West Virginia University, USA

Cristina Calleja-García, Jorge Suárez-Baraza and Enrique Mencía-Gutiérrez
Ophthalmology Department, 12 de Octubre Hospital, Complutense University, 28041 Madrid, Spain

Laurentino Biccas Neto
Ocular Oftalmologia, Vitória, Brazil

José Z. Pulido
Department of Oncology, Hospital Evangélico, Cachoeiro do Itapemirim, Brazil

Gustavo B. Melo
Hospital de Olhos de Sergipe, Aracaju, Brazil
Department of Ophthalmology, Universidade Federal de São Paulo, São Paulo, Brazil

Eduardo B. Rodrigues
Department of Ophthalmology, Universidade Federal de São Paulo, São Paulo, Brazil
Department of Ophthalmology, Saint Louis University School of Medicine, Saint Louis, MO, USA

Luiz H. Lima
Department of Ophthalmology, Universidade Federal de São Paulo, São Paulo, Brazil

Mónica Gimeno-Carrero, María-Jesús Suárez-Fernández, Beatriz Alonso-Martín and Almudena de-Pablo-Cabrera
Ophthalmology Department, 12 de Octubre Hospital, Complutense University, 28041 Madrid, Spain

María-Concepción Garrido-Ruíz
Pathology Department, 12 de Octubre Hospital, Complutense University, 28041 Madrid, Spain

Samreen Khanam, Ayushi Agarwal, Neha Rathie, Akash Raut, Shweta Raghav, Sumit Kumar, Mohit Chhabra, Sonam Singh and Sushil Kumar
Guru Nanak Eye Centre, Maulana Azad Medical College, New Delhi, India

Sukhmandeep Kaur
Touro College of Osteopathic Medicine, Harlem, USA

Zachary Raphael Teibel
Department of Medicine, Hackensack Meridian Health Palisades Medical Center, USA

Nada Farhat
Department of Pathology, Mount Sinai Health System, USA

Adam Atoot
Department of Medicine, Hackensack Meridian Health Palisades Medical Center, Riverside Medical Group, USA

Brett Bielory
Department of Ophthalmology, New York Eye and Ear infirmary of Mount Sinai School of Medicine, Hackensack University Medical Center, Riverside Medical Group, USA

Nicholas Hadjokas, Robert Swan and Samuel Alpert
Department of Ophthalmology and Visual Sciences, SUNY Upstate Medical University, Syracuse, NY, USA

Han Y. Yin
Department of Ophthalmology and Visual Sciences, SUNY Upstate Medical University, Syracuse, NY, USA
Herbert Wertheim College of Medicine, Florida International University, Miami, FL, USA

Kanish Mirchia
Department of Pathology, SUNY Upstate Medical University, Syracuse, NY, USA

Carsten Faber, Steffen Heegaard and Jens Folke Kiilgaard
Department of Ophthalmology, University Hospital Copenhagen, Rigshospitalet, Denmark

Megha Kotecha
Department of Ophthalmology, Dr. D.Y. Patil Medical College and Hospital, Pimpri, Pune, Maharashtra, India

Sarang Gotecha, Ashish Chugh and Prashant Punia
Department of Neurosurgery, Dr. D.Y. Patil Medical College and Hospital, Pimpri, Pune, Maharashtra, India

Manami Misawa, Hironobu Tampo and Shinji Makino
Department of Ophthalmology, Jichi Medical University, Tochigi, Shimotsuke, Japan

Khalid Alrubaie
King Khaled Eye Specialist Hospital, Riyadh, Saudi Arabia

Nasser G. Alsaedi
King Khaled Eye Specialist Hospital, Riyadh, Saudi Arabia
King Abdullah Medical City, Makkah, Saudi Arabia

Melih Akıdan
Department of Ophthalmology, Antalya Kepez State Hospital, Antalya, Turkey

Mehmet Bulut, Lütfiye Yaprak, Muhammet Kazım Erol and Elcin Suren
Department of Ophtalmology, Antalya Education and Research Hospital, Antalya, Turkey

Belghmaidi Sarah, Ghazza Ahmed, Boutgayout Saloua, Hajji Ibtissam and Moutaouakil Abdeljalil
Ophthalmology Department, Mohammed VI University Hospital, Marrakech, Morocco

Dref Maria, Fakhri Anass and Raiss Hanane
Histopathology Department, Mohammed VI University Hospital, Marrakech, Morocco

Kepa Balparda
Department of Cornea and Refractive Surgery, Clínica de Oftalmología Sandiego, Medellín, Colombia

Claudia Marcela Vanegas-Ramírez
Department of Ophthalmology, Universidad Ponticia Bolivariana, Medellín, Colombia

Laura Segura-Muñoz and Manuela Gómez-Londoño
School of Medicine, Universidad Ponticia Bolivariana, Medellín, Colombia

Hilal Kilinç Hekimsoy and Mehmet Ali Şekeroğlu
University of Health Sciences, Ulucanlar Eye Training and Research Hospital, Ophthalmology Clinic, Ankara, Turkey

Lisa Pohl, Lisa Strudel, Spyridon Dimopoulos and Focke Ziemssen
Center for Ophthalmology, Eberhard Karl University, Tuebingen, Germany

Keiichi Aomatsu
Department of Ophthalmology, Nara Hospital, Kindai University Faculty of Medicine, Nara, Japan

Shunji Kusaka
Department of Ophthalmology, Kindai University Faculty of Medicine, Osaka, Japan

Toyo Ikebukuro, Tsutomu Igarashi, Takeshi Arima, Tomoyuki Kunishige and Hiroshi Takahashi
Department of Ophthalmology, Nippon Medical School, 1-1-5 Sendagi, Bunkyo-ku, Tokyo, Japan

Shuhei Kameya
Department of Ophthalmology, Nippon Medical School Chiba Hokusoh Hospital, 1715 Kamagari, Inzai, Chiba, Japan

Augusto Magalhães, Ana Maria Cunha, Rodrigo Vilares-Morgado and Jorge Breda
Department of Ophthalmology, Centro Hospitalar Universitário de São João, Porto, Portugal

Manuel Falcão, Ângela Carneiro and Fernando Falcão-Reis
Department of Ophthalmology, Centro Hospitalar Universitário de São João, Porto, Portugal
Department of Surgery and Physiology, Faculty of Medicine of University of Porto, Porto, Portugal

Elisa Leão-Teles and Esmeralda Rodrigues
Pediatric Department, Reference Centre of Inherited Metabolic Diseases, Centro Hospitalar Universitário de São João, Porto, Portugal

Fariba Ghassemi, Nazanin Ebrahimiadib, Hamid Riazi-Esfahani, Hassan Khojasteh and Zahra Mahdizad
Translational Ophthalmology Research Center, Farabi Eye Hospital, Tehran University of Medical Sciences, Tehran, Iran

Masumi G. Asahi
Western University of Health Sciences, 309 E 2nd St., Pomona, CA 91766, USA

Peggy Bouzika, Ilias Georgalas, Maria-Evanthia Sotirianakou, Aristotelis Karamaounas, Chrysanthos Symeonidis, Konstantinos Tyrlis, Stylianos Blounas, Ekaterini Mani and Tryfon Rotsos
Retina Service, 1st Department of Ophthalmology, National and Kapodistrian University of Athens, General Hospital of Athens"G. Gennimatas", Athens, Greece

Krishi Peddada
Drexel University College of Medicine, 219 N. Broad St., 3rd Floor, Philadelphia, PA 19107, USA

Stephanie J. Weiss
Drexel University College of Medicine, 219 N. Broad St., 3rd Floor, Philadelphia, PA 19107, USA
Weill Cornell Medical College, 1305 York Ave., New York, NY 10021, USA

Deepika Malik
Drexel University College of Medicine, 219 N. Broad St., 3rd Floor, Philadelphia, PA 19107, USA
Moore Eye Institute, 100 W Sproul Rd., Springfield, PA 19064, USA
Philadelphia College of Osteopathic Medicine, 4170 City Ave., Philadelphia, PA 19131, USA

Ana Sofia Lopes, Rita Basto, Susana Henriques, Luísa Colaço, Filomena Costa e Silva and Isabel Prieto
Department of Ophthalmology of Professor Doutor Fernando Fonseca E.P.E. Hospital (Amadora-Sintra), Lisbon, Portugal

Francisco Guerreiro
Underwater and Hyperbaric Medicine Center, Armed Forces Hospital—Lisbon Pole, Lisbon, Portugal

Hannah Schellhase, Matthias Fuest, David Kuerten, Peter Walter and Niklas Plange
Department of Ophthalmology, Universitätsklinikum Aachen, Pauwelsstr. 30, 52057 Aachen, Germany

Index

R

S

T

V

X

www.ingramcontent.com/pod-product-compliance
Lightning Source LLC
LaVergne TN
LVHW082232200926
848484LV00008B/2339